Hepatitis B Virus Update

Editor

TAREK I. HASSANEIN

CLINICS IN
LIVER DISEASE

www.liver.theclinics.com

Consulting Editor
NORMAN GITLIN

August 2019 • Volume 23 • Number 3

ELSEVIER

1600 John F. Kennedy Boulevard • Suite 1800 • Philadelphia, Pennsylvania, 19103-2899

http://www.theclinics.com

CLINICS IN LIVER DISEASE Volume 23, Number 3
August 2019 ISSN 1089-3261, ISBN-13: 978-0-323-68228-2

Editor: Kerry Holland
Developmental Editor: Meredith Madeira

Clinics in Liver Disease (ISSN 1089-3261) is published quarterly by Elsevier Inc., 360 Park Avenue South, New York, NY 10010-1710. Months of issue are February, May, August, and November. Business and Editorial Offices: 1600 John F. Kennedy Blvd., Ste. 1800, Philadelphia, PA 19103-2899. Customer Service Office: 3251 Riverport Lane, Maryland Heights, MO 63043. Periodicals postage paid at New York, NY and additional mailing offices. Subscription prices are $304.00 per year (U.S. individuals), $100.00 per year (U.S. student/resident), $542.00 per year (U.S. institutions), $409.00 per year (international individuals), $200.00 per year (international student/resident), $672.00 per year (international institutions), $343.00 per year (Canadian individuals), $200.00 per year (Canadian student/resident), and $672.00 per year (Canadian institutions). Foreign air speed delivery is included in all *Clinics* subscription prices. All prices are subject to change without notice. **POSTMASTER:** Send address changes to *Clinics in Liver Disease*, Elsevier Health Sciences Division, Subscription Customer Service, 3251 Riverport Lane, Maryland Heights, MO 63043. **Customer Service: Telephone: 1-800-654-2452 (U.S. and Canada); 314-447-8871 (outside U.S. and Canada). Fax: 314-447-8029. E-mail: journalscustomer service-usa@elsevier.com (for print support); journalsonlinesupport-usa@elsevier.com (for online support).**

Reprints. For copies of 100 or more of articles in this publication, please contact the Commercial Reprints Department, Elsevier Inc., 360 Park Avenue South, New York, NY 10010-1710. Tel.: 212-633-3874; Fax: 212-633-3820; E-mail: reprints@elsevier.com.

Clinics in Liver Disease is covered in *MEDLINE/PubMed (Index Medicus)*, Science Citation Index Expanded, Journal Citation Reports/Science Edition, and Current Contents/Clinical Medicine.

Contributors

CONSULTING EDITOR

NORMAN GITLIN, MD, FRCP (LONDON), FRCPE (EDINBURGH), FAASLD, FACP, FACG
Head of Hepatology, Southern California Liver Centers, San Clemente, California, USA

EDITOR

TAREK I. HASSANEIN, MD, FACP, FACG, AGAF, FAASLD
Professor of Medicine, University of California, San Diego (UCSD), San Diego, California, USA; Southern California Liver Centers, Southern California Research Center, Coronado, California, USA

AUTHORS

RASHED ABDELAAL, BS
Departments of Surgery and Transplant Hepatology, University of California, Los Angeles, California State University, Los Angeles, Los Angeles, California, USA

NOHA ABDELGELIL, MBBCh
Southern California Research Center, Coronado, California, USA

ALICIA M. CRYER, DO
Department of Gynecology and Obstetrics, Loma Linda Medical Center, Loma Linda, California, USA

BEN L. DA, MD
Digestive Diseases Branch, National Institute of Diabetes and Digestive and Kidney Diseases, National Institutes of Health, Bethesda, Maryland, USA

PETER DE CRUZ, MBBS, PhD, FRACP
University of Melbourne, Melbourne, Victoria, Australia

JOSEPH DOYLE, MBBS, MPH, PhD, FRACP, FAFPHM
The Alfred and Monash University, Burnet Institute, Melbourne, Victoria, Australia

MOHAMED EL KABANY, MD
Departments of Surgery, Transplant Hepatology, and Medicine, University of California, Los Angeles, Los Angeles, California, USA

MARC G. GHANY, MD, MHSc
Investigator, Liver Diseases Branch, National Institute of Diabetes and Digestive and Kidney Diseases, National Institutes of Health, Bethesda, Maryland, USA

ROBERT G. GISH, MD
Division of Gastroenterology and Hepatology, Department of Medicine, Stanford University, Stanford University Medical Center, Stanford, California, USA; Division of Gastroenterology and Hepatology, Stanford Health Care, Palo Alto, California, USA

JEFFREY S. GLENN, MD, PhD
Departments of Medicine, and Medicine Microbiology and Immunology, Division of Gastroenterology and Hepatology, Stanford University School of Medicine, Stanford, California, USA

CHANTAL GOMES, MD
Department of Medicine, Division of Gastroenterology and Hepatology, Endoscopy Unit, Alameda Health System, Highland Hospital, Oakland, California, USA

ANDREW GRIGG, MBBS, FRACP, FRCPA, MD
Olivia Newton John Cancer Research Institute, Austin Hospital, Heidelberg, Victoria, Australia

TAREK I. HASSANEIN, MD, FACP, FACG, AGAF, FAASLD
Professor of Medicine, University of California, San Diego (UCSD), San Diego, California; Southern California Liver Centers, Southern California Research Center, Coronado, California, USA

PETER D. HUGHES, MBBS, PhD, FRACP
Peter Doherty Institute for Infection and Immunity, University of Melbourne, Melbourne, Victoria, Australia; Royal Melbourne Hospital, Parkville, Victoria, Australia

JOANNE C. IMPERIAL, MD, FAASLD
Transplant Hepatologist, Southern California Liver Center, San Diego, California, USA

FARAH KASSAMALI, MD
St. Mary's Medical Center, San Francisco, California, USA

CHRISTOPHER KOH, MD, MHSc
Liver Diseases Branch, National Institute of Diabetes and Digestive and Kidney Diseases, National Institutes of Health, Bethesda, Maryland, USA

SENG LEE LIM, MBBS, FRACP, FRCP, MD
National University of Singapore, Singapore

ALISA LIKHITSUP, MD
Fellow, Division of Gastroenterology and Hepatology, University of Michigan, Ann Arbor, Michigan, USA

ANNA S. LOK, MD
Professor of Medicine, Division of Gastroenterology and Hepatology, Department of Internal Medicine, University of Michigan, Ann Arbor, Michigan, USA

URI LOPATIN, MD
Assembly Biosciences, South San Francisco, California, USA

MICHAELA LUCAS, MD, Dr Med, FRACP, FRCPA
University of Western Australia, Crawley, Western Australia, Australia

GEOFF McCOLL, MBBS, BMedSc, MEd, PhD, FRACP
University of Queensland Oral Health Centre, Queensland, Australia

SUE ANNE McLACHLAN, MBBS, MSc, FRACP
St Vincent's Hospital, Fitzroy, Victoria, Australia

MARION G. PETERS, MD, MBBS
University of California, San Francisco, San Francisco, California, USA

JAMES RICKARD, MBBS (Hons), PhD
Olivia Newton John Cancer Research Institute, Austin Hospital, Heidelberg, Australia

JOE SASADEUSZ, MBBS, PhD, FRACP
Peter Doherty Institute for Infection and Immunity, University of Melbourne, Melbourne, Victoria, Australia

NICHOLAS SHACKEL, BSc Hons (Medal), MB, BS (Hons), FRACP, PhD
Ingham Institute, Liverpool, Sydney, New South Wales, Australia

MONICA SLAVIN, MBBS, FRACP, MD
Royal Melbourne Hospital, Parkville, Victoria, Australia; Victorian Comprehensive Cancer Centre, Melbourne, Victoria, Australia

IDREES SULIMAN, MD
Blake Medical Center, Internal Medicine, Bradenton, Florida, USA

VIJAYA SUNDARARAJAN, MD, MPH, FACP
University of Melbourne, Melbourne, Victoria, Australia; St Vincent's Hospital, Fitzroy, Victoria, Australia; Department of Public Health, La Trobe University, Bundoora, Victoria, Australia

ALEXANDER THOMPSON, MBBS (hons), PhD, FRACP
University of Melbourne, Melbourne, Victoria, Australia; St Vincent's Hospital, Fitzroy, Victoria, Australia

KUMAR VISVANATHAN, MBBS, PhD, FRACP
University of Melbourne, Melbourne, Victoria, Australia; St Vincent's Hospital, Fitzroy, Victoria, Australia

ANUSHA VITTAL, MD
Liver Diseases Branch, National Institute of Diabetes and Digestive and Kidney Diseases, National Institutes of Health, Bethesda, Maryland, USA

ROBERT J. WONG, MD, MS
Assistant Clinical Professor of Medicine, Director of Research and Education, Department of Medicine, Division of Gastroenterology and Hepatology, Endoscopy Unit, Alameda Health System, Highland Hospital, Oakland, California, USA

DAVID L. WYLES, MD, FIDSA
Professor of Medicine, Division of Infectious Diseases, University of Colorado School of Medicine, Aurora, Colorado, USA; Chief, Division of Infectious Diseases, Denver Health Medical Center, Denver, Colorado, USA

BESHOY YANNY, MD
Health Sciences Clinical Instructor of Medicine, Department of Medicine, Division of Digestive Diseases and Hepatology, David Geffen School of Medicine, University of California, Los Angeles, Los Angeles, California, USA

Contents

Hepatitis B virus (HBV) infection is a global health burden. The chronicity of this infection leads to complication such as cirrhosis and hepatocellular carcinoma, making it a leading cause of morbidity and mortality world-wide. Chronic infection commonly develops among those who acquire infection during childhood, hence the importance of effective implementation of HBV vaccination policies designed to eradicate chronic HBV. This article provides updated estimates of worldwide HBV disease prevalence and discusses how implementation of vaccination policies has affected HBV epidemiology.

Hepatitis B virus (HBV) infection is the most common chronic viral infection worldwide and remains a significant global health problem. Chronic HBV infection can progress to cirrhosis, liver failure, and hepatocellular carcinoma. Outcome of chronic HBV infections depends on the host, virus, and environmental factors. Although effective prophylactic vaccines and antiviral therapies exist, curative treatment is not yet available. Intense research into a cure for HBV is ongoing and proposed definitions of cure and endpoints for clinical trials evaluating "curative" therapy are discussed.

The prevalence of chronic hepatitis B (CHB) differs globally. CHB is responsible for 30% of all deaths from cirrhosis and 40% from hepatocellular carcinoma. The WHO developed guidelines in 2015 on prevention, care, and treatment of chronic HBV infection targeted to program managers in all health care settings, particularly in low- and middle-income countries. Several of the recommendations differ from those of the major Liver Societies, including the American Association for the Study of Liver Diseases (AASLD). This review highlights key differences between the AASLD and WHO guidelines and discusses the impact on management of CHB.

Fatty liver prevalence is increasing and becoming a global health burden. Chronic hepatitis B infection (CHB) is one of the most common chronic viral infections. Steatosis in CHB patients increases risk of cirrhosis and hepatocellular carcinoma. Data from studies on the interaction between CHB and nonalcoholic fatty liver disease are not conclusive. Liver biopsy is the gold standard for diagnosis of fatty liver; however, noninvasive diagnostic tests have been developed to diagnose and predict fibrosis in CHB/NAFLD. Treatment guidelines are not clear.

Chronic hepatitis B is a global health problem affecting approximately 350 million to 400 million individuals worldwide, and mother to child transmission remains the major mode of transmission. Approximately 50% of chronically infected individuals acquire infection, either perinatally or early in childhood, predominantly in areas where hepatitis B virus (HBV) is endemic. Management of HBV in pregnancy presents a unique set of challenges. All infants born of hepatitis B surface antigen–positive mothers should receive postexposure immune prophylaxis with hepatitis B immunoglobulin and HBV vaccination within 24 hours of birth and need close follow-up for the first few years of life.

Epidemiologic studies suggest that 10% to 15% of patients infected with hepatitis C virus (HCV) are coinfected with hepatitis B virus (HBV) in the United States as a result of the shared modality of transmission, but the true prevalence is not known. The progression of liver disease to cirrhosis and hepatocellular carcinoma is generally faster in patients who are coinfected, and HCV is usually more predominant. Immunosuppression of the host or eradication of hepatitis C can change this paradigm, causing hepatitis B reactivation. This review describes HCV-HBV viral interactions, risks for reactivation, screening, and society guidelines for surveillance and treatment.

Hepatitis B virus (HBV) coinfection is common in persons with human immunodeficiency virus (HIV) infection, contributing significantly to morbidity and mortality. Many currently used HIV antiretroviral therapy (ART) regimens provide potent anti-HBV activity and it is recommended that HBV-HIV coinfected persons be treated with ART regimens containing tenofovir. ART has multiple benefits, including increasing rates of HBV clearance after initial infection and potent suppression of HBV DNA in chronic infection. Nevertheless, long-term studies have yet to demonstrate a profound positive impact of ART on HBV-related fibrosis progression and development of endstage liver disease.

> Because of the relatively high prevalence of both hepatitis B infection and various forms of autoimmune inflammatory diseases treated with aggressive immunotherapy, reactivation of hepatitis B occurs in a substantial number of patients. The risk of reactivation depends on the degree and duration of immunosuppression. A large number of drug treatments have resulted in reactivation of hepatitis B virus infection and, based on the mechanisms and extent of immunosuppression, recommendations for some of the newer classes of immunosuppressive drugs are provided.

> Chronic hepatitis B remains a significant cause of morbidity and mortality worldwide. Most hepatitis B virus (HBV)-infected individuals are neither diagnosed nor treated. In those treated, nucleos(t)ide polymerase inhibitors persistently suppress viremia to the limits of quantitation; however, few achieve a "functional cure," defined as sustained off-treatment loss of detectable serum HBV DNA with or without loss of hepatitis B surface antigen. The low cure rate has been attributed to an inability to eliminate the viral reservoir of covalently closed circular DNA from hepatocytes. This review focuses on the diverse therapeutic approaches currently under development that may contribute to the goal of HBV cure.

> Chronic hepatitis D (CHD) results from an infection with the hepatitis B virus and hepatitis D virus (HDV). CHD is the most severe form of human viral hepatitis. Current treatment options consist of interferon alfa, which is effective only in a minority of patients. Study of HDV molecular virology has resulted in new approaches entering clinical trials, with phase-3 studies the most advanced. These include the entry inhibitor bulevirtide, the nucleic acid polymer REP 2139-Ca, the farnesyltransferase inhibitor lonafarnib, and pegylated interferon lambda. This article summarizes the available data on these emerging therapeutics.

CLINICS IN LIVER DISEASE

THE CLINICS ARE AVAILABLE ONLINE!
Access your subscription at:
www.theclinics.com

Preface

Hepatitis B Virus Update

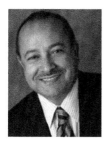

Tarek I. Hassanein, MD, FACP, FACG, AGAF, FAASLD
Editor

Hepatitis B virus (HBV) continues to be a worldwide prevalent virus with global impact on the health of individuals and health economies of many countries, particularly in the Asia-Pacific regions and Africa. Entering an era of worldwide collaborations in health management, and a time of conceivable success to control or even eradicate liver viruses, we gathered a group of thought leaders and investigators to update the knowledge of HBV prevalence, management, and current status of new therapies.

Drs Gomes, Wong, and Gish summarized the updated global prevalence of HBV infection and the current vaccination policies, implementation, and challenges around the world.

Drs Likhitsup and Lok briefly reviewed the natural history of HBV and elaborated on the new goals of viral therapy and its surrogate markers, a field that is in pertinent development.

To coordinate the global policies for HBV containment, the World Health Organization (WHO) published its guidelines for prevention, care, and treatment of HBV-infected individuals. Drs Vittal and Ghany addressed the WHO guidelines from the US perspective since the WHO guidelines were more focused on low- and middle-income countries.

The increase in obesity rates around the world with its concurrent fatty liver overlaps with the spread of HBV infection. The interaction between these 2 maladies is reviewed by Drs Suliman, Abdelgelil, Kassamali, and Hassanein.

The prevention of HBV spread starts with preventing HBV infection in newborn babies. Drs Cryer and Imperial addressed the management of HBV in pregnant women and the prevention of HBV transmission to the newborn.

Reactivation of HBV and the clinical flare seen as a result of increased replication of HBV are becoming a major clinical issue important not only to Hepatologists but also to Gastroenterologists, Oncologists, Rheumatologists, and other specialists using other antivirals or immune modulators.

Clin Liver Dis 23 (2019) xiii–xiv
https://doi.org/10.1016/j.cld.2019.05.002
1089-3261/19/© 2019 Published by Elsevier Inc.

liver.theclinics.com

Drs Abdelaal, Yanny, and Kabany summarized the evolving data of HBV reactivation in patients who are receiving direct-acting agents for hepatitis C virus infection.

Dr Wyles reviewed the impact of human immunodeficiency virus (HIV) on the natural history of HBV and the effects of HIV antiretrovirals on HBV therapy.

The topic of HBV reactivation in patients treated with immunosuppression medications for different indications is addressed in 4 articles authored by an international group of thought leaders who simplified and skillfully addressed the topic in respect to screening, early diagnosis, and management of patients with hematologic or solid organ malignancies as well as patients who receive immunosuppressive therapy for other immune diseases and organ transplantation. These 4 articles, by Drs Sasadeusz, Grigg, Hughes, Lim, Lucas, McColl, McLachlan, Peters, Shackel, Slavin, Sundararajan, Thompson, Doyle, Rickard, De Cruz, Gish, and Visvanathan, are a resource for all health care providers to assess and manage their patients with or without active HBV infection before and during treatment with immunosuppression. I would like to give special thanks to Dr Gish for coordinating the publication of the 4 articles.

To end this issue with the most recent developments in therapies, Dr Lopatin simplified the current and planned new therapies to combat HBV. Drs Koh, Da, and Glenn reviewed the role of emerging therapeutic options for HBV and hepatitis D virus coinfection.

I am very grateful to all our authors and contributors who enthusiastically updated and taught us about the current status and the future of HBV infection and the efforts to combat this complex virus; many thanks to the editorial team who saved no effort in putting this issue together.

Tarek I. Hassanein, MD, FACP, FACG, AGAF, FAASLD
Southern California Liver Centers
131 Orange Avenue, Suite 101
Coronado, CA 92118, USA

E-mail address:
thassanein@livercenters.com

Global Perspective on Hepatitis B Virus Infections in the Era of Effective Vaccines

Chantal Gomes, MD[a], Robert J. Wong, MD, MS[a],*,
Robert G. Gish, MD[b]

KEYWORDS

- Hepatitis B • Vaccination • Seroprevalence • Global prevalence
- Birth dose vaccine • Vaccine implementation

KEY POINTS

- Hepatitis B virus (HBV) infection remains a leading cause of morbidity and mortality worldwide.
- HBV vaccination implementation contributes to significant declines in incident HBV infections as well as HBV-related liver cancer and mortality, particularly among infants and children.
- However, effective implementation of HBV vaccination programs is not uniform across all world regions.
- Globally, birth dose vaccination is currently universal in only 101 countries.
- A significant number of countries within the African and European regions continue to lack universal HBV birth dose administration.

INTRODUCTION

Hepatitis B virus (HBV) is a leading cause of morbidity and mortality worldwide.[1] Viral hepatitis deaths have increased globally from 0.89 million to 1.45 million between 1990 and 2013.[1] According to the World Health Organization (WHO) there were 887,000 deaths from HBV in 2015, particularly caused by complications such as cirrhosis and hepatocellular carcinoma (HCC).

Although understanding the global prevalence of HBV is important epidemiologically to provide accurate estimates of disease burden and disease risk associated with HBV and its associated complications, accurate estimation of HBV prevalence is complex. The complexity is driven by 3 major issues. First, disease prevalence is

Disclosure: See last page of article.
[a] Department of Medicine, Division of Gastroenterology and Hepatology, Endoscopy Unit, Alameda Health System, Highland Hospital, Highland Hospital Campus, Highland Care Pavilion 5th Floor, 1411 East 31st Street, Oakland, CA 94602, USA; [b] Division of Gastroenterology and Hepatology, Stanford Health Care, 300 Pasteur Drive, Palo Alto, CA 94304, USA
* Corresponding author.
E-mail address: Rowong@alamedahealthsystem.org

Clin Liver Dis 23 (2019) 383–399
https://doi.org/10.1016/j.cld.2019.04.001
1089-3261/19/© 2019 Elsevier Inc. All rights reserved.

not uniform across all regions. For example, most of the worldwide HBV is concentrated in African and Asia-Pacific regions, whereas Europe and the Americas have lower prevalence.[2] Second, even within a region such as the United States, HBV prevalence varies across demographics, with the highest prevalence seen in African and Asian immigrants, thus making accurate assessments of national prevalence challenging. Third, although most worldwide HBV is seen in Asia and Africa, there is limited high-quality published epidemiology from African regions.

As a result of these limitations, HBV prevalence is underestimated in many regions. Furthermore, HBV incidence and prevalence are dynamic and are directly affected by implementation of public health initiatives designed to eradicate chronic HBV, such as HBV vaccination policies and education and awareness campaigns.[3] However, the implementation of such vaccination policies and educational campaigns is not uniform across all regions, and accurately identifying regions where such programs are lacking can further stimulate public policies in those regions to strive for HBV eradication. In addition, it is essential to accurately capture HBV disease prevalence given that HBV can contribute to long-term clinical consequences, including cirrhosis, HCC, and end-stage liver disease. These data will help clinicians understand not only the clinical burden but also the long-term economic burden of HBV worldwide. This article provides updated estimates of worldwide HBV disease prevalence with a focus on understanding which regions have implemented effective vaccination policies and how implementation of vaccination policies have affected HBV epidemiology in each of these regions.

Natural History and Routes of Transmission

The highest rate of chronic HBV infection is seen among individuals that were infected at less than 6 years of age via either perinatal infection or horizontal infection early in childhood. Chronic infection develops in 80% to 90% of infants that are infected in the first year of life and in 30% to 50% of children who are infected before the age of 6 years. In contrast, chronic infection develops in only 5% of healthy individuals that are infected as adults. However, adults infected via horizontal infection typically develop acute HBV infection and are therefore at increased risk of developing fulminant hepatitis. Overall, the largest burden of chronic HBV infection stems from vertical transmission and horizontal infection of early childhood.[2]

Routes of transmission vary by region, with vertical transmission usually in highly endemic regions and horizontal transmission in low endemic regions. In the Asia-Pacific regions, transmission is largely vertical.[4] Although the African region has extensive vertical transmission, the main route is parenteral horizontal transmission.[5] Transmission of HBV infection in Europe is largely horizontal, although vertical transmission in Europe does play a significant role in chronic infection as well.[6] Transmission in the Americas does tend to be horizontal but, in areas that have a large foreign-born population, particularly from Asia, vertical transmission is prevalent.[7] Overall, reducing vertical transmission and horizontal infection of early childhood is vital to reducing chronic infection, because the risk of developing chronic infection is highest among children.

Hepatitis B Virus Vaccination

The ultimate goal, set by the WHO, is to eliminate both hepatitis C virus (HCV) and HBV by 2030. The most effective way to achieve this goal is via effective vaccination programs. It is of particular interest to reduce prevalence in infants via vaccination because they are the leading source of new chronic HBV. Studies show that new chronic infections can be reduced by 90% and mortality by 65% if there is improvement in the rate of infant/neonate vaccination, peripartum antiviral use where appropriate, and more of the test/treat approach in the general population.[8] The inadequate use of screening, prophylaxis, and treatment challenges the path to HBV elimination. Therefore, developing programs, like US and global hepatitis B vaccination programs, with specific guidelines, are key to elimination.

HBV vaccine was licensed in 1981 and became available for use in 1982 but there was limited application in low-income and middle-income countries because of the cost of the vaccine and operationalizing the injection process.[8] However, by the early 2000s vaccine coverage increased because of the efforts of the Global Alliance for Vaccines and Immunization (GAVI). Another factor that has improved vaccine availability is proof that it can be safely stored at room temperature.[9] It is also important to understand that there was not a standard global vaccine schedule; it was country specific. Therefore, despite early introduction of the vaccine, the administration schedule varied among different countries. Vaccination schedules can be divided into those that include the birth dose and those that do not. Birth dose vaccination schedules include a dose at birth followed by 2 additional doses or 3 additional doses. Non–birth dose vaccine schedules involve 3 separate doses after birth.[10] Given the variation in vaccination schedules between countries, by 2015, global coverage reached 84% with the third dose of HBV vaccine but coverage with the initial birth dose vaccine was still low at 39%.[11]

Timely administration of the HBV birth dose vaccine with at least 2 additional doses given early in infancy can prevent about 90% of perinatal infections.[12] Furthermore, Jourdain and colleagues[13] found that mother-to-child HBV transmission was not significantly lower with the additional maternal use of tenofovir disoproxil fumarate versus administration of hepatitis B immune globulin and hepatitis B vaccine among infants born to hepatitis B e-antigen (HBeAg)–positive mothers. Therefore, birth dose vaccination is highly recommended but administration varies by country. Not all countries with birth dose vaccine follow universal administration (administer to all newborns); instead, they screen all pregnant women and only administer vaccine to infants born to HBV surface antigen (HBsAg)–positive women. In 2000 only 26% of WHO represented countries had a universal HBV birth dose policy but by 2016 this increased to 52%. Despite this improvement, worldwide there are still a significant number of countries without universal HBV birth dose administration. For instance, in 2016 only 19% of countries in the African region and 49% in the Americas and Europe had universal HBV birth dose administration. These percentages are significantly low compared with the 73% administration in the southeast Asia region and 93% in the western Pacific region.[12]

An added benefit to the HBV vaccine is prevention of hepatitis D virus (HDV). HDV requires HBV for replication and 5% of people with chronic HBV infection are coinfected with HDV. The most severe form of chronic viral hepatitis is HDV-HBV coinfection. Many countries do not report HDV prevalence but it is highly endemic in Africa, Asia, the Middle East, Eastern Europe, South America, and Greenland. The only form of HDV prevention is the HBV vaccine. Overall, HDV worldwide incidence has declined as a result of vaccination programs.[14]

The cost of the HBV vaccine varies by region and dose. According to the WHO in 2016 the cost of hepatitis B vaccine was as high as $55.45 in the European region for each dose of the adult vaccine to as low as $0.17 in the African and southeast Asian regions for 10 doses of the pediatric vaccine and the western Pacific region for 10 doses of the adult vaccine.[15] New in 2018 is HEPLISAV-B, a 2-dose adult HBV vaccine by Dynavax that costs $115 per dose.[16] However, this vaccine has been recognized by the US Centers for Disease Control and Prevention as being effective with the 2 doses administered over just 1 month.[17]

Overall, effective vaccination is ideal because it aids in decreasing both vertical and horizontal transmission. Implementation of effective national vaccination policies across world regions is a critical step to achieve the WHO's goal of global HBV elimination. Current goals aim for 90% third-dose childhood vaccination coverage and 50% birth dose coverage by 2020, with the overall goal to eliminate HBV infection by 2030.

HEPATITIS B VIRUS EPIDEMIOLOGY BY WORLD REGIONS

HBV endemicity can be determined with HBsAg seroprevalence: low endemicity is less than 2% HBsAg seroprevalence, low-intermediate endemicity is 2% to 4.99% HBsAg seroprevalence, high-intermediate endemicity is 5% to 7.99% HBsAg seroprevalence, and high endemicity is greater than 8% HBsAg seroprevalence.

The Polaris Observatory Collaborators progression model estimates the 2016 global prevalence of HBV infection to be 3.9%. According to the same model, as of 2016 the African and Western Pacific regions were high-intermediate endemicity, the southeast Asia region was low-intermediate endemicity, and the European and pan-American regions were low endemicity.[8]

Asia-Pacific Regions

Based on The Polaris Observatory Collaborators progression model, the estimated 2016 HBsAg prevalence in the western Pacific region was 5.7% and in the southeast Asia region was 3.5%.[8] According to the same model, the countries within these regions with high endemicity (seroprevalence>8%) include Turkmenistan (9.5%), Uzbekistan (8.0%), Taiwan (9.4%), Myanmar (8.3%), Philippines (9.8%), and Vietnam (8.2%). Those countries with high-intermediate endemicity (seroprevalence 5%–7.99%) include Kyrgyzstan (6.3%), Tajikistan (6.7%), China (6.1%), Hong Kong (6.4%), and Indonesia (6.8%) (WHO specific countries in **Tables 1 and 2**).[8]

An estimated 50% of the global burden of chronic HBV infection is in the western Pacific region.[4] Vertical transmission is the primary route of infection in this region, and thus the particular importance of screening and implementation of vaccination policies in this region. As of 2016 the southeast Asia region had 47% coverage with timely HBV birth dose vaccine and the western Pacific region had 88% coverage.[8]

Globally, the western Pacific region has the highest mortality from viral hepatitis at 24.1 deaths per 100 000, and similarly the southeast Asia region has 21.2 death per 100,000.[11] This article particularly focuses on vaccine efficacy within China and Taiwan because these are the countries within the Asia-Pacific region that have been heavily studied with significant results.

China

Licensure of the HBV recombinant vaccine was established in 1992 in China. By 2005 all newborn HBV vaccines and injections were free and provided by the government.[4] Free screening for mothers and immunoglobulin for infants born to HBsAg-positive mothers were started in 2012 by the national program to prevent mother-to-child transmission. Despite availability, successful implementation of birth dose vaccination was limited by the high prevalence of home childbirths. However, with promotion of facility-based childbirth along with the GAVI HBV project, which encouraged the birth dose policy, facility-based childbirths increased from 44% in 1985 to 99% in 2013 and birth dose vaccination increased from 22% in 1992 to 94% in 2013.[18] Despite reaching 94% coverage of the 3-dose infant vaccine, new mother-to-child transmission rates in China

Table 1
Hepatitis B virus surface antigen seroprevalence and year hepatitis B virus vaccine introduced in the World Health Organization southeast Asia region

Country	(A) Year Hepatitis B Vaccine Introduced	Birth Dose Vaccine Introduction	(B) 2016 Prevalence Estimate (%)
Bangladesh	2005	No	4.8% (3.3%–6.2%)
Bhutan	1997	Yes	—
India	2011 (2002)[a]	Yes	2.5% (2.2%–2.7%)
Indonesia	2003 (1992)[a]	Yes	6.8% (6.3%–8.2%)
Maldives	1995	Yes	—
Myanmar	2005 (2003)[a]	Yes	8.3% (4.6%–9.4%)
Nepal	2005 (2002)[a]	No	—
Sri Lanka	2005 (2003)[a]	No	—
Thailand	1992 (1988)[a]	Yes	3.5% (1.6%–4.0%)
SEARO	—	—	3.5% (2.9%–4.0%)

Column (A) represents the year the 3-dose HBV was introduced to the entire country, and this includes countries with both birth and nonbirth vaccination schedules.[29]

Abbreviation: SEARO, South-East Asia Regional Office.

[a] Year of HBV vaccine introduction in part of the country. Column (B) is 2016 HBsAg seroprevalence estimates based on The Polaris Observatory Collaborators.[8]

Data from Polaris Observatory Collaborators. Global prevalence, treatment, and prevention of hepatitis B virus infection in 2016: a modelling study. Lancet Gastroenterol Hepatol 2018;3:383–403; and Data, statistics and graphics. World Health Organization. http://www.who.int/immunization/monitoring_surveillance/data/en/. Published 2018. Accessed September 23, 2018.

were still 40% to 50%, partly because of mothers with high viral load who did not receive antiviral treatment during pregnancy.[4] Also, infant deaths that occurred after vaccination administration led to a decline in overall HBV vaccination rates in 2013 to 2014.[19]

Overall, the HBV prevention policy was very successful at reducing HBsAg prevalence. Compared with the prevaccine era, China has reduced chronic HBV infection in children less than 15 years of age by 90% (from 10.5% to 0.8%) and among children less than 5 years old by 97% (from 9.9% to 0.3%). Among those less than 30 years of age, HBsAg prevalence declined 46% (from 10.1% to 5.5%) between 1992 and 2006 and 52% (from 5.5% to 2.6%) between 2006 and 2014. This progress has resulted in China's transition to becoming a high-intermediate endemic area from being a high-endemic area.[4,18]

Taiwan

Before the national immunization program, 90% of the Taiwan population less than 40 years of age was infected with HBV.[20] In July 1984, Taiwan implemented the nationwide HBV immunization program for newborns. In 1986 the program covered all newborns, and each year HBV vaccination coverage continued to expand from preschool children to health care workers and eventually all primary school children. As a direct result of this nationwide HBV vaccination program, overall HBsAg prevalence declined from 10.5% in 1989 to 0.8% in 2007.[4] The Polaris Observatory Collaborators report that the estimated 2016 HBsAg prevalence in children aged 5 years was 0.3% in Taiwan.[8] Although the reduced HBsAg prevalence is evidence of their success, it is also important to note that, by 2015, the second dose of the infant vaccine reached 98.7% coverage and third dose reached 97.8% coverage in Taiwan.[5] Also, according to The Polaris Observatory Collaborators, the timely birth dose vaccine reached 92% coverage in 2016.[8]

Table 2
Hepatitis B virus surface antigen seroprevalence and year hepatitis B virus vaccine introduced in the World Health Organization western Pacific region

Country	(A) Year Hepatitis B Vaccine Introduced	Birth Dose Vaccine Introduction	(B) 2016 Prevalence Estimate (%)
Australia	2000	Yes	1.0% (0.9%–1.0%)
Brunei Darussalam	1988 (1983)[a]	Yes	—
Cambodia	2006 (2001)	Yes	3.0% (2.9%–5.1%)
China	2002 (licensed 1992)	Yes	6.1% (5.5%–6.9%)
Fiji	1995 (1989)[a]	Yes	2.0% (1.8%–2.3%)
Japan	2016	No	0.6% (0.5%–0.6%)
Kiribati	1995 (1990)[a]	Yes	9.1% (6.2%–10.5)
Laos	2004 (2001)[a]	Yes	3.7% (3.3%–4.6%)
Malaysia	1989	Yes	0.9% (0.5%–1.0%)
Marshall Islands	1988 (1983)[a]	Yes	—
Federated States of Micronesia	1989	Yes	—
Mongolia	1991 (1987)[a]	Yes	4.1% (3.1%–4.8%)
Nauru	Before 1998	Yes	—
New Zealand	1988 (1985)[a]	Yes	2.0% (1.4%–3.4%)
Niue	1986	No	—
Palau	1988	Yes	—
Papua New Guinea	1989	Yes	6.6% (6.0%–7.7%)
Philippines	1992	Yes	9.8% (8.8%–10.9%)
South Korea	1995 (1983)[a]	Yes	2.4% (2.3%–3.0%)
Samoa	1990	Yes	—
Singapore	1987 (1985)[a]	Yes	2.4% (2.1%–2.7%)
Solomon Islands	1991	Yes	—
Tonga	1988	Yes	—
Tuvalu	1993	Yes	—
Vanuatu	1995 (1993)[a]	yes	—
Vietnam	2003 (1997)[a]	Yes	8.2% (7.3%–10.3%)
WPRO	2000	Yes	5.7% (5.1%–6·6%)

Column (A) represents the year the 3-dose hepatitis B vaccine was introduced to the entire country and this includes countries with both birth and nonbirth vaccination schedules.[29]
Abbreviation: WRPO, Western Pacific Regional Office.
[a] Year of HBV vaccine introduction in part of the country. Column (B) is 2016 HBsAg seroprevalence estimates based on The Polaris Observatory Collaborators.[8]
Data from Polaris Observatory Collaborators. Global prevalence, treatment, and prevention of hepatitis B virus infection in 2016: a modelling study. Lancet Gastroenterol Hepatol 2018;3:383–403; and Data, statistics and graphics. World Health Organization. http://www.who.int/immunization/monitoring_surveillance/data/en/. Published 2018. Accessed September 23, 2018.

Additional studies show the significant clinical long-term impact of this successful vaccination policy. Chien and colleagues[20] reported that the incidence of HCC was significantly lower among vaccinated children aged 6 to 29 years compared with unvaccinated children (64 hepatocellular cancers among vaccinees in 37,709,304 person-years vs 444 cancers in unvaccinated persons in 78,496,406 person-years, showing an age-adjusted and sex-adjusted relative risk of 0.31, *P*<.001, for persons vaccinated at birth). Furthermore, according to Chien and colleagues, the age-adjusted and sex-adjusted rate ratios, using Poisson regression models, for HCC incidence, chronic liver disease (CLD), and HCC mortality declined for birth cohorts after implementation of the vaccine program. Using prevaccination era birth years 1977 to 1980 as the reference, the age-adjusted and sex-adjusted rate ratio in 2001 to 2004 was 0.20 (95% confidence interval [CI], 0.06–0.65) for HCC incidence, 0.11 (95% CI, 0.02–0.08) for CLD mortality, and 0.08 (95% CI, 0.02–0.34) for HCC mortality.[8] In addition, Shan and colleagues[4] reported that after the launch of the immunization program there was a 68% decline (95% CI, 58–76; $P<.001$) in fulminant hepatitis mortality among infants by 1998, which led to a reduction in fulminant hepatitis-related mortalities from 5.4 (95% CI, 2.9–6.9) in 1975 to 1984 to 1.7 (95% CI, 0.3–4.6) in 1985 to 1998.

African Regions

Based on The Polaris Observatory Collaborators progression model, the estimated 2016 HBsAg prevalence in Africa was 7.2%.[8] Africa also has one of the highest mortalities from viral hepatitis, slightly less than the Asia-Pacific regions, at 13.7 deaths per 100,000.[11]

The highest prevalence of chronic HBV infection in Africa is within the sub-Saharan countries, including Nigeria, Gabon, Namibia, Cameroon, and Burkina Faso.[5] A recent study by The Polaris Observatory Collaborators estimates that the countries in the African region with high HBV endemicity in 2016 include Angola (10.2), Central African Republic (12.1%), Zimbabwe (8.5%), Chad (10.5%), Côte d'Ivoire (8.9%), Ghana (10.3%), Mauritania (9.3%), Nigeria (11.2%), and Senegal (8.1%) (**Table 3**).[8] Also, according to Zampino,[5] in 1990, western sub-Saharan African countries had the highest HBV prevalence of 12% among children and adolescents (up to age 19 years) in the world. Therefore, most of the disease burden is within western sub-Saharan Africa. Despite this high prevalence, there exist limited high-quality epidemiologic data to provide accurate estimates of HBV incidence and prevalence in many African regions.

In the African region, of those infected at childhood, about 20% to 30% of them become chronic carriers but, unlike Asia, only 10% of them remain HBeAg positive. Also, HBsAg-positive pregnant women are often HBeAg negative, and therefore there are low rates of vertical transmission. However, there is still high risk of HBV infection for children in African countries, with the highest rate being 15.7% in South Africa among children 5 and 6 years old. HBV infection of children in African countries is usually acquired between parents or siblings via parenteral horizontal transmission. Daily practices that account for this mode of transmission include cutting, scraping, and scratching.[5] Because of high disease burden in sub-Saharan Africa, this article focuses on details from countries within this region. It particularly emphasizes The Gambia, because the first screen-and-treat program for monoinfected people in sub-Saharan Africa, Prevention of Liver Fibrosis and Cancer in Africa, was started there. It also touches on South Africa given the high rate of HBV infection among children there.

Sub-Saharan Africa

The first country in sub-Saharan Africa to implement the HBV birth dose vaccine was The Gambia in 1990. Other countries did not implement the birth dose vaccine until the 2000s, and some planned for as late as 2017 to 2018, including Cameroon, Congo, Côte d'Ivoire, Ghana, and Sierra Leone. Barriers in sub-Saharan Africa to administration of the birth dose vaccine include cost, because of lack of funding; home births; and storage, because there is concern about access to refrigeration and security. Overall, there are limited published data on the vaccine efficacy in sub-Saharan African countries.[21]

Table 3
Hepatitis B virus surface antigen seroprevalence and year hepatitis B virus vaccine introduced in the World Health Organization African region

Country	(A) Year Hepatitis B Vaccine Introduced	Birth Dose Vaccine Introduction	(B) 2016 Prevalence Estimate (%)
Algeria	2001	Yes	1.5% (1.4%–1.7%)
Angola	2006	Yes	10.2% (9.3%–11.4%)
Benin	2002	No	—
Botswana	1994	Yes	—
Burkina Faso	2006	No	6.1% (5.4%–6.6%)
Burundi	2004	No	2.8% (2.6%–3.3%)
Cameroon	2005 (2003)[a]	No	6.8% (6.5%–7.4%)
Cape Verde	2002	Yes	—
Central African Republic	2008	No	12.1% (11.0%–13.5%)
Chad	2008	No	10.5% (8.2%–12.3%)
Congo	2007	No	
Côte d'Ivoire	2003 (1999)[a]	No	8.9% (5.5%–9.4%)
Democratic Republic of the Congo	2007	No	—
Equatorial Guinea	2013	No	—
Eritrea	2002	No	—
Eswatini	1996	No	—
Ethiopia	2007	No	7.7% (7.0%–8.1%)
Gabon	2004	No	5.1% (3.2%–6.0%)
Gambia	1995 (1990)[a]	Yes	4.8% (4.4%–5.2%)
Ghana	2002	No	10.3% (6.9%–11.4%)
Guinea	2006	No	—
Kenya	2001	No	1.2% (0.9%–1.5%)
Liberia	2008	No	—
Madagascar	2002	No	5.5% (4.7%–6.4%)
Malawi	2002	No	3.2% (2.7%–3.9%)
Mali	2002	No	5.2% (4.9%–5.9%)
Mauritania	2005	Yes	9.3% (8.7%–10.2%)
Mozambique	2001	No	7.5% (5.6%–8.7%)
Namibia	2009	Yes	—
Niger	2008	No	—
Nigeria	2004	Yes	11.2% (10.1%–12.8%)
Rwanda	2002	No	3.4% (2.2%–4.3%)
Senegal	2004	Yes	8.1% (7.5%–9.0%)
Seychelles	1995	No	—
Sierra Leone	2007	No	—
South Africa	1995	No	—
South Sudan	2014	No	5.3% (4.2%–6.2%)
Togo	2008	No	—
Uganda	2002	No	5.5% (4.5%–6.0%)

(continued on next page)

Table 3 (continued)			
Country	(A) Year Hepatitis B Vaccine Introduced	Birth Dose Vaccine Introduction	(B) 2016 Prevalence Estimate (%)
Tanzania	2002	No	4.1% (3.2%–5.4%)
Zambia	2005	No	3.3% (3.0%–3.6%)
Zimbabwe	1994	No	8.5% (7.9%–9.7%)
AFRO	—	—	7.2% (6.2%–8·2%)

Column (A) represents the year the 3-dose hepatitis B vaccine was introduced to the entire country and this includes countries with both birth and nonbirth vaccination schedules.[29]

Abbreviation: AFRO, Regional Office for Africa.

[a] Year of HBV vaccine introduction in part of the country. Column (B) is 2016 HBsAg seroprevalence estimates based on The Polaris Observatory Collaborators.[8]

Data from Polaris Observatory Collaborators. Global prevalence, treatment, and prevention of hepatitis B virus infection in 2016: a modelling study. Lancet Gastroenterol Hepatol 2018;3:383–403; and Data, statistics and graphics. World Health Organization. http://www.who.int/immunization/monitoring_surveillance/data/en/. Published 2018. Accessed September 23, 2018.

Poor access to screening, vaccination, and treatment of those with chronic HBV infection limits the goal of HBV eradication in this region. For instance, the only place to receive free screening was in the blood bank, but this option lacked an effective linkage to care plan for those with newly diagnosed chronic HBV. Low levels of knowledge and awareness among individuals at risk for chronic HBV within this region also challenged the effective implementation of these programs.[22]

In addition to limited awareness, the cost for screening and treatment in the setting of minimal trained health care professionals and poor infrastructure also contribute to the challenge of eliminating HBV in sub-Saharan Africa. Potential solutions include integration of HBV screening with already-established screening programs, like human immunodeficiency virus, and using generic prices for treatment options.[23]

To improve screening and treatment in sub-Saharan Africa, The Prevention of Liver Fibrosis and Cancer in Africa (PROLIFICA), the first screen-and-treat program, was created in 2011 and started in The Gambia. Lemoine and colleagues[22] studied the effectiveness of the program in The Gambia and found that individuals who were screened and positive were compliant with treatment and 91.5% achieved virologic response at 1 year.

The Gambia

The Gambia Hepatitis Intervention Study (GHIS) was one of the first HBV intervention studies in The Gambia and ultimately led to widespread HBV vaccination. GHIS, a trial of the HBV vaccine, began in 1986, and focused on the effectiveness in preventing HCC with the infant HBV vaccination. GHIS led to the introduction of the Expanded Program of Immunization (EPI) in The Gambia, which resulted in vaccine coverage for the entire country by 1990. The GHIS trial ended in 1990 and was replaced by the national infant HBV vaccination program.[24] This program provided the HBV birth dose along with the 3-dose infant regimen. Peto and colleagues[25] studied the efficacy of GHIS and HBV vaccination in reducing HBsAg prevalence. The study was based on a 2007 to 2008 cross-sectional survey on both vaccinated and unvaccinated young adults born during 1986 to 1990 (during GHIS). The prevalence of HBsAg in those fully vaccinated (3 or 4 doses of infant vaccine) was 0.8%, in those unvaccinated it was 12.4%, and among those partially vaccinated it was 17.9%. Overall, there was

94% vaccine efficacy comparing HBsAg prevalence between those vaccinated and unvaccinated.

Furthermore, the GHIS and the national vaccination program were linked to The Gambia National Cancer Registry with the goal of determining the impact of HBV vaccination in prevention of HCC. These data are still being collected, but the expectation is that the reductions in HCC may be similar to those in studies performed in Asia regions.

South Africa

The 3-dose HBV vaccine was introduced into the national EPI of South Africa in 1995 by the South African National Department of Health. South Africa has yet to implement the birth dose vaccine. After introduction of the universal HBV vaccine, the seroprevalence of HBsAg in children younger than 5 years decreased from 12.8% in 1995 to 3% in 2009.[21] Also, Burnett and colleagues[26] reported that a study based on an Eastern Cape cohort showed that none of the 1213 12-month-olds to 25-month-olds born after 1995 that were fully vaccinated were HBsAg positive. In contrast, of those 12 to 25 months old born before 1995 who were unvaccinated, 7.8% (39 of 498) of them were HBsAg positive. Furthermore, although it is still too early to determine the efficacy of HBV vaccine on HCC prevalence in South African adults, Burnett and colleagues[26] described a national audit in children less than or equal to 14 years of age that is promising. The national audit found that between 1988 to 2003 and 1988 to 2006 there was a decrease in HCC malignant liver tumors from 35% (68 of 194) to 27% (77 of 274).

Europe

Based on The Polaris Observatory Collaborators progression model, the estimated 2016 HBsAg prevalence in Europe was 1.6%. Central Europe and Eastern Europe had higher prevalence than Western Europe at 1.7%, 1.5%, and 0.6% respectively. European countries with the highest prevalences include Albania (6.9%), Bulgaria (3.2%), Romania (3.4%), and Belarus (4.3%) (**Table 4**).[8] Overall, Europe is a region with low HBV endemicity. According to the WHO, there are 36,000 deaths from HBV per year in Europe.[27]

According to the 2016 European Center for Disease and Control (ECDC) report, most HBV infections were reported as chronic at 60%, and the most common routes of transmission were nosocomial and mother to child (32.6% and 31.6% respectively).[6]

The first introduction of HBV vaccine in Europe was in Italy in 1982. The earliest implementation of the universal HBV vaccination in Europe was in Cyprus in 1990, and then in Spain, Italy, Bulgaria, and San Marino in 1991 and in Israel in 1992. By 2012, 47 (89%) of the 53 countries within the European WHO region introduced universal HBV vaccination.[28] As of 2017, Hungary, Denmark, Switzerland, and Finland have yet to introduce HBV vaccine, whereas Norway and the United Kingdom have recently introduced it (see **Table 4**).[8,29]

Universal HBV vaccine efficacy in Europe has mainly been studied in countries that implemented the vaccine early on. For instance, in 1987, before implementation of the universal HBV vaccine in Italy, the incidence of acute HBV infection was 11 per 100,000 compared with 0.9 per 100,000 in 2010.[30] Also, based on a seroepidemiologic survey in 2011, Boccalini and colleagues[31] found that HBsAg prevalence in Tuscany decreased from 5.1% in prevaccination cohorts (aged 41–50 years) to 0% in children 1 to 10 years old, and 0.6% in individuals 11 to 20 years old in 2011. In addition, a 2002 study by Salleras and colleagues[32] observed that the global prevalence of HBsAg in Catalonia, Spain, has decreased from 1.5% in 1989, prevaccination, to 0.7%

Table 4
Hepatitis B virus surface antigen seroprevalence and year hepatitis B virus vaccine introduced in the World Health Organization European region

Country	(A) Year Hepatitis B Vaccine Introduced	Birth Dose Vaccine Introduction	(B) 2016 Prevalence Estimate (%)
Albania	1994	Yes	6.9% (4.7%–9.3%)
Austria	1997	No	—
Azerbaijan	2001	Yes	1.8% (1.5%–2.1%)
Belarus	1996	Yes	4.3% (3.9%–4.8%)
Belgium	1996	No	0.6% (0.5%–0.7%)
Bosnia and Herzegovina	2001 (1999)[a]	No	—
Bulgaria	1991	Yes	3.2% (1.9%–5.6%)
Croatia	1999	Yes	0.6% (0.5%–1.0%)
Cyprus	1989	No	—
Czech Republic	2001	No	0.4% (0.2%–0.5%)
Denmark	—	No	0.3% (0.2%–0.3%)
Estonia	2003 (1999)[a]	Yes	0.5% (0.5%–0.6%)
Finland	—	No	0.2% (0.2%–0.2%)
France	1994	No	0.5% (0.4%–0.7%)
Georgia	2001	Yes	2.5% (1.9%–3.0%)
Germany	1995	No	0.3% (0.2%–0.6%)
Greece	2000	No	1.8% (1.5%–2.0%)
Hungary	—	No	0.4% (0.4%–0.5%)
Iceland	—	No	—
Ireland	2008	No	0.1% (0.1%–0.1%)
Israel	Before 1998	Yes	—
Italy	1982	No	0.6% (0.3%–0.7%)
Kazakhstan	1998	Yes	2.7% (1.9%–3.6%)
Kyrgyzstan	2001 (1999)[a]	Yes	6.3% (4.1%–8.5%)
Lithuania	1998	Yes	—
Netherlands	2011	No	0.3% (0.1%–0.4%)
Norway	2017	No	0.3% (0.3%–0.4%)
Poland	1997 (1995)[a]	Yes	0.9% (0.7%–1.1%)
Portugal	1994	Yes	1.2% (0.9%–1.5%)
Moldova	1995	Yes	—
Romania	1995	Yes	3.4% (3.2%–3.7%)
Russia	2000	Yes	1.4% (0.6%–1.7%)
San Marino	1995	No	—
Serbia	2006 (2002)[a]	Yes	—
Slovakia	1998	No	1.6% (0.7%–1.8%)
Slovenia	—	No	1.0% (0.4%–1.1%)
Spain	1996 (1991)[a]	Yes	0.6% (0.4%–0.9%)
Sweden	2016 (2014)[a]	No	0.2% (0.1%–0.2%)
Switzerland	—	No	0.5% (0.3%–0.9%)
Tajikistan	2002	Yes	6.7% (5.6%–8.6%)

(continued on next page)

	(A) Year Hepatitis B	Birth Dose Vaccine	(B) 2016 Prevalence
Country	Vaccine Introduced	Introduction	Estimate (%)
Turkey	1998	Yes	2.6% (1.9%–3.5%)
Ukraine	2003 (2001)[a]	Yes	—
United Kingdom	2017	No	0.7% (0.5%–0.9%)
Uzbekistan	2001 (1997)[a]	Yes	8.0% (4.1%–11.7%)
EURO	—	—	1.6% (1.1%–2.1%)

Table 4
(continued)

Column (A) represents the year the 3-dose hepatitis B vaccine was introduced to the entire country and this includes countries with both birth and nonbirth vaccination schedules.[29]

Abbreviation: EURO, Regional Office for Europe.

[a] Year of HBV vaccine introduction in part of the country. Column (B) is 2016 HBsAg seroprevalence estimates based on The Polaris Observatory Collaborators.[8]

Data from Polaris Observatory Collaborators. Global prevalence, treatment, and prevention of hepatitis B virus infection in 2016: a modelling study. Lancet Gastroenterol Hepatol 2018;3:383–403; and Data, statistics and graphics. World Health Organization. http://www.who.int/immunization/monitoring_surveillance/data/en/. Published 2018. Accessed September 23, 2018.

after vaccination implementation. The European Vaccine Action Plan 2015–2020 is in effect and aims to improve immunization programs and access.

Americas

Based on The Polaris Observatory Collaborators progression model, the estimated 2016 HBsAg prevalence of the WHO pan-American region was 0.4%, making it a region of low endemicity. However, 2 countries in the Caribbean are still within the low-intermediate/high-intermediate endemicity: Haiti at 2.9% and Jamaica at 5.0% HBsAg prevalence in 2016 (**Table 5**).[8] The American region has the lowest viral hepatitis mortality (11.2 per 100,000).[11]

Within the Americas the earliest implementation of the 3-dose infant vaccine was in 1991 in the United States. The last few countries in the Americas to implement the 3-dose HBV vaccine were Saba, Haiti, and Bonaire in 2012. By 2016, 69% (35 of 51) of the countries within the Americas had HBV birth dose vaccination.[33] As of 2017, Chile, Nicaragua, Haiti, Barbados, Bolivia, Canada, and Jamaica have yet to introduce birth dose vaccination (see **Table 5**).[29]

South America

Significant data on HBV vaccine efficacy in South America have been collected in Colombia and Peru. For instance, a seroepidemiologic survey by Hoz and colleagues[34] based on children of the Colombian Amazon found that HBsAg prevalence of children aged 5 to 9 years decreased from 7% in 1992 (prevaccine) to 2% in 1999 (postvaccine). Another study, by Ramírez-Soto and colleagues,[35] used death certificate data from a hyperendemic province, Abancay, in Peru and compared mortalities after (1991–2012) the HBV vaccine was implemented with rates before (1960–1990) the vaccine. Overall, they found decreases in mortalities of HBV-related fulminant hepatitis from 34.8 to 1.28 per 100,000 population, cirrhosis from 16.0 to 6.3 per 100,000 population, and HCC from 9.20 to 3.30 per 100,000 population.

North America

North America is considered an area of low endemicity. The 2016 estimated HBsAg prevalence was 0.6% in Canada and 0.3% in United States.[8] However, it is important

Table 5
Hepatitis B virus surface antigen seroprevalence and year hepatitis B virus vaccine introduced in the World Health Organization region of the Americas

Country	(A) Year Hepatitis B Vaccine Introduced	Birth Dose Vaccine Introduction	(B) 2016 Prevalence Estimate (%)
Argentina	2000	Yes	0.2% (0.1%–0.3%)
Barbados	2000	No	—
Belize	2000	Yes	1.4% (0.6%–1.7%)
Bolivia	2000	No	—
Brazil	1998 (1989)[a]	Yes	0.4% (0.2%–0.6%)
Canada	1998 (1992)[a]	No	0.6% (0.4%–1.1%)
Chile	2005	No	0.1% (<0.1%–0.2%)
Colombia	1994	Yes	0.3% (0.1%–2.2%)
Costa Rica	2000	Yes	0.2% (0.1%–0.2%)
Cuba	1990	Yes	0.6% (0.5%–0.7%)
Dominican Republic	1994	Yes	1.7% (1.1%–2.0%)
Ecuador	1999	Yes	—
Guatemala	2005	Yes	0.6% (0.4%–0.7%)
Haiti	2012	No	2.9% (2.7%–4.1%)
Jamaica	2001	No	5.0% (2.4%–5.7%)
Mexico	1999	Yes	0.1% (0.1%–0.2%)
Nicaragua	1999	No	0.8% (0.4%–0.9%)
Panama	1999	Yes	—
Peru	2005 (1998)[a]	Yes	0.3% (0.3%–0.4%)
Suriname	2003	Yes	—
United States	1991 (1982)[a]	Yes	0.3% (0.2%–0.3%)
Venezuela	2000	Yes	1.2% (1.1%–1.8%)
PAHO	—	—	0.4% (0.3%–0.6%)

Column (A) represents the year the 3-dose hepatitis B vaccine was introduced to the entire country and this includes countries with both birth and nonbirth vaccination schedules.[29]
Abbreviation: PAHO, Pan American Health Organization.
[a] Year of HBV vaccine introduction in part of the country. Column (B) is 2016 HBsAg seroprevalence estimates based on The Polaris Observatory Collaborators.[8]
Data from Polaris Observatory Collaborators. Global prevalence, treatment, and prevention of hepatitis B virus infection in 2016: a modelling study. Lancet Gastroenterol Hepatol 2018;3:383–403; and Data, statistics and graphics. World Health Organization. http://www.who.int/immunization/monitoring_surveillance/data/en/. Published 2018. Accessed September 23, 2018.

to understand that data based on a selective population likely underestimate the actual prevalence. For instance, neglecting to observe the prevalence of HBV in the Asian and sub-Saharan African immigrant populations, incarcerated, homeless, and undocumented immigrants in America results in a substantial underestimation. An example is the National Health and Nutrition Survey (NHANES), which underestimated the US prevalence of HBV by only using data on noninstitutionalized US residents and may not accurately capture ethnic minorities or immigrant populations that have the highest risks of HBV in the United States.[36]

Ghany and colleagues[7] evaluated 1265 adults in the United States with chronic HBV and observed that transmission was largely vertical (60%), especially among Asians, who also held the highest prevalence, compared with horizontal transmission, which comprised 40% of infections. Horizontal transmission was mainly via sexual and medical exposure and was more common among white and black people.

In 1985, HBV vaccine was implemented via the health worker's vaccination program in the United States. However, it was not until 1991 that there was routine infant vaccination and then by 1995 routine adolescent vaccination.[37] By 2012 there was about 93% HBV vaccine coverage among adolescents (13–17 years old).[38] The 2016 estimate for 3-dose infant vaccination coverage in the United States was 93% and timely birth dose coverage was 64%.[8]

Despite NHANES underestimation of the total US prevalence, studies on HBV vaccination efficacy in the United States are typically based on NHANES participants. For instance, Wasley and colleagues[39] found that the age-adjusted prevalence of past and present HBV infection exposure (using anti–hepatitis B core) among children 6 to 19 years of age decreased from 1.9% (95% CI, 1.2–2.7) in NHANES 1988 to 1994 to 0.6% (95% CI, 0.4–0.9) in NHANES 1999 to 2006.

SUMMARY

Routine vaccination programs have reduced the global burden of HBV infection, because they have been particularly successful in decreasing HBsAg prevalence among infants and children. For instance, China has shown significant success because it has transitioned from a high endemic area to a high-intermediate endemic area because of vaccine implementation. However, there is still room for improvement and global challenges remain with effective implementation of universal HBV birth dose administration. Globally, birth dose vaccination is currently universal in only 101 countries.[40] A significant number of countries within the African and European regions continue to lack universal HBV birth dose administration.

Future advancements reside within the Global Health Sector Strategy, passed by the World Health Assembly in 2016, which has set goals toward elimination of both HBV and HCV by 2030. The plan is to reach specific targets, in 2020 and 2030, for global coverage of the childhood and birth dose vaccinations. This initiative has also set targets for population-wide testing and treatment. According to The Polaris Observatory Collaborators progression model, as of 2016 infant vaccination was already effective at a global level, with 94 of the modeled countries having already reached 1% HBsAg prevalence in children aged 5 years, the 2020 target, and 46 countries had already reach 0.1% prevalence, the 2030 target.[8]

Overall, the goal in eliminating HBV infection hinges on the ability to effectively implement and mobilize HBV vaccination programs. Achieving this goal involves expanding birth dose vaccination coverage and increasing awareness, at both the provider and public level, about the global burden of HBV infection and vaccine effectiveness.

DISCLOSURE

C. Gomes has nothing to disclose. R.J. Wong: research funding, advisory board, consulting, speaker's bureau for Gilead; research funding from Abbvie; speaker's bureau for Salix, Bayer. R.J. Wong is also funded by an American Association for the Study of Liver Diseases Foundation Clinical and Translational Research Award in Liver Diseases. R.G. Gish has received grants/research support from AbbVie, Benitec Biopharma, Gilead Sciences, and Merck. Dr R.J. Gish has performed as consultant and/or advisor to (in the last 2 years) Abbot, AbbVie, Alexion, Arrowhead, Bayer AG, Bristol-Myers Squibb Company, Contravir, Eiger, Enyo, eStudySite, Genentech, Gilead Sciences, HepaTX, HepQuant, Hoffmann-LaRoche, Intellia, Intercept, Ionis

Pharmaceuticals, Janssen, MedImmune, Merck, Shionogi, Transgene, and Trimaran. Dr R.G. Gish has current activity with the scientific or clinical advisory boards of AbbVie, Merck, Arrowhead, Bayer, Contravir, Dova Pharmaceuticals, Eiger, Enyo, Janssen, Medimmune, Janssen/J&J, Intercept, Shionogi, and Spring Bank. Dr R.G. Gish is a member of the Speakers Bureau for AbbVie, Bristol-Myers Squibb, Gilead Sciences, and Merck. Dr R.G. Gish is a minor stock shareholder of Cocrystal Pharma.

REFERENCES

1. Stanaway JD, Flaxman AD, Naghavi M, et al. The global burden of viral hepatitis from 1990 to 2013: findings from the Global Burden of Disease Study. Lancet 2013. https://doi.org/10.1016/s0140-6736(16)30579-7.
2. Hepatitis B. World Health Organization. 2018. Available at: http://www.who.int/news-room/fact-sheets/detail/hepatitis-b. Accessed September 9, 2018.
3. CEVHAP strategy 2017-2021 booklet FIN.pdf. Dropbox. 2018. Available at: https://www.dropbox.com/s/fkdlpwggcasihqi/CEVHAP%20Strategy%202017-2021%20booklet%20FIN.pdf?dl=0. Accessed September 9, 2018.
4. Shan S, Cui F, Jia J. How to control highly endemic hepatitis B in Asia. Liver Int 2018;38:122–5.
5. Zampino R. Hepatitis B virus burden in developing countries. World J Gastroenterol 2015;21(42):11941.
6. Hepatitis B. European Centre for Disease Prevention and Control. 2018. Available at: http://ecdc.europa.eu/en/hepatitis-b. Accessed August 28, 2018.
7. Ghany MG, Perrillo R, Li R, et al. Characteristics of adults in the hepatitis B research network in North America reflect their country of origin and hepatitis B virus genotype. Clin Gastroenterol Hepatol 2015;13:183–92.
8. Polaris Observatory Collaborators. Global prevalence, treatment, and prevention of hepatitis B virus infection in 2016: a modelling study. Lancet Gastroenterol Hepatol 2018;3:383–403.
9. FDA.gov. 2018. Available at: https://www.fda.gov/downloads/biologicsblood vaccines/vaccines/approvedproducts/ucm110114.pdf. Accessed October 4, 2018.
10. Who.int. 2018. Available at: http://www.who.int/immunization/topics/WHO_position_paper_HepB.pdf. Accessed September 23, 2018.
11. Global hepatitis report, 2017. World Health Organization. 2018. Available at: http://www.who.int/hepatitis/publications/global-hepatitis-report2017/en/. Accessed August 28, 2018.
12. LI X, Dumolard L, Patel M, et al. Implementation of hepatitis B birth dose vaccination – worldwide, 2016. Wkly Epidemiol Rec 2018;93(07):61–72.
13. Jourdain G, Ngo-Giang-Huong N, Harrison L, et al. Tenofovir versus placebo to prevent perinatal transmission of hepatitis B. N Engl J Med 2018;378:911–23.
14. Hepatitis D. World Health Organization. 2018. Available at: http://www.who.int/news-room/fact-sheets/detail/hepatitis-d. Accessed October 3, 2018.
15. MI4A information repository. World Health Organization. 2018. Available at: http://www.who.int/immunization/programmes_systems/procurement/v3p/platform/module2/en/. Accessed October 21, 2018.
16. Dynavax announces HEPLISAV-B™ is now available in the United States for the prevention of hepatitis B in adults. Dynavax Technologies Corporation; 2018. Available at: http://investors.dynavax.com/news-releases/news-release-details/dynavax-announces-heplisav-btm-now-available-united-states. Accessed October 21, 2018.

17. Schillie S, Harris A, Link-Gelles R, et al. Recommendations of the advisory committee on immunization practices for use of a hepatitis B vaccine with a novel adjuvant. MMWR Morb Mortal Wkly Rep 2018;67(15):455–8.
18. Cui F, Shen L, Li L, et al. Prevention of chronic hepatitis B after 3 decades of escalating vaccination policy, China. Emerg Infect Dis 2017;23(5):765–72.
19. Yu W, Liu D, Zheng J, et al. Loss of confidence in vaccines following media reports of infant deaths after hepatitis B vaccination in China. Int J Epidemiol 2016;45:441–9.
20. Chien Y. Nationwide hepatitis B vaccination program in Taiwan: effectiveness in the 20 Years after it was launched. Epidemiol Rev 2006;28(1):126–35.
21. Spearman C, Afihene M, Ally R, et al. Hepatitis B in Sub-Saharan Africa: strategies to achieve the 2030 elimination targets. Lancet Gastroenterol Hepatol 2017;2(12):900–9.
22. Lemoine M, Shimakawa Y, Njie R, et al. Acceptability and feasibility of a screen-and-treat programme for hepatitis B virus infection in the Gambia: the prevention of liver fibrosis and cancer in Africa (PROLIFICA) study. Lancet Glob Health 2016; 4(8):e559–67.
23. Nayagam S, Conteh L, Sicuri E, et al. Cost-effectiveness of community-based screening and treatment for chronic hepatitis B in the Gambia: an economic modelling analysis. Lancet Glob Health 2016;4(8):e568–78.
24. Shimakawa Y, Lemoine M, Mendy M, et al. Population-based interventions to reduce the public health burden related with hepatitis B virus infection in the Gambia, West Africa. Trop Med Health 2014;42(2 Suppl):S59–64.
25. Peto T, Mendy M, Lowe Y, et al. Efficacy and effectiveness of infant vaccination against chronic hepatitis B in the Gambia Hepatitis Intervention Study (1986–90) and in the nationwide immunisation program. BMC Infect Dis 2014;14:7.
26. Burnett R, Kramvis A, Dochez C, et al. An update after 16 years of hepatitis B vaccination in South Africa. Vaccine 2012;30:C45–51.
27. Data and statistics. Euro.who.int. 2018. Available at: http://www.euro.who.int/en/health-topics/communicable-diseases/hepatitis/data-and-statistics. Accessed September 19, 2018.
28. Lernout T, Hendrickx G, Vorsters A, et al. A cohesive European policy for hepatitis B vaccination, are we there yet? Clin Microbiol Infect 2014;20:19–24.
29. Data, statistics and graphics. World Health Organization; 2018. Available at: http://www.who.int/immunization/monitoring_surveillance/data/en/. Accessed September 23, 2018.
30. Romano L, Paladini S, Van Damme P, et al. The worldwide impact of vaccination on the control and protection of viral hepatitis B. Dig Liver Dis 2011;43(suppl 1):S2–7.
31. Boccalini S, Pellegrino E, Tiscione E, et al. Sero-epidemiology of hepatitis B markers in the population of Tuscany, central Italy, 20 years after the implementation of universal vaccination. Hum Vaccin Immunother 2013;9:1–6.
32. Salleras L, Dominguez A, Bruguera M, et al. Declining prevalence of hepatitis B virus infection in Catalonia (Spain) 12 years after the introduction of universal vaccination. Vaccine 2007;25:8726–31.
33. Ropero Álvarez A, Pérez-Vilar S, Pacis-Tirso C, et al. Progress in vaccination towards hepatitis B control and elimination in the Region of the Americas. BMC Public Health 2017;17(1):325.
34. Hoz F, Perez L, Neira M, et al. Eight years of hepatitis B vaccination in Colombia with a recombinant vaccine: factors influencing hepatitis B infection and effectiveness. Int J Infect Dis 2008;12:183–9.

35. Ramírez-Soto M, Ortega-Cáceres G, Cabezas C. Trends in mortality burden of hepatocellular carcinoma, cirrhosis, and fulminant hepatitis before and after roll-out of the first pilot vaccination program against hepatitis B in Peru: an analysis of death certificate data. Vaccine 2017;35(31):3808–12.
36. Gish R, Cohen C, Block J, et al. Data supporting updating estimates of the prevalence of chronic hepatitis B and C in the United States. Hepatology 2015;62(5): 1339–41.
37. Centers for Disease Control and Prevention (CDC). Hepatitis B vaccination–United States, 1982-2002. 2018. Available at: https://www.ncbi.nlm.nih.gov/pubmed/12118536. Accessed October 1, 2018.
38. Walker T, Smith E, Fenlon N, et al. Characteristics of pregnant women with hepatitis B virus infection in 5 US public health Jurisdictions, 2008-2012. Public Health Rep 2016;131(5):685–94.
39. Wasley A, Kruszon-Moran D, Kuhnert W, et al. The prevalence of hepatitis B virus infection in the United States in the era of vaccination. J Infect Dis 2010;202(2): 192–201.
40. Hutin Y, Desai S, Bulterys M. Preventing hepatitis B virus infection: milestones and targets. Bull World Health Organ 2018;96(7):443-443A.

Understanding the Natural History of Hepatitis B Virus Infection and the New Definitions of Cure and the Endpoints of Clinical Trials

Alisa Likhitsup, MD[a], Anna S. Lok, MD[b],*

KEYWORDS

- Cirrhosis • Hepatocellular carcinoma • Hepatitis B e Antigen
- Hepatitis B surface antigen • Hepatitis B virus DNA • Immunotherapy
- Antiviral therapy

KEY POINTS

- Currently available treatments are effective in inhibiting HBV replication, but rarely achieve the goal of HBsAg clearance.
- Several definitions of HBV cure have been proposed. Currently, the consensus definition of HBV "cure" is HBsAg clearance or functional cure.
- To achieve HBV cure, combination of antiviral therapies targeting multiple steps in the HBV lifecycle and immune-mediated therapies are necessary.

INTRODUCTION

Chronic hepatitis B virus (HBV) infection can cause cirrhosis, liver failure, hepatocellular carcinoma (HCC), and death. Worldwide, approximately 257 million people are chronically infected. Mortality due to viral hepatitis increased from 1.1 million in 2000 to 1.34 million in 2015, surpassing deaths from tuberculosis, HIV, and

Conflict of Interest: Dr A. Likhitsup has nothing to disclose. Dr A.S. Lok receives research grants from Assembly, Bristol-Myers Squibb, Gilead, and TARGET PharmaSolution; and serves as advisor for Gilead, Roche, Spring Bank, TARGET PharmaSolution, and Viravaxx.
[a] Division of Gastroenterology and Hepatology, Department of Internal Medicine, University of Missouri – Kansas City, St. Luke's Liver Disease and Transplant Specialist, 4320 Wornall Road, Suite 240, Kansas City, MO 64111, USA; [b] Division of Gastroenterology and Hepatology, Department of Internal Medicine, University of Michigan, 3912 Taubman Center, SPC 5362, 1500 East Medical Center Drive, Ann Arbor, MI 48109, USA
* Corresponding author.
E-mail address: aslok@med.umich.edu

malaria; prompting the World Health Organization to declare goals to eliminate hepatitis B and C by 2030.[1]

The goal of treatment of chronic HBV infection is to improve quality of life and survival in infected persons by preventing disease progression. Currently available treatments are effective in inhibiting HBV replication, reversing liver inflammation and fibrosis, and decreasing risk of cirrhosis and HCC.[2–7] However, these treatments do not eradicate HBV and rarely result in clearance of hepatitis B surface antigen (HBsAg). Thus, most patients need to receive long durations and often lifelong treatment. The success of hepatitis C cure has renewed enthusiasm in the search of a cure for hepatitis B. This article reviews the natural history of HBV infection, proposed definitions of HBV cure, and endpoints of clinical trials to evaluate potentially curative therapies.

NATURAL HISTORY OF HEPATITIS B VIRUS INFECTION

Acute HBV infection in adults is usually clinically inapparent. Most immunocompetent adults will spontaneously recover with HBsAg to hepatitis B surface antibody (anti-HBs) seroconversion, and only 1% to 5% will develop chronic infection. However, the risk of developing chronic HBV infection is 90% if infection is acquired at birth and 16% to 30% if infection is acquired in childhood.[8,9]

In acute HBV infection, serum HBV DNA level declines before the onset of clinical hepatitis.[10] There is no or minimal infiltration of immune cells in the liver suggesting a process of noncytolytic clearance of HBV during the early phase of acute infection.[11] Cytokine-mediated inhibition of HBV replication by virus-specific CD8+ T cells play a key role in recovery from acute HBV infection but other immune responses including B cells and innate immunity may also contribute.[11]

Although persons who have recovered from acute HBV infection are protected against reinfection, HBV persists in the liver of these persons, as demonstrated by detection of HBV DNA in the liver up to 10 years from the acute infection, reports of HBV reactivation with HBsAg seroreversion in persons receiving potent immunosuppressive therapy, and reports of HBV transmission when livers from these persons are transplanted into HBV nonimmune recipients.[12–15] Furthermore, it has been suggested that persistence of high titer anti-HBs decades after the initial infection may be maintained by continued stimulation of immune response from small amounts of residual virus.[16]

PHASES OF CHRONIC HEPATITIS B VIRUS INFECTION

The natural course of chronic HBV infection is variable and depends on the complex interplay between the individual's immune response and the virus (**Fig. 1**). Four clinical phases have been defined by hepatitis B e antigen (HBeAg) status, serum HBV DNA, and alanine aminotransferase (ALT) level.[7,17,18]

The first phase is characterized by the presence of HBeAg, very high HBV DNA level, and normal ALT. This phase has been termed "immune tolerant" based on absence of clinical and histologic evidence of liver disease in the face of high serum HBV DNA levels. This phase is more frequent and prolonged in persons infected perinatally. The concept of immune tolerance has recently been challenged because HBV-specific T-cell response in this phase although weak is not significantly different from that in the immune active phase.[19,20] It has been suggested that this phase be renamed as "HBeAg-positive non-inflammatory phase" or "HBeAg-positive chronic HBV infection." The notion that patients in this phase are not immune tolerant to HBV has prompted calls for expanding treatment

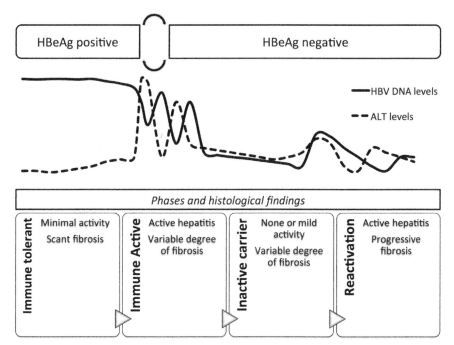

Fig. 1. Phases of chronic hepatitis B infection.

recommendations to include these patients who are at an early stage of chronic HBV infection, before irreversible liver damage and malignant transformation of hepatocytes. However, currently available treatments have low efficacy in patients in the immune tolerant phase. In 1 study of 126 HBeAg-positive adults with serum HBV DNA greater than 1.7×10^7 IU/mL and normal ALT, who received tenofovir disoproxil fumarate (TDF) with or without emtricitabine for 4 years, serum HBV DNA remained $\geq$69 IU/mL in 45% who received TDF and 24% who received combination of TDF and emtricitabine, and only 3 (5%) patients cleared HBeAg, and none cleared HBsAg.[21] Virologic relapse occurred in all patients when treatment was stopped. Two studies, 1 in adults and 1 in children in the immune tolerant phase treated with lead-in entecavir followed by combination of pegylated interferon (PEG-IFN) α2a and entecavir for 1 year also found very low rates of response.[22,23] Furthermore, although viral relapse occurred in all patients when treatment was stopped, it was not accompanied by ALT flares, supporting that immune response to HBV in this phase is weak and different from that in immune active phases.

The second phase, HBeAg-positive chronic hepatitis or HBeAg-positive immune active phase, is characterized by the presence of HBeAg, high serum HBV DNA levels, and elevated ALT. Exacerbations of chronic hepatitis or ALT flares are common during this phase and may reflect heightened immune clearance of infected hepatocytes as some flares are followed by HBeAg clearance.[24,25] However, many flares only lead to transient decrease in serum HBV DNA levels and do not result in HBeAg clearance. Recurrent flares may increase the risk of cirrhosis and HCC, and some flares may lead to hepatic decompensation.

After varying periods, most patients achieve HBeAg to hepatitis B e antibody (anti-HBe) seroconversion, serum HBV DNA levels decrease to low or undetectable levels and ALT levels normalize. Most patients who clear HBeAg enter the inactive carrier phase but some proceed directly to HBeAg-negative chronic hepatitis. Factors associated with higher rates of spontaneous HBeAg clearance include older age, higher ALT, race (Whites vs Asians), and HBV genotype (B > C).[18,25,26]

The third phase, HBeAg-negative chronic infection or inactive carrier phase, is characterized by absence of HBeAg and presence of anti-HBe, low serum HBV DNA level, and normal ALT. These patients have low risk of liver disease progression if they remain in this phase and their prognosis is excellent if they have not incurred significant liver damage before entering this phase.[27] Patients who remain in this phase may also undergo spontaneous HBsAg clearance. The annual rate of spontaneous HBsAg clearance has been estimated to be 1%, but the rate is not linear, with very low rates during the first 4 decades and more rapid increase afterward.[28–30] Progression to HBeAg-negative chronic hepatitis B may occur with an estimated annual risk of 0.37% to 3.3%.[31–33]

The fourth phase, HBeAg-negative chronic hepatitis or HBeAg-negative immune active phase, is characterized by absence of HBeAg and presence of anti-HBe, moderate to high serum HBV DNA levels, and elevated ALT. Exacerbations of chronic hepatitis can be observed during this phase. A recent study found that a 1-time testing of quantitative serum HBsAg levels is as reliable as 2 to 3 tests for HBV DNA and ALT levels over a 1-year period in differentiating patients in the inactive period of this phase versus those who are truly inactive carriers.[34] Continued HBV replication in the absence of HBeAg is often explained by the presence of mutations in the precore and/or basal core promoter regions of HBV that abolish or downregulate HBeAg production.

In patients who cleared HBsAg, ALT levels normalize and liver histology markedly improves.[12,35] Hepatitis B core antibody (anti-HBc, immunoglobulin G) persists in serum and most have detectable HBV DNA in the liver, although HBV DNA is seldom detected in serum.[12] These patients are considered to have occult HBV infection.[36] In 1 study, none of 146 patients without hepatitis C virus (HCV) or hepatitis D virus (HDV) coinfection or cirrhosis, who achieved HBsAg clearance developed cirrhosis or HCC after 63 months of follow-up, whereas cirrhosis and HCC occurred in 6 (4%) patients in the matched control group who did not clear HBsAg.[37,38] Overall, the long-term outcomes are favorable in patients with no concurrent HCV or HDV infection if HBsAg clearance is achieved before age 50 or before cirrhosis has developed.[38–40] Factors associated with higher rates of HBsAg clearance include age over 40 years and HBeAg negativity.[37]

OUTCOMES OF CHRONIC INFECTION

Among persons with untreated chronic HBV infection, the lifetime risks of HCC and liver-related mortality have been estimated to be 40% to 50% for men and 15% for women.[41] It should be noted that these estimates were based on studies in Asia where most people with chronic HBV infection were infected perinatally or during early childhood, and similar data for people with adult-acquired HBV infection are not available.

The annual incidence rate for developing liver cirrhosis is 2% to 6% for HBeAg-positive patients and 8% to 10% for HBeAg-negative patients.[26] Factors associated with risk of cirrhosis development include older age, male sex, obesity, persistent presence of HBeAg, persistently high HBV DNA level, high HBsAg levels, HBV genotype C > B, coinfection with HIV, HCV, or HDV, and heavy alcohol use.[18,26]

The annual risk of developing HCC is less than 1% in patients without and 2% to 5% in those with cirrhosis.[42] Factors associated with increased risk of HCC include: host (older age, Asian race or Blacks born in Africa, male sex, obesity, diabetes, family history of HCC), virus (persistently high HBV DNA level, persistent presence of HBeAg, core promoter variants, HBV genotype C > B, coinfection with HIV, HCV, or HDV), liver (ALT elevation, presence of cirrhosis), and environmental factors (carcinogens such as aflatoxin, tobacco, and heavy alcohol use).[18,42–47] Recent studies also showed that high serum HBsAg levels are associated with increased risks of HCC and cirrhosis, particularly for patients with low viremia (HBV DNA <2000 IU/mL).[48]

Several models have been developed to predict the risk of HCC, cirrhosis, and liver-related outcomes in untreated patients with chronic HBV infection.[46,47,49–51] These models may be used to guide disease monitoring and to inform treatment decisions. Recently, some models have incorporated liver stiffness measurements as indicators of liver fibrosis.[51] Furthermore, new models have been derived for patients who are receiving oral antiviral therapy[52,53] (**Table 1**).

CURRENT HEPATITIS B VIRUS TREATMENT
Efficacy and Safety of Current Treatments

The ultimate goal of treatment is to prevent cirrhosis, HCC, and death. Surrogate markers used to assess efficacy of treatment include: HBV DNA suppression, ALT normalization, HBeAg clearance, and HBsAg clearance.

Currently available antiviral treatments are limited to PEG-IFN and nucleos/tide analogs (NAs). Both are effective in inhibiting HBV replication but rarely achieve the goal of HBsAg clearance.

In HBeAg-positive patients who received PEG-IFN for 52 weeks, seroconversion to anti-HBe occurred in 39% of patients and HBsAg clearance in 6% to 8% after a mean follow-up period of 3 years.[54] HBV genotype A, high ALT levels, low HBV DNA levels, female sex, older age, and absence of previous interferon therapy were significantly associated with higher rates of seroconversion to anti-HBe as well as HBsAg loss[55] In HBeAg-negative patients who received PEG-IFN-based treatment for 48 weeks, HBsAg clearance was achieved in 8.7%, after a mean follow-up period of 3 years.[56] Baseline ALT was significantly associated with virologic response 3 years after treatment. HBV DNA and younger age were significant predictors of virologic response at 6 months after treatment but did not reach significant level as independent predictors of response 3 years after treatment.[56] Common adverse events of PEG-IFN include flu-like symptoms, fever, fatigue, depression, and exacerbation or unmasking of autoimmune illnesses.

NAs that have been approved for HBV treatment include lamivudine, adefovir dipivoxil, entecavir, telbivudine, TDF, and tenofovir alafenamide. Entecavir or tenofovir monotherapy are preferred because they have potent antiviral activity and high barrier to antiviral resistance. Although NAs are more effective in suppressing HBV replication than PEG-IFN, rates of HBsAg clearance with NAs is lower, 0% to 1% for HBeAg-negative patients and 4% to 10% for HBeAg-positive patients after 5 years of continuous treatment.[7] Virologic relapse is common when NAs are stopped. Guidelines recommend that NAs may be stopped in selected patients with no cirrhosis. For HBeAg-positive patients, NAs may be stopped in those who achieved HBeAg seroconversion and completed at least 1 year of consolidation therapy but viral and clinical relapses can still occur. For HBeAg-negative patients, NAs may be stopped in patients who cleared HBsAg but some guidelines now recommend NA withdrawal in patients with virus suppression for at least 2 to 3 years if they agree to close monitoring after treatment discontinuation.[17,57] These new recommendations are based on data from recent studies suggesting that NA withdrawal after 2 to 5 years treatment may

Table 1
Prediction models for hepatocellular carcinoma in chronic hepatitis B patients

Risk Score	Cohorts, n (%Cirrhosis)	Variables	5-y Prediction	10-y Prediction
GAG-HCC score[46]	Training: 820 (15%) Validation: not available	Sex Age HBV DNA Cirrhosis	Cut-off: 100 AUC: 0.87 Sensitivity: 70% Specificity: 88% PPV: 21% NPV: 98%	Cut-off: 82 AUC: 0.88 Sensitivity: 100% Specificity: 75% PPV: 22% NPV: 100%
CU-HCC score[47]	Training: 1005 (38%) Validation: 424 (16%)	Age Albumin Bilirubin HBV DNA Cirrhosis	Cut-off: 5 AUC: 0.76 Sensitivity: 78% Specificity: 73% PPV: 14% NPV: 98%	Cut-off: 5 AUC: 0.78 Sensitivity: 81% Specificity: 76% PPV: 27% NPV: 97%
REACH-B score[49]	Training: 3584 (0) Validation: 1505 (18%)	Sex Age ALT HBeAg HBV DNA	AUC: 0.79 Nomogram for predicted risk	AUC: 0.77 Nomogram for predicted risk
REVEAL[50]	Training: 2227 (0) Validation: 1113 (0)	Age Sex ALT Family history of HCC HBeAg HBV DNA Quantitative HBsAg HBV genotype	AUC: 0.89 Nomogram for predicted risk	AUC: 0.86 Nomogram for predicted risk
LSM-HCC score[51]	Training: 1035 (32%) Validation: 520 (31%)	Age Albumin HBV DNA Liver stiffness	Cut-off: 11 AUC: 0.83 Sensitivity: 92% Specificity: 71% PPV: 8% NPV: 100%	
PAGE-B score[a,52]	Training: 1325 (20%) Validation: 490 (48%)	Platelets Age Gender	Cut-off:10 C-index: 0.82 Sensitivity: 100% Specificity: 41% PPV: 10% NPV: 100% Nomogram for predicted risk	

Abbreviations: ALT, alanine aminotransferase; AUC, area under receiver operating characteristic curve; HBeAg, hepatitis B e antigen; HBsAg, hepatitis B surface antigen; HBV, hepatitis B virus; HCC, hepatocellular carcinoma; LSM, liver stiffness measurement; NPV, negative predictive value; PPV, positive predictive value.
    [a] Chronic hepatitis B patients under entecavir/tenofovir therapy.

result in higher rates of HBsAg clearance compared with patients who continued NAs.[17,58–60] These data need to be validated as most studies were retrospective and the only randomized study was small with a total of 42 patients. Furthermore, decompensation and death were reported in 1 study that included patients with cirrhosis.[60]

Despite the low rates of HBsAg loss, maintained suppression of HBV replication during long-term NA treatment can reverse liver fibrosis and even cirrhosis, and decrease risks of cirrhosis, HCC and liver-related mortality.[3–5]

LIMITATIONS OF CURRENT TREATMENTS

PEG-IFN and NAs inhibit HBV replication but they do not eradicate HBV and rarely achieve the goal of HBsAg clearance.[7] In addition, whereas the risk of HCC is reduced it is not eliminated.

A longer duration of PEG-IFN therapy may lead to a higher rate of HBsAg loss but many patients cannot tolerate PEG-IFN, and IFN is contraindicated in patients with decompensated cirrhosis and must be used with caution in patients with compensated cirrhosis.

NAs have few side effects, but long-term and often lifelong treatment is needed to maintain virus suppression. Extending the duration of NA treatment has very little impact on HBsAg clearance. Indeed, 1 study based on mathematical modeling estimated that median duration of NA treatment needed to achieve HBsAg clearance is 52 years.[61]

BARRIERS TO HEPATITIS B VIRUS CURE

Persistent presence of cccDNA and integrated HBV DNA in infected hepatocytes is a barrier to eradication of HBV. cccDNA serves as the template for transcription of pregenomic RNA, which is reverse transcribed into HBV DNA, and messenger RNAs, which are translated into viral proteins. There are 2 sources of cccDNA—incoming virions and recycling of nucleocapsids newly synthesized in the hepatocyte cytoplasm. Thus cccDNA may be replenished without the need for entry of new viruses. Furthermore, cccDNA seems to have a long half-life and seems to be mainly eliminated through hepatocyte turnover. Currently available NAs inhibit reverse transcription of pregenomic RNA to HBV DNA but do not inhibit cccDNA formation. In vitro studies suggest that PEG-IFN may enhance cccDNA degradation, but it is unclear if this occurs in patients receiving PEG-IFN.[62]

HBV DNA can be integrated into the host genome. Previous studies found that integrated HBV DNA frequently has deletions and rearrangements and is likely to be replication defective and may not contribute to production of functional viral proteins. However, recent studies suggest that integrated HBV DNA may be a major source of HBsAg in HBeAg-negative patients.[63] Although it is unclear if HBsAg translated from integrated HBV DNA is functional, it can be detected with serologic assays used in clinical practice, and will affect assessment of treatment endpoint based on HBsAg clearance.

Robust immune response is important to clear infections. Patients with chronic HBV infection have impaired innate as well as T-cell responses to HBV. It has been suggested that T cells are exhausted due to chronic exposure to large amounts of circulating HBsAg. Several studies showed that T-cell response to HBV is restored in patients with HBeAg or HBsAg clearance spontaneously or after treatment with PEG-IFN or NA. Thus, whereas previous immune modulatory therapies have failed to stimulate adequate T-cell response leading to decrease in HBV DNA or HBsAg levels, new approaches including blocking inhibitory pathways and engineered T cells, which have revolutionized oncology treatment might be more effective in restoring immune response in patients with chronic HBV infection, particularly after antiviral therapy has suppressed HBV replication and reduced HBsAg production.[64]

NEW DEFINITIONS OF CURE

With renewed interest in developing HBV cure, the American Association for the Study of Liver Diseases and the European Association for the Study of the Liver in collaboration with the United States Food and Drug Administration and the European Medicines Agency held a joint workshop in September 2016 to discuss definitions of HBV cure and design of clinical trials aimed at hepatitis B cure.[65] Several definitions of HBV cure were proposed (**Table 2**).

Complete or sterilizing cure is defined as sustained loss of HBsAg in serum and complete eradication of HBV DNA including intrahepatic cccDNA and integrated HBV DNA. Achievement of sterilizing cure would simulate persons who have never been infected. The consensus was that this goal although ideal is not feasible.

Functional cure is defined as sustained loss of HBsAg and HBV DNA in serum with or without seroconversion to anti-HBs after completion of a finite course of treatment. This scenario does not require eradication of cccDNA or integrated HBV DNA but will require that cccDNA production be decreased and rendered transcriptionally inactive. Two levels of functional cure were proposed, 1 simulating recovery after transient acute HBV infection (idealistic) and the other simulating spontaneous or IFN- or NA-induced HBsAg loss after years or decades of chronic HBV infection (realistic). The difference between these 2 scenarios is that in the former, there would be no liver injury and no increased risk of HCC, whereas, in the latter, there would be residual liver damage that is inactive and over time fibrosis would regress and the risk of HCC would decrease.

Functional cure as determined by HBsAg clearance is currently accepted as the definition of HBV cure and the goal for new HBV therapies.[65] Thus, it is crucial to have HBsAg assays that are capable of detecting extremely low levels of HBsAg, common HBV S gene variants and HBsAg bound to anti-HBs as immune complexes; and can differentiate HBsAg translated from integrated HBV DNA versus cccDNA. The lower limit of detection of commercially available immunoassays is 0.05 IU/mL. One study found that 20 of 2043 serum samples from patients who were negative for HBsAg using the Abbott Architect assay tested positive using a Lumipulse assay with a detection limit of 0.005 IU/mL.[66] Six of these 20 samples had detectable HBV DNA ranging from 32 to 600 IU/mL highlighting the need for more sensitive HBsAg assays. HBV S gene variants have been detected in infants born to HBsAg-positive mothers, who were infected despite prophylaxis with hepatitis B immune globulin and HBV vaccine; and in patients with liver transplantation for hepatitis B, who had recurrent HBV despite prophylaxis with hepatitis B immune globulin. HBV S gene variants have also been detected in other persons who have not been exposed to hepatitis B immune globulin. Although these variants are rare, some result in alteration of the dominant S epitopes and may escape detection in serologic assays for HBsAg that rely on monovalent antibodies. Clearance of HBsAg may be accompanied by development of anti-HBs and immune complex formation. HBsAg in these complexes may not be detected until it has been dissociated from anti-HBs, a step that is, not included in commercially available HBsAg assays. Recent data suggest that integrated HBV DNA may be the predominant source of circulating HBsAg in HBeAg-negative patients, and HBsAg may persist even after cccDNA has been rendered transcriptionally inactive or eliminated. Validating this finding is important and, if confirmed, HBsAg clearance may not be an achievable endpoint unless integrated HBV DNA can be eradicated. Another issue that needs to be resolved is whether seroconversion to anti-HBs is necessary for durable HBsAg clearance. Clinical experience suggests that HBsAg clearance if confirmed

Table 2
Definitions of HBV cure

Clinical Scenario	Complete/Sterilizing Cure Never Infected	Idealistic Functional Cure Recovery After Acute HBV	Realistic Functional Cure Chronic HBV with HBsAg Loss	Partial "Cure" Inactive Carrier Off Treatment
HBsAg	Negative	Negative	Negative	Positive
Anti-HBs	Negative	Positive	Positive/negative	Negative
HBeAg	Negative	Negative	Negative	Negative
Serum HBV DNA	Not detected	Not detected	Not detected	Low level or not detected
Hepatic cccDNA, transcription	Not detected Not active	Detected Not active	Detected Not active	Detected Low level
Integrated HBV DNA	Not detected	Detected?	Detected	Detected
Liver disease	None	None	Inactive, fibrosis regress over time	Inactive
Risk of HCC	Not increased	Not increased	Declines with time	Risk lower vs active hepatitis

on repeat testing at least 6 months apart is sustained in greater than 90% of cases regardless of anti-HBs seroconversion. Studies to verify this observation is important because the interval between HBsAg clearance and detection of anti-HBs is variable and may be up to a few years making it difficult to use HBsAg seroconversion as endpoint in clinical trials.

Partial cure is defined as persistent detection of HBsAg but not HBeAg and low or undetectable HBV DNA in serum after completion of a finite course of treatment, simulating an inactive carrier state. Although this is not ideal, it may be a reasonable intermediate endpoint if it can be sustained without the need for continued treatment.

NOVEL HEPATITIS B VIRUS TREATMENT

To achieve HBV cure, combination of antiviral therapies targeting multiple steps in the HBV lifecycle and immune-mediated therapies are necessary.

POTENTIAL ANTIVIRAL TARGETS

Several new classes of antiviral therapies are currently in early-phase clinical trials. Entry inhibitors target HBV receptor—sodium taurocholate cotransporting polypeptide. A prime example is Myrucldex B, which is being evaluated for hepatitis B, and D. Two types of core particle assembly modifiers are in phase 2 clinical trials. These compounds lead to empty or dysfunctional core particles preventing reverse transcription of pregenomic RNA to HBV DNA, recycling of nucleocapsids to replenish cccDNA, production of virions, and possibly also reduce HBsAg translation.

Eradication of cccDNA is the Achilles heel to HBV cure. Several approaches have been proposed.[67] They include: (1) decrease production by blocking infection using entry inhibitors or by blocking conversion of relaxed circular DNA to cccDNA[68]; (2) decrease cccDNA amplification by blocking intracellular entry of new capsids with core particle assembly modulators or NAs; (3) decrease persistence of cccDNA by increasing turnover of infected hepatocytes or increase degradation of cccDNA directly using CRISPR or gene editing or indirectly using PEG-IFN; and (4) decrease transcription of cccDNA through epigenetic modification or hepatitis B X protein inhibitors.[69,70]

Another class of novel antiviral therapy targets viral transcripts with small interfering RNAs. Preliminary results of phase 2 trials showed promising results but optimal drug delivery remains challenging.[63]

Abundance of circulating HBsAg has been attributed to be a major cause of immune exhaustion. Thus, some antiviral approaches aimed to decrease HBsAg production or secretion. Nucleic acid polymers target host factors involved in assembly or secretion. Trials of REP 2055 and REP 2139 used in monotherapy followed by combination with PEG-IFN or TDF induced a marked decline in circulating HBsAg levels and viremia and anti-HBs seroconversion in some patients.[71,72] However, these results need to be validated in larger studies and long-term safety remains to be established as retention of viral proteins in hepatocytes can cause liver injury and severe hepatitis flares were observed in clinical trials of REPs.

POTENTIAL APPROACHES TO RESTORE IMMUNE RESPONSE TO HEPATITIS B VIRUS

Patients with chronic HBV infection have impaired immune response to HBV. Studies of patients who cleared HBsAg spontaneously or after PEG-IFN or NA treatment showed that immune response can be restored indicating that immune modulatory therapy may enhance immune recovery and in combination with antiviral therapy may increase the likelihood of achieving HBV cure.

At present clinical trials of immune modulatory therapies with or without antiviral therapy have not been successful. However, newer approaches such as use of check-point inhibitors and engineered T cells that have revolutionized oncology treatment are worth exploring. It is also possible that therapeutic vaccines or pharmacologic activation of the innate immune response may also be effective if used in combination with antiviral therapies that not only inhibit HBV replication but also reduce HBsAg production.

ENDPOINTS OF CLINICAL TRIALS

Currently, the consensus definition of HBV "cure" is HBsAg clearance. Clinical trials aimed at HBV cure should demonstrate that a higher proportion of treated patients can achieve HBsAg clearance than currently available therapies. These new treatments need to be safe and easy to administer given the excellent safety profile and ease of administration of NAs, and HBsAg clearance should be sustained after a finite duration (1–2 years) of treatment.[65] Although HBsAg clearance should be the endpoint for phase 3 trials, it may not be realistic for phase 2 trials, which are shorter in duration. Thus, other endpoints such as decrease in quantitative HBsAg, serum HBV RNA, or hepatitis B core-related antigen (HBcrAg) levels, and serum HBV DNA levels if NAs are not used in combination may need to be used in phase 2 trials.[65] However, the reliability of these markers as surrogates for HBsAg clearance has not been established and standardized assays for serum HBV RNA and HBcrAg are not available. Although it would be ideal to demonstrate that cccDNA is decreased or eradicated, assessment of cccDNA concentration or activity requires access to liver tissue and standardized assays, which is not practical or feasible. For immune modulatory therapy trials, it would be ideal to demonstrate that immune response to HBV is enhanced but there is currently no consensus on which immune response is critical. Furthermore, immunologic assays are not standardized and complex. Thus, clinical trials of immune modulatory therapies would also rely on virological endpoints.

Given the fluctuating nature of chronic HBV infection and that it is unlikely that all traces of HBV can be eradicated, timing of assessment of treatment response is critical in clinical trials. Appropriate time to assess treatment response depends on mechanism of action of the drug tested; virologic response occurs earlier with direct antiviral agents, whereas response to immune modulatory therapy may be delayed. Time to assess treatment outcomes also depends on phase of trial; antiviral activity should be assessed during and at the end of treatment in phase 2 studies, and sustained antiviral activity ≥ 6 months off treatment should be assessed in phase 3 studies, and posttreatment monitoring for at least 3 to 5 years should be conducted to confirm durability of response and impact on clinical outcomes.

Endpoints of clinical trials of new HBV treatment should also include safety assessment. A major concern is hepatitis flare but other adverse events such as antiviral drug resistance, off-target effects, and immune-mediated organ damage may also prevent new therapies from approval even if they prove to be efficacious.

WHAT TO EXPECT IN THE FUTURE

Improved knowledge about HBV life cycle and immune response has led to the development of many new antiviral and immune modulatory therapies aimed at HBV cure.

Different strategies may need to be deployed depending on the phase of chronic HBV infection. Combination therapies will likely be required to achieve cure. Safety is paramount and validation of surrogate markers of cure is urgently needed. Concerted efforts of researchers, clinicians, diagnostic and therapeutic companies, and regulatory agencies can make the possibility of HBV cure a reality.

REFERENCES

1. Global Hepatitis Report 2017, Geneva: World Health Organization; 2017. Licence: CC BY-NC-SA 3.0 IGO.
2. Chang TT, Liaw YF, Wu SS, et al. Long-term entecavir therapy results in the reversal of fibrosis/cirrhosis and continued histological improvement in patients with chronic hepatitis B. Hepatology 2010;52(3):886–93.
3. Liaw YF, Sung JJ, Chow WC, et al. Lamivudine for patients with chronic hepatitis B and advanced liver disease. N Engl J Med 2004;351(15):1521–31.
4. Marcellin P, Gane E, Buti M, et al. Regression of cirrhosis during treatment with tenofovir disoproxil fumarate for chronic hepatitis B: a 5-year open-label follow-up study. Lancet 2013;381(9865):468–75.
5. Papatheodoridis GV, Idilman R, Dalekos GN, et al. The risk of hepatocellular carcinoma decreases after the first 5 years of entecavir or tenofovir in Caucasians with chronic hepatitis B. Hepatology 2017;66(5):1444–53.
6. Lok AS, McMahon BJ, Brown RS Jr, et al. Antiviral therapy for chronic hepatitis B viral infection in adults: a systematic review and meta-analysis. Hepatology 2016; 63(1):284–306.
7. Terrault NA, Lok ASF, McMahon BJ, et al. Update on prevention, diagnosis, and treatment of chronic hepatitis B: AASLD 2018 hepatitis B guidance. Hepatology 2018;67(4):1560–99.
8. Beasley RP, Hwang LY, Lee GC, et al. Prevention of perinatally transmitted hepatitis B virus infections with hepatitis B immune globulin and hepatitis B vaccine. Lancet 1983;2(8359):1099–102.
9. McMahon BJ. Natural history of chronic hepatitis B. Clin Liver Dis 2010;14(3): 381–96.
10. Webster GJ, Reignat S, Maini MK, et al. Incubation phase of acute hepatitis B in man: dynamic of cellular immune mechanisms. Hepatology 2000;32(5):1117–24.
11. Xia Y, Stadler D, Lucifora J, et al. Interferon-gamma and tumor necrosis factor-alpha produced by T cells reduce the HBV persistence form, cccDNA, without cytolysis. Gastroenterology 2016;150(1):194–205.
12. Ahn SH, Park YN, Park JY, et al. Long-term clinical and histological outcomes in patients with spontaneous hepatitis B surface antigen seroclearance. J Hepatol 2005;42(2):188–94.
13. Hsu C, Tsou HH, Lin SJ, et al. Chemotherapy-induced hepatitis B reactivation in lymphoma patients with resolved HBV infection: a prospective study. Hepatology 2014;59(6):2092–100.
14. Seto WK, Chan TS, Hwang YY, et al. Hepatitis B reactivation in occult viral carriers undergoing hematopoietic stem cell transplantation: a prospective study. Hepatology 2017;65(5):1451–61.
15. Yuki N, Nagaoka T, Yamashiro M, et al. Long-term histologic and virologic outcomes of acute self-limited hepatitis B. Hepatology 2003;37(5):1172–9.
16. Rehermann B, Ferrari C, Pasquinelli C, et al. The hepatitis B virus persists for decades after patients' recovery from acute viral hepatitis despite active maintenance of a cytotoxic T-lymphocyte response. Nat Med 1996;2(10):1104–8.

17. European Association for the Study of the Liver, Electronic address, e.e.e. and L. European Association for the Study of the Liver. EASL 2017 clinical practice guidelines on the management of hepatitis B virus infection. J Hepatol 2017; 67(2):370–98.

18. Yim HJ, Lok AS. Natural history of chronic hepatitis B virus infection: what we knew in 1981 and what we know in 2005. Hepatology 2006;43(2 Suppl 1): S173–81.

19. Kennedy PTF, Sandalova E, Jo J, et al. Preserved T-cell function in children and young adults with immune-tolerant chronic hepatitis B. Gastroenterology 2012; 143(3):637–45.

20. Park JJ, Wong DK, Wahed AS, et al. Hepatitis B virus-specific and global T-cell dysfunction in chronic hepatitis B. Gastroenterology 2016;150(3):684–95.e5.

21. Chan HL, Chan CK, Hui AJ, et al. Effects of tenofovir disoproxil fumarate in hepatitis B e antigen-positive patients with normal levels of alanine aminotransferase and high levels of hepatitis B virus DNA. Gastroenterology 2014;146(5):1240–8.

22. Feld JJ, Terrault N, Lin HS. Entecavir and peginterferon alfa-2a in adults with HBeAg-positive immune tolerant chronic hepatitis B virus infection. Hepatology 2018. https://doi.org/10.1002/hep.30417.

23. Rosenthal P, Ling SC, Belle SH, et al. Combination of entecavir/peginterferon alfa-2a in children with HBeAg-positive immune tolerant chronic hepatitis B virus infection. Hepatology 2018. https://doi.org/10.1002/hep.30312.

24. Lok AS, Lai CL. Acute exacerbations in Chinese patients with chronic hepatitis B virus (HBV) infection. Incidence, predisposing factors and etiology. J Hepatol 1990;10(1):29–34.

25. Liaw YF, Pao CC, Chu CM, et al. Changes of serum hepatitis B virus DNA in two types of clinical events preceding spontaneous hepatitis B e antigen seroconversion in chronic type B hepatitis. Hepatology 1987;7(1):1–3.

26. Fattovich G, Bortolotti F, Donato F. Natural history of chronic hepatitis B: special emphasis on disease progression and prognostic factors. J Hepatol 2008; 48(2):335–52.

27. Manno M, Cammà C, Schepis F, et al. Natural history of chronic HBV carriers in northern Italy: morbidity and mortality after 30 years. Gastroenterology 2004; 127(3):756–63.

28. Liu J, Yang HI, Lee MH, et al. Incidence and determinants of spontaneous hepatitis B surface antigen seroclearance: a community-based follow-up study. Gastroenterology 2010;139(2):474–82.

29. Chu CM, Liaw YF. HBsAg seroclearance in asymptomatic carriers of high endemic areas: appreciably high rates during a long-term follow-up. Hepatology 2007;45(5):1187–92.

30. Yeo YH, Ho HJ, Yang HI, et al. Factors associated with rates of HBsAg seroclearance in adults with chronic HBV infection: a systematic review and meta-analysis. Gastroenterology 2018;156(3):635–46.e9.

31. Chu CM, Liaw YF. Predictive factors for reactivation of hepatitis B following hepatitis B e antigen seroconversion in chronic hepatitis B. Gastroenterology 2007; 133(5):1458–65.

32. Chen YC, Chu CM, Liaw YF. Age-specific prognosis following spontaneous hepatitis B e antigen seroconversion in chronic hepatitis B. Hepatology 2010;51(2): 435–44.

33. Wu JF, Chiu YC, Chang KC, et al. Predictors of hepatitis B e antigen-negative hepatitis in chronic hepatitis B virus-infected patients from childhood to adulthood. Hepatology 2016;63(1):74–82.

34. Liu J, Yang HI, Lee MH, et al. Serum levels of hepatitis B surface antigen and DNA can predict inactive carriers with low risk of disease progression. Hepatology 2016;64(2):381–9.

35. Yuen MF, Wong DK, Sablon E, et al. HBsAg seroclearance in chronic hepatitis B in the Chinese: virological, histological, and clinical aspects. Hepatology 2004; 39(6):1694–701.

36. Raimondo G, Navarra G, Mondello S, et al. Occult hepatitis B virus in liver tissue of individuals without hepatic disease. J Hepatol 2008;48(5):743–6.

37. Liaw YF, Sheen IS, Chen TJ, et al. Incidence, determinants and significance of delayed clearance of serum HBsAg in chronic hepatitis B virus infection: a prospective study. Hepatology 1991;13(4):627–31.

38. Chen YC, Sheen IS, Chu CM, et al. Prognosis following spontaneous HBsAg seroclearance in chronic hepatitis B patients with or without concurrent infection. Gastroenterology 2002;123(4):1084–9.

39. Huo TI, Wu JC, Lee PC, et al. Sero-clearance of hepatitis B surface antigen in chronic carriers does not necessarily imply a good prognosis. Hepatology 1998;28(1):231–6.

40. Yuen MF, Wong DK, Fung J, et al. HBsAg Seroclearance in chronic hepatitis B in Asian patients: replicative level and risk of hepatocellular carcinoma. Gastroenterology 2008;135(4):1192–9.

41. Beasley RP, Lin CC, Chien CS, et al. Geographic distribution of HBsAg carriers in China. Hepatology 1982;2(5):553–6.

42. Raffetti E, Fattovich G, Donato F. Incidence of hepatocellular carcinoma in untreated subjects with chronic hepatitis B: a systematic review and meta-analysis. Liver Int 2016;36(9):1239–51.

43. Iloeje UH, Yang HI, Jen CL, et al. Risk and predictors of mortality associated with chronic hepatitis B infection. Clin Gastroenterol Hepatol 2007;5(8):921–31.

44. Yang JD, Mannalithara A, Piscitello AJ, et al. Impact of surveillance for hepatocellular carcinoma on survival in patients with compensated cirrhosis. Hepatology 2018;68(1):78–88.

45. Chen CJ, Yang HI, Su J, et al. Risk of hepatocellular carcinoma across a biological gradient of serum hepatitis B virus DNA level. JAMA 2006;295(1):65–73.

46. Yuen MF, Tanaka Y, Fong DY, et al. Independent risk factors and predictive score for the development of hepatocellular carcinoma in chronic hepatitis B. J Hepatol 2009;50(1):80–8.

47. Wong VW, Chan SL, Mo F, et al. Clinical scoring system to predict hepatocellular carcinoma in chronic hepatitis B carriers. J Clin Oncol 2010;28(10):1660–5.

48. Tseng TC, Liu CJ, Yang HC, et al. Serum hepatitis B surface antigen levels help predict disease progression in patients with low hepatitis B virus loads. Hepatology 2013;57(2):441–50.

49. Yang HI, Yuen MF, Chan HL, et al. Risk estimation for hepatocellular carcinoma in chronic hepatitis B (REACH-B): development and validation of a predictive score. Lancet Oncol 2011;12(6):568–74.

50. Lee MH, Yang HI, Liu J, et al. Prediction models of long-term cirrhosis and hepatocellular carcinoma risk in chronic hepatitis B patients: risk scores integrating host and virus profiles. Hepatology 2013;58(2):546–54.

51. Wong GL, Chan HL, Wong CK, et al. Liver stiffness-based optimization of hepatocellular carcinoma risk score in patients with chronic hepatitis B. J Hepatol 2014;60(2):339–45.

52. Papatheodoridis G, Dalekos G, Sypsa V, et al. PAGE-B predicts the risk of developing hepatocellular carcinoma in Caucasians with chronic hepatitis B on 5-year antiviral therapy. J Hepatol 2016;64(4):800–6.

53. Kim JH, Kim YD, Lee M, et al. Modified PAGE-B score predicts the risk of hepatocellular carcinoma in Asians with chronic hepatitis B on antiviral therapy. J Hepatol 2018;69(5):1066–73.

54. Buster EH, Flink HJ, Cakaloglu Y, et al. Sustained HBeAg and HBsAg loss after long-term follow-up of HBeAg-positive patients treated with peginterferon alpha-2b. Gastroenterology 2008;135(2):459–67.

55. Buster EH, Hansen BE, Lau GK, et al. Factors that predict response of patients with hepatitis B e antigen-positive chronic hepatitis B to peginterferon-alfa. Gastroenterology 2009;137(6):2002–9.

56. Marcellin P, Bonino F, Lau GK, et al. Sustained response of hepatitis B e antigen-negative patients 3 years after treatment with peginterferon alpha-2a. Gastroenterology 2009;136(7):2169–79.e1-4.

57. Sarin SK, Kumar M, Lau GK, et al. Asian-Pacific clinical practice guidelines on the management of hepatitis B: a 2015 update. Hepatol Int 2016;10(1):1–98.

58. Berg T, Simon KG, Mauss S, et al. Long-term response after stopping tenofovir disoproxil fumarate in non-cirrhotic HBeAg-negative patients - FINITE study. J Hepatol 2017;67(5):918–24.

59. Hadziyannis SJ, Sevastianos V, Rapti I, et al. Sustained responses and loss of HBsAg in HBeAg-negative patients with chronic hepatitis B who stop long-term treatment with adefovir. Gastroenterology 2012;143(3):629–36.e1.

60. Jeng WJ, Chen YC, Chien RN, et al. Incidence and predictors of hepatitis B surface antigen seroclearance after cessation of nucleos(t)ide analogue therapy in hepatitis B e antigen-negative chronic hepatitis B. Hepatology 2018;68(2):425–34.

61. Chevaliez S, Hézode C, Bahrami S, et al. Long-term hepatitis B surface antigen (HBsAg) kinetics during nucleoside/nucleotide analogue therapy: finite treatment duration unlikely. J Hepatol 2013;58(4):676–83.

62. Lucifora J, Xia Y, Reisinger F, et al. Specific and nonhepatotoxic degradation of nuclear hepatitis B virus cccDNA. Science 2014;343(6176):1221–8.

63. Wooddell CI, Yuen MF, Chan HL, et al. RNAi-based treatment of chronically infected patients and chimpanzees reveals that integrated hepatitis B virus DNA is a source of HBsAg. Sci Transl Med 2017;9(409) [pii:eaan0241].

64. Fisicaro P, Valdatta C, Massari M, et al. Antiviral intrahepatic T-cell responses can be restored by blocking programmed death-1 pathway in chronic hepatitis B. Gastroenterology 2010;138(2):682–93, 693.e1-4.

65. Lok AS, Zoulim F, Dusheiko G, et al. Hepatitis B cure: from discovery to regulatory approval. J Hepatol 2017;67(4):847–61.

66. Yang R, Song G, Guan W, et al. The Lumipulse G HBsAg-Quant assay for screening and quantification of the hepatitis B surface antigen. J Virol Methods 2016;228:39–47.

67. Levrero M, Subic M, Villeret F, et al. Perspectives and limitations for nucleo(t)side analogs in future HBV therapies. Curr Opin Virol 2018;30:80–9.

68. Blank A, Markert C, Hohmann N, et al. First-in-human application of the novel hepatitis B and hepatitis D virus entry inhibitor myrcludex B. J Hepatol 2016;65(3):483–9.

69. Lucifora J, Arzberger S, Durantel D, et al. Hepatitis B virus X protein is essential to initiate and maintain virus replication after infection. J Hepatol 2011;55(5):996–1003.

70. Lucifora J, Protzer U. Attacking hepatitis B virus cccDNA – the holy grail to hepatitis B cure. J Hepatol 2016;64(1 Suppl):S41–8.

71. Al-Mahtab M, Bazinet M, Vaillant A. Safety and efficacy of nucleic acid polymers in monotherapy and combined with immunotherapy in treatment-naive Bangladeshi patients with HBeAg+ chronic hepatitis B infection. PLoS One 2016;11(6): e0156667.

72. Bazinet M, Pantea V, Placinta G. Preliminary safety and efficacy of REP 2139-Mg or REP 2165-Mg used in combination with tenofovir disoproxil fumarate and pegylated interferon alpha 2a in treatment naive Caucasian patients with chronic HBeAg negative HBV infection. Hepatology 2016;64:LB–L7.

WHO Guidelines for Prevention, Care and Treatment of Individuals Infected with HBV

A US Perspective

Anusha Vittal, MD[a], Marc G. Ghany, MD, MHSc[b],*

KEYWORDS

- Chronic hepatitis B virus Infection • WHO guidelines • AASLD guidelines

KEY POINTS

- The 2016 WHO guidelines on testing for HBV are the first global evidence-based guidelines that complement the 2015 guidelines on prevention, care, and treatment of chronic HBV infection.
- Screening and linkage to care are key steps to management of chronic hepatitis B.
- Prevention of chronic hepatitis B through vaccination and postexposure prophylaxis remains the cornerstone for reducing the incidence of the disease and its related mortality.

INTRODUCTION

More than 2 billion people have been exposed to the hepatitis B virus (HBV) of whom an estimated 257 million people have chronic infection.[1] Chronic HBV infection occurs globally but the seroprevalence of hepatitis B surface antigen (HBsAg), the marker of chronicity, varies geographically, with the highest rates noted in sub-Saharan Africa and East Asia and the lowest rates in North America, western Europe, and Australia (**Fig. 1**).[2] Despite the availability of a safe and effective vaccine and antiviral therapy, chronic HBV infection continues to be a substantial public health burden, accounting for 30% of all deaths from cirrhosis and 40% of all deaths related to hepatocellular carcinoma globally.[3] As a consequence, in 2016 the World Health Organization (WHO) issued guidance to eliminate chronic viral hepatitis as a public health problem by 2030,

Financial Disclosure: The authors are employees of the US Government and have no financial conflicts of interest to disclose.
Funding: This work was supported by the Intramural Research Program of NIDDK, NIH.
[a] Liver Diseases Branch, NIDDK, NIH, Building 10, Room10/4-5722, 10 Center drive, MSC 1614, Bethesda, MD 20892-1800, USA; [b] Liver Diseases Branch, NIDDK, NIH, Building 10, Room 9B-16, 10 Center Drive, MSC 1800, Bethesda, MD 20892-1800, USA
* Corresponding author.
E-mail address: marcg@intra.niddk.nih.gov

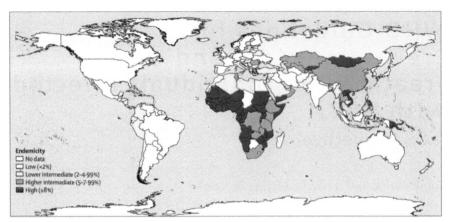

Fig. 1. Global estimates of the prevalence of hepatitis B surface antigen (HBsAg). *Reprinted with permission from* Elsevier (Schweitzer A, Horn J, Mikolajczyk RT. Estimations of worldwide prevalence of chronic hepatitis B virus infection: a systematic review of data published between 1965 and 2013. Lancet. 2015 Oct 17;386:1546–55).

by reducing the incidence of chronic HBV infection by 90% and mortality by 65%.[4] As part of this strategy, the WHO developed guidelines to provide evidence-based advice for the prevention, care, and treatment of persons affected by chronic HBV infection.[5] A driving force for development of these guidelines was to provide a global consensus on the principles of hepatitis B prevention, care, and treatment, to country program managers in all health care settings, particularly in low- and middle-income countries (LMICs). Because these guidelines were developed to target LMICs, several of the recommendations differ from those of the major Liver Societies, the American Association for the Study of Liver Diseases (AASLD), Asian Pacific Association for the Study of Liver Diseases (APASL), and the European Association for the Study of Liver Diseases (EASL). This review highlights key differences between the AASLD and WHO guidelines and discusses the impact on management of chronic hepatitis B.[6,7]

PREVENTION AND SCREENING
Screening

Screening for chronic HBV infection is performed by testing for serum HBsAg. The presence of HBsAg for a period of at least 6 months defines chronic HBV infection. Anti-HBs should be included in screening so that unexposed persons can be identified and offered HBV vaccination. AASLD guidelines recommend screening of persons born in regions of high or intermediate HBV endemicity (HBsAg prevalence of ≥2%), United States–born persons not vaccinated as an infant whose parents were born in regions with HBV endemicity ≥8%, pregnant women, people needing immunosuppressive medications including chemotherapy, blood donors, and patients with end-stage renal disease. The WHO recommends universal screening in countries with an HBsAg seroprevalence of 2% or greater. They also recommend routine testing of all pregnant women presenting to antenatal clinics and high-risk groups including sexual and household contacts of persons with chronic HBV infection, HIV-infected persons, persons who inject drugs, men who have sex with men, sex workers, indigenous peoples, persons who are incarcerated, and transgender persons. Blood and organ donors, and adults presenting with signs and symptoms suspicious of viral infection, should be screened for HBsAg. A complete list of groups at high risk for HBV infection and who should be screened is provided in **Table 1**.

Table 1
Comparison of recommendations for screening of patients at risk for acquiring HBV (differences between the AASLD and WHO guidelines are in italics)

WHO	AASLD
• Household and sexual contacts of persons with HBV • Persons infected with HIV • Persons who inject drugs • Men who have sex with men • Persons who are incarcerated • Blood and organ donors • Pregnant women • General population screening in countries with high HBV endemicity	• *Persons born in regions of high or intermediate HBV endemicity (HBsAg prevalence of ≥2%)* • *US-born persons not vaccinated as an infant whose parents were born in regions with HBV endemicity ≥8%* • Men who have sex with men • Intravenous drug users • *Individuals needing immunosuppressive therapy, including chemotherapy, immunosuppression related to transplantation, and immunosuppression for various disorders* • *Persons with elevated ALT or AST of unknown etiology* • Organ, plasma, blood, tissue or semen donors • End-stage renal disease patients needing dialysis • All pregnant women and infants born to HBsAg mothers • Persons infected with hepatitis C and HIV • Household and sexual contacts of HBsAg-positive persons • *Persons requesting evaluation/treatment of sexually transmitted disease or have multiple sexual partners* • *Health care staff, public safety workers, and staff of facilities for developmentally disabled persons* • *Persons traveling to countries with intermediate or high HBV prevalence* • Inmates of correctional facilities • *Unvaccinated persons with diabetes with age of 19–59 y*

Primary Prevention

HBV is transmitted primarily through parental exposure. In endemic countries, vertical and perinatal transmission is the most important cause of chronic infection, and efforts to interrupt this mode of transmission will have the greatest impact on reducing the incidence and prevalence of chronic HBV infection.[8] Primary prevention of HBV infection is achieved through HBV vaccination, which is 90% to 95% effective in preventing HBV infection and transmission. Implementation of universal HBV infant vaccination programs has resulted in a dramatic decline in the incidence and prevalence of HBV and hepatocellular carcinoma (HCC) in children.[9,10] Therefore, in 2009 the WHO recommended that all countries, even those with low HBV prevalence, introduce universal hepatitis B birth dose (HepB-BD) vaccination, whereby the first dose of hepatitis B vaccine should be given as soon as possible (<24 hours) after birth, even in low-birth-weight infants and low-endemicity countries. Despite WHO recommendations, in 2014 only 96 (49%) out of 194 countries reported offering HepB-BD as part of their national immunization program and less than 38% of babies born worldwide received HepB-BD within 24 hours after birth (**Fig. 2**).

The WHO released its updated recommendations for the use of HBV vaccine in 2017.[11] AASLD recommendations mirror those of the Centers for Disease Control and Prevention (CDC) guidelines, released in 2012.[12] The WHO recommends a 3- to 4-dose schedule with doses separated by 4 weeks. At present there are no data supporting the administration of booster doses after the completion of vaccination series. Vaccination given to premature and low-birth-weight infants (birth weight <2000 g) does not count toward the vaccination series, and these infants should receive 3 additional doses to complete the vaccination schedule.

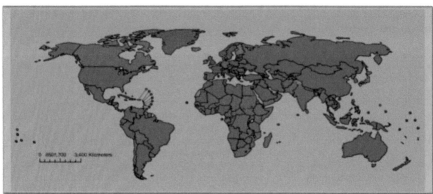

HepB-BD is part of national immunization schedule (95 countries or 49%)
HepB-BD only for infants born to HBsAg-positive mothers (22 countries or 11%)
HepB-BD in national immunization schedule but not HepB-BD
HepB-BD only for risk groups or adolescents

Fig. 2. Countries providing hepatitis B birth dose (HepB-BD) in 2016. In 2016 only, half of all countries globally had adopted HepB-BD as part of their national immunization program and less than 38% of babies born worldwide received HepB-BD within the recommended time frame. (*Data from* WHO/IVB Database as at 05 September 2016 and ECDC published data at http://vaccine-schedule.ecdc.europa.eu/Pages/Scheduler.aspx.)

Catch-up Vaccination

Catch-up vaccination of individuals who are not immune to hepatitis B hastens the development of population-based immunity, thereby decreasing the incidence of HBV. Immunity to hepatitis B can be determined by measurement of HBsAg and anti-HBs titers. WHO and AASLD guidelines both recommend vaccination of high-risk groups including household and sexual contacts of HBsAg-positive patients, health care workers, persons with multiple sex partners, and men who have sex with men. Recently, HEPLISAV-B, a two-dose vaccination series given at 0 and 1 months, was approved for use in adults in the United States.[13] AASLD guidelines also recommend vaccination of patients who are negative for anti-HBs in the following groups: people injecting intravenous drugs, patients with hepatitis C virus and HIV co-infection, people with elevated alanine aminotransferase (ALT) and aspartate amino-transferase (AST) levels of unknown etiology, patients seeking evaluation or treatment of sexually transmitted diseases, patients with diabetes mellitus aged 19 to 59 years, prisoners, people traveling to countries of high HBV endemicity, and residents and staff of facilities for developmentally disabled people.

Postexposure Prophylaxis

AASLD guidelines recommend that infants born to HBsAg-positive mothers should receive immunoprophylaxis with the combination of hepatitis B immune globulin (HBIg)[14,15] along with HBV vaccine within 24 hours of delivery, regardless of the mother's HBeAg status. The vaccine is given as a 3-dose series at 0, 1, and 6 months or as a 4-dose schedule administered at 0, 7, 21, and 30 days followed by a dose at 12 months if combined with the hepatitis A vaccine. The AASLD also recommends that infants born to HBsAg-positive mothers should undergo postvaccination serologic testing at 9 to 15 months of age to determine the response to vaccine series. Nonresponders to the initial vaccine series should receive a repeat 3-dose vaccination series. By contrast, WHO guidelines only recommend the combination of HBIg with HBV vaccination to infants born to mothers who are both HBsAg- and HBeAg-positive. HBV vaccination only is recommended in children of HBsAg-positive, HBeAg-negative mothers, owing to concerns for low supply and high cost of HBIg. This is a reasonable recommendation in LMICs, given that most vaccine failures occur when the maternal viral load is greater than 10^7 IU/mL and that these viral levels would be uncommon in an HBeAg-negative mother.

Mother-to-Child Transmission

In countries with high endemicity, the most common mode of HBV transmission is mother-to-child transmission, usually from exposure to maternal blood and body fluids at the time of delivery.[16] Transmission of HBV occurring early in life carries a much higher risk of developing chronic infection; therefore, measures to prevent mother-to-child transmission will have the greatest impact on reducing the burden of chronic infection. Both WHO and AASLD guidelines recommend treating HBsAg-positive pregnant women if they meet the standard criteria for initiation of antiviral treatment. Breastfeeding is not contraindicated in HBV-infected mothers on antiviral therapy. There are, however, some major differences between the 2 guidelines regarding recommendations to prevent mother-to-child HBV transmission. The AASLD recommends administration of antiviral therapy (tenofovir is preferred) in the third trimester of pregnancy to women with serum HBV DNA levels greater than 200,000 IU/mL until 4 weeks postpartum. This advice is based on the results of 2 recent randomized controlled trials comparing tenofovir with no antiviral treatment in the third trimester, which demonstrated a significant reduction in risk of mother-to-child transmission of HBV in highly viremic mothers.[17,18] The WHO has not made any recommendations on the use of antiviral therapy in the third trimester to prevent mother-to-child transmission. The WHO guidelines cited the lack of evidence on the effectiveness and safety of antiviral therapy at the time of writing of the guidelines as the reason for not recommending antiviral therapy. Given the availability of updated data, the complete absence of mother-to-child transmission in women receiving antiviral therapy, the fact that therapy is administered for only short duration, and the low rates of HepB-BD vaccine in LMICs, updating the WHO guidance would have a great impact on reducing the prevalence of chronic HBV infection. Both treated and untreated HBsAg-positive pregnant women should be monitored for at least 6 months postpartum for hepatitis flares and seroconversion.[19,20] The AASLD suggests that HBV-infected pregnant patients with cirrhosis should be managed in a tertiary care center where high-risk obstetric services are readily available. This recommendation is unlikely to be adopted by the WHO given the limited availability of these resources in LMICs. A comparison of recommendations for the prevention of HBV is provided in **Table 2**.

TREATMENT
Who to Treat?

The outcome of chronic HBV infection is variable, ranging from mild fibrosis to cirrhosis and decompensated liver disease. It is estimated that 20% to 30% of those with chronic HBV infection will be at risk for progressive liver fibrosis, leading to cirrhosis and an increased risk of HCC. However, most patients will not require antiviral therapy. The primary goal of antiviral therapy is to suppress HBV DNA levels to undetectable, as this end point is associated with improvement in liver inflammation and fibrosis and reversal of cirrhosis, a lower risk of HCC, and reduced liver-related mortality.[21] However, none of the currently available therapies is curative, and once treatment is started it must usually be continued lifelong. Therefore, treatment guidelines emphasize the importance of careful patient selection, initiating therapy only in those would derive the greatest benefit. Identifying which patients benefit the most

Table 2
Comparison of recommendations for prevention of hepatitis B

	WHO	AASLD
Primary prevention	Universal HBV vaccination to all infants	Universal HBV vaccination to all infants
Catch-up vaccination	HBV vaccination of nonimmune high-risk groups	HBV vaccination of nonimmune high-risk groups
Prevention of mother-to-child transmission	HBIG + HBV vaccination to all infants born to HBsAg/HBeAg-positive mothers HBV vaccination to all infants born to HBsAg-positive/HBeAg-negative mothers Antiviral therapy not recommended for highly viremic mothers	HBIG + HBV vaccination within 12 h of birth to all infants born to HBsAg-positive mothers Antiviral therapy (tenofovir) initiated at 28–32 wk of gestation for pregnant women with serum HBV DNA levels >200,000 IU/mL until 4 wk postpartum

from therapy is challenging. The pretreatment assessment is based on the level of viral replication (HBeAg status and HBV DNA level), degree of inflammation (serum ALT level), and stage of disease (noninvasive test of fibrosis or liver biopsy), and additional factors such as a family history of cirrhosis and HCC, age, and presence of comorbid medical conditions.

There is general consensus between the AASLD and WHO guidelines that all patients with compensated or decompensated cirrhosis require treatment independent of HBeAg status, HBV DNA, and ALT levels.[22] The diagnosis of cirrhosis can be made clinically by the presence of hepatosplenomegaly, reversal of AST/ALT ratio, and low albumin level and low platelet count, or through the use of noninvasive tests of liver fibrosis. Alternatively, more accurate tests such as liver biopsy or vibration-controlled transient elastography may be used to diagnose cirrhosis, if available. The WHO recommends using an AST-to-platelet-ratio index (APRI) cutoff of greater than 2.0 or elevated vibration-controlled elastography reading, if available, to start treatment. Tests such as vibration-controlled transient elastography and liver biopsy are not widely available in LMICs, which poses a challenge to accurately diagnosing cirrhosis.

For patients without cirrhosis, the objective criteria used to determine the need for treatment differs between the 2 guidelines mainly because specialized testing may not be available, as highlighted in **Table 3** and **Figs. 3** and **4**. For HBeAg-positive patients without cirrhosis, the AASLD recommends initiating treatment in patients with HBV DNA levels greater than 20,000 IU/mL and ALT greater than 2-times the upper limit of normal (ULN) using a cutoff ALT of 35 for men and 25 for women as normal (see **Fig. 3**). For HBeAg-positive patients with lower HBV DNA and ALT levels, the decision to treat should be individualized and based on the presence of additional risk factors and results of a liver biopsy or noninvasive assessment of fibrosis. HBeAg-positive patients with HBV DNA levels greater than 20,000 IU/mL with normal ALT levels are not candidates for therapy. Among HBeAg-negative patients, the AASLD recommends treatment for patients with HBV DNA levels greater than 2000 IU/mL and an elevated ALT greater than 2× ULN (see **Fig. 3**). For HBeAg-negative patients with lower levels of ALT elevation (1–2× ULN), treatment should be individualized based on results of a liver biopsy or noninvasive test of fibrosis. HBeAg-negative patients with normal ALT levels and HBV DNA less than 2000 IU/mL are not treatment candidates.

Table 3
Comparison of recommendations for treatment and monitoring of chronic hepatitis B

	WHO	AASLD
Who to treat	• All compensated and decompensated cirrhotics • All adults >30 y with chronic HBV without clinical evidence of cirrhosis (based on APRI score ≤2 and physical examination) but have persistently abnormal ALT levels and evidence of HBV DNA >20,000 IU/mL (if available) regardless of HBeAg status	• All compensated and decompensated cirrhotics • HBeAg-positive patients with HBV DNA >20,000 IU/mL and ALT >2× ULN • HBeAg-negative patients with HBV DNA >2000 IU/mL and ALT >2× ULN
Criteria used for deciding treatment	• Age • ALT levels • Fibrosis staging based on APRI score	• HBV DNA levels • ALT level • HBeAg status • Fibrosis staging based on liver biopsy or noninvasive tests including vibration-controlled transient elastography
Upper limit of normal for ALT	Laboratory-defined upper limit of normal	• Men: ALT of 35 U/L • Women: ALT of 25 U/L
What drugs to treat with	• Tenofovir disoproxil fumarate • Entecavir	• Tenofovir disoproxil fumarate • Entecavir • Tenofovir alafenamide • Peginterferon-α-2a
When to stop treatment	• Cirrhosis—continue treatment indefinitely • No cirrhosis—consider discontinuing nucleos(t)ides if there is HBeAg seroconversion or HBsAg loss and treatment consolidation for at least 12 mo	• Cirrhosis—continue treatment indefinitely • No cirrhosis—consider discontinuing nucleos(t)ides if there is HBeAg seroconversion or HBsAg loss and treatment consolidation for at least 12 mo
Treatment failure	• Lamivudine, adefovir, telbivudine, and entecavir resistance—switch to tenofovir	Lamivudine, adefovir, telbivudine, and entecavir resistance—switch to tenofovir/tenofovir alafenamide/add tenofovir/ tenofovir alafenamide to ongoing therapy Tenofovir resistance—switch/add entecavir
Screening for hepatocellular carcinoma	Ultrasound + α-fetoprotein every 6 mo	Ultrasound ± α-fetoprotein every 6 mo

In LMICs, access to nucleic acid and serologic testing may be limited. To circumvent this issue, the WHO recommends using age, ALT level, and noninvasive testing in the decision algorithm to start treatment (see **Fig. 4**). For patients without cirrhosis (APRI <2.0) where specialized testing is unavailable, the WHO recommends treating all adults older than 30 years who have persistently abnormal ALT levels. Persistently

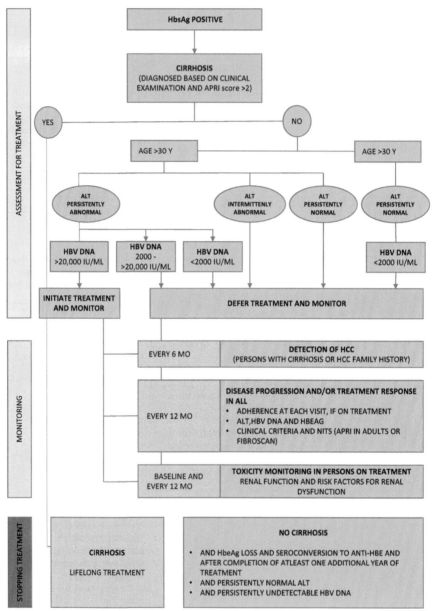

Fig. 3. Algorithm of WHO recommendations on the management of persons with chronic hepatitis B infection. Chronic hepatitis B is defined as persistence of HBsAg for 6 months or more. ALT, alanine aminotransferase level; APRI, aspartate aminotransferase-to-platelet-ratio index; HBsAg, Hepatitis B surface antigen; NITs, noninvasive tests; WHO, World Health Organization. [a] Clinical features of decompensated cirrhosis (ascites, variceal hemorrhage, and hepatic encephalopathy), coagulopathy, or jaundice. Other clinical features of cirrhosis include hepatomegaly, splenomegaly, pruritus, fatigue, arthralgias, palmar erythema, and peripheral edema. [b] The age cutoff of greater than 30 years is not absolute and some persons with chronic hepatitis B for less than 30 years may also meet criteria for antiviral treatment. [c] ALT levels fluctuate in persons with chronic hepatitis B and require

A

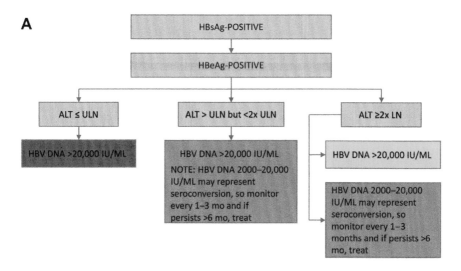

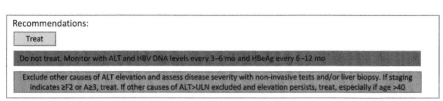

Fig. 4. (*A*) AASLD guidelines on management of persons with HBeAg-positive chronic hepatitis B. (*B*) AASLD guidelines on management of persons with HBeAg-negative chronic hepatitis B. Treatment algorithm for patients with HBeAg-positive and HBeAg-negative chronic hepatitis B based on AASLD guidelines. ULN, upper limit of normal. (*Adapted from* Terrault NA, Lok AS, McMahon BJ, et al. Update on prevention, diagnosis, and treatment and of chronic hepatitis B: AASLD 2018 hepatitis B guidance. Hepatology 2018; 67(4):1560–99; with permission.)

---

longitudinal monitoring to determine the trend. Upper limits for normal ALT have been defined as less than 30 U/L for men and 19 U/L for women, although local laboratory normal ranges should be applied. Persistently normal/abnormal may be defined as 3 ALT determinations below or above the ULN, made at unspecified intervals during a 6- to 12-month period or predefined intervals during 12-month period. [d] Where HBV DNA testing is not available, treatment may be considered based on persistently abnormal ALT levels, but other common causes of persistently raised ALT levels such as impaired glucose tolerance, dyslipidemia, and fatty liver should be excluded. [e] All persons with chronic hepatitis B should be monitored regularly for disease activity/progression and detection of hepatocellular carcinoma (HCC), and, after stopping treatment, for evidence of reactivation. More frequent monitoring may be required in those with more advanced liver disease, during the first year of treatment or when adherence is a concern, and in those with abnormal ALT and HBV DNA levels greater than 2000 IU/mL, not yet on treatment. [f] Before initiation, assessment should be done of renal function: serum creatinine level, estimated glomerular filtration rate, urine dipsticks for proteinuria and glycosuria, risk factors for renal dysfunction (decompensated cirrhosis, CrCl <50 mL/min, poorly controlled hypertension, proteinuria, uncontrolled diabetes, active glomerulonephritis, concomitant nephrotoxic drugs, solid organ transplantation, older age, body mass index <18.5 kg/m^2 (or body weight <50 kg), concomitant use of nephrotoxic drugs, or a boosted protease inhibitor for HIV. Monitoring should be more frequent in those at higher risk of renal dysfunction. (*Adapted from* WHO. Guidelines for the prevention, care and treatment of persons with chronic hepatitis B infection. 2015.)

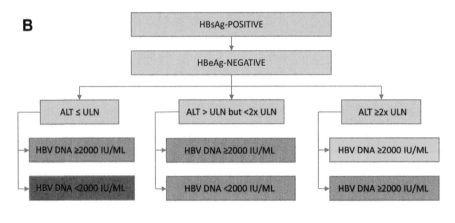

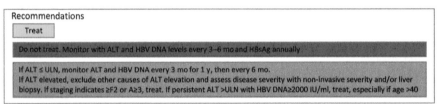

Fig. 4. (*continued*).

abnormal ALT levels are defined as 3 ALT determinations above the ULN made at unspecified intervals during a 6- to 12-month period or predefined intervals during a 12-month period. Of note, the WHO uses laboratory-defined upper limits whereas the AASLD uses gender-specific ALT cutoffs. If HBV DNA testing is available, the cutoffs to begin treatment are the same as those for AASLD. The WHO acknowledges that the evidence supporting the recommendations are imprecise and that relying solely on age and ALT may mean that some patients with chronic hepatitis B with ALT elevations attributable to other causes may be inadvertently exposed to HBV treatment without direct benefit; moreover, the requirement for 3 ALT levels over 6 to 12 months may mean there is a delay in initiating treatment. However, the rationale of the WHO recommendations was to strike a balance between the potential benefits of treatment against the need for long-term therapy and the associated toxicities. Recently a simple score consisting of HBeAg and 4 categories of ALT was shown to correctly identify 82% to 85% of patients meeting the international treatment criteria based on the conventional reference tests (serum HBV DNA and liver biopsy or vibration-controlled elastography), and 77% to 78% of patients who do not meet treatment criteria.[23] It is anticipated that advances in rapid detection technology[24] will improve care by providing greater access to testing and will allow on-treatment monitoring to better align the management of patients in LMICs with those in developed countries.

Which Drugs to Treat With?

Currently there are 8 drugs approved for the treatment of chronic hepatitis B, which can be categorized into 2 main classes: interferon preparations (standard interferon-α-2b, peginterferon-α-2a) and nucleos(t)ide analogs (lamivudine, adefovir, entecavir, telbivudine, tenofovir disoproxil fumarate, and tenofovir alafenamide). Both guidelines recommend initiating treatment with a potent agent that has a high barrier to resistance and a low rate of antiviral resistance. Thus, entecavir and tenofovir are recommended as first-line therapy for treatment of chronic HBV infection. Entecavir is licensed for use in children older than 2 years and tenofovir in children aged 12 years and older. AASLD guidelines also include tenofovir alafenamide, which is an orally available prodrug of tenofovir with similar antiviral efficacy but lower renal and bone toxicity.[25,26] Peginterferon-α-2a, which is also considered a first-line option in the AASLD guidelines in patients with suitable pretreatment characteristics, is not recommended in the WHO guidelines because of the need for additional monitoring and toxicity.

When to Stop Treatment?

Peginterferon-α-2a is administered for a fixed duration of 48 weeks when used for treatment of chronic HBV infection. Early stopping rules at weeks 12 and 24 exist for HBeAg-positive and HBeAg-negative patients based on tolerability, HBV genotype, and decline in HBsAg and HBV DNA levels. Stopping nucleoside analog therapy requires careful consideration of the benefits and risks of doing so. Benefits include reduced financial burden and the need to take a medication daily that carries a risk of drug toxicity and antiviral resistance. Risks include virologic relapse, hepatic decompensation, HCC, and death. Both guidelines recommend careful selection of patients after consideration of the risk/benefit ratio, the patients' ability to comply with the additional monitoring in the initial 6 months of stopping treatment, and the need for lifelong monitoring.

AASLD and WHO guidelines recommend that all patients with compensated and decompensated cirrhosis treated with a nucleos(t)ide analog require lifelong therapy and should not discontinue treatment, to avoid the risk of HBV reactivation leading to hepatic decompensation and death.[27] Both guidelines recommend discontinuation of treatment in patients who achieve HBsAg loss or HBeAg-positive patients who undergo HBeAg seroconversion and who receive a minimum of 12 months of treatment consolidation, and have normal ALT levels and persistently undetectable HBV DNA levels.

It is imperative that if treatment is stopped, patients are carefully monitored every 3 months or more frequently as necessary for at least a year to detect episodes of recurrent viremia, ALT flares, clinical decompensation, and HBsAg and HBeAg seroreversion. Both the AASLD and WHO recommend lifelong treatment of patients with HBeAg-negative chronic hepatitis B unless they achieve HBsAg loss.[28] Recently, there has been a recommendation by the EASL and APASL to consider discontinuing therapy in selected patients with HBeAg-negative chronic hepatitis B without cirrhosis who have maintained undetectable HBV DNA and normal ALT levels for a period of 2 to 3 years. Small series have reported rates of HBsAg loss around 20%, but ~ 50% of patients require reinitiation of therapy and 10% to 20% may experience withdrawal flares with or without hepatic decompensation. Given the need for close surveillance and frequent testing after stopping treatment, this approach is not recommended for LMICs.

MANAGEMENT OF TREATMENT FAILURE

Primary treatment failure is defined as the failure to reduce HBV DNA levels by $\geq 1 \times \log_{10}$ IU/mL within 3 months from the start of therapy. Secondary treatment failure is defined as increase of HBV DNA by $\geq 1 \times \log_{10}$ IU/mL from baseline in persons with initial treatment response ($\geq 1 \times \log_{10}$ IU/mL reduction in HBV DNA). An increase in HBV DNA levels on treatment may signify noncompliance or antiviral resistance. In these clinical circumstances it is important to review medication compliance with the patient and if adherence is confirmed, antiviral resistance testing should be considered. In LMICs, access to HBV DNA testing remains a limiting factor in diagnosing antiviral resistance. In settings without access to HBV DNA testing or antiviral resistance testing, assessment of resistance is largely based on clinical suspicion and should be considered in the following circumstances: (1) patients receiving antiviral drugs with low barrier to resistance in combination with poor adherence; (2) increase in levels of serum aminotransferases; and (3) evidence of progression in liver disease based on physical examination or APRI score. Clinical relapse manifested by elevation in ALT levels tends to lag virological relapse and is therefore not a sensitive marker of resistance.

Primary treatment failure is rarely seen in patients who are adherent to treatment with entecavir and tenofovir, and adherence to treatment should be reinforced.[29] If antiviral resistance to lamivudine, adefovir, telbivudine, or entecavir is suspected or confirmed, the preferred management strategy of both guidelines is switching to tenofovir; tenofovir alafenamide is an alternative option in the AASLD guidelines.[30,31] The AASLD also recommends adding tenofovir to the ongoing nucleos(t)ide analog. However, the WHO does not recommend this option as of all the available nucleos(t)ide analogs, tenofovir is associated with the highest probability at 1 year of achieving low or undetectable HBV DNA levels. For patients with resistance to tenofovir, switching to or adding entecavir to ongoing tenofovir are recommended options. The AASLD recommends that patients with low-level viremia on entecavir of tenofovir should continue monotherapy regardless of ALT levels. Both guidelines emphasize the importance of counseling patients regularly during clinic visits about treatment adherence, because noncompliance is a major contributor to antiviral resistance.

MONITORING
Monitoring of Patients Receiving Treatment

Patients on antiviral treatment require monitoring to assess compliance and efficacy of treatment, progression of liver disease, development of antiviral resistance, and complications of treatment. Treatment efficacy is best assessed by monitoring HBV DNA levels. There are no clear-cut guidelines regarding the frequency of testing HBV DNA levels. However, given the excellent efficacy and low rate of antiviral resistance in adherent patients receiving entecavir and tenofovir, monitoring can be relatively infrequent. The AASLD recommends testing HBV DNA levels every 3 months for the first 6 months of therapy to establish efficacy and then increase the testing interval to every 3 to 6 months, and also recommends obtaining ALT, HBeAg, anti-HBe, and HBsAg every 6 to 12 months. In patients at risk for renal toxicity, creatinine clearance, serum phosphate, urine glucose, and protein should be assessed annually. A bone density study should be considered at baseline and periodically during treatment in patients with a history of fracture or at risk for osteopenia. Lactic acid levels should be tested if there is clinical suspicion of mitochondrial injury.

WHO guidelines advise, at a minimum, annual monitoring of ALT, HBsAg, HBeAg, HBV DNA levels (if available), and APRI score to assess for the presence of cirrhosis in those without cirrhosis at baseline, along with baseline and annual testing of renal function with urine dipstick and creatinine measurement. The WHO additionally recommends frequent monitoring of these parameters for at least 3 months for the first year in patients with cirrhosis and HIV coinfection. Tests to assess bone density are not widely available in LMICs.

Monitoring of Untreated Patients

Chronic HBV is a dynamic disorder with a fluctuating course of disease.[32] The primary goal of monitoring is to identify clinical changes that might indicate disease progression necessitating treatment. In general, the frequency of monitoring should be appropriate for activity and stage of the liver disease. It is therefore important to remind untreated patients of the need for lifelong monitoring. Patients who do not presently require treatment may need treatment in the future because of change in the clinical status, which can be recognized by elevated ALT and HBV DNA levels. AASLD guidelines recommend that patients who are inactive carriers and those with immune-tolerant disease, the 2 groups in whom treatment is not recommended, should be tested periodically for disease transition and HBeAg (if applicable) and HBsAg loss. Inactive carriers should be monitored with HBV DNA and ALT every 3 months for first year and every 6 to 12 months thereafter, and HBsAg tested annually. Patients with immune-tolerant disease should be monitored with HBV DNA and ALT levels and HBeAg at least every 6 months. WHO guidelines recommend annual monitoring of HBeAg, HBsAg, serum ALT, HBV DNA levels, and APRI scores for all patients without cirrhosis at baseline who do not qualify for treatment.

Screening for Hepatocellular Carcinoma

HBV accounts for the largest proportion of HCCs globally. In LMICs with high HBV seroprevalence, patients are sometimes diagnosed with HBV only after they present with advanced HCC. In patients with HBV, HCC can occur even in the absence of cirrhosis.[33] Therefore, surveillance is required even in patients without cirrhosis to detect HCC at an early stage to increase the chances of survival. AASLD and WHO guidelines recommend a screening ultrasound scan every 6 months for patients with cirrhosis and family history of HCC. The WHO recommends obtaining an α-fetoprotein measure in addition to ultrasonography,[34,35] whereas α-fetoprotein testing is optional in AASLD guidelines. Where ultrasound is not available, screening with α-fetoprotein every 6 months is recommended. There are minor differences in the age to initiate screening between the 2 guidelines. The WHO recommends screening for HCC in all patients older than 40 years with HBV DNA levels greater than 2000 IU/mL. The AASLD recommends HCC screening only for Asian or African American men older than 40 years and to begin screening Asian women at 50 years of age.[36] The screening interval recommended by the WHO is appropriate for the prevalence of HBV-related HCC in LMICs. The inclusion of α-fetoprotein in the WHO recommendations may result in unnecessary and costly interventions and the need for additional screening visits because of false-positive results. In LMICs, for surveillance to be effective in improving survival there must be access to treatment of early-stage HCC, which includes alcohol injection, ablation, chemoembolization, and resection. However, there is limited access to these interventions in LMICs and this is a challenge that must be addressed.

SUMMARY

The 2016 WHO guidelines on testing for HBV are the first global evidence-based guidelines that complement the 2015 guidelines on prevention, care, and treatment of chronic HBV infection. Their main focus is to target LMICs to improve their regional and national testing strategies. Unlike the other clinician-focused international guidelines from the AASLD, APASL, and EASL,[37,38] the target audience for the WHO guidelines are national program managers and health policy makers who are responsible for the development of national hepatitis testing and treatment policies.[39]

The WHO guidelines are created around the limitations of resources, accessibility, and affordability to measure of HBV DNA levels. This expensive assay requires highly advanced equipment and facilities. However, HBV DNA is a major predictor for development of HBV-related diseases including HCC and a key marker for identifying response to treatment and deciding on eligibility for antiviral therapy. In the absence of HBV DNA assays, the WHO relies on serial ALT measurements, which is problematic because it requires several blood tests and medical visits before a decision to treat can be made. With the increasing availability of HBV DNA testing and novel rapid detection technology, patients around the world will be able to be screened, treated, and monitored more effectively. However, under the present circumstances, prevention of chronic hepatitis B through vaccination and postexposure prophylaxis remains the cornerstone for reducing the incidence of the disease and its related mortality.

REFERENCES

1. Schweitzer A, Horn J, Mikolajczyk RT, et al. Estimations of worldwide prevalence of chronic hepatitis B virus infection: a systematic review of data published between 1965 and 2013. Lancet 2015;386(10003):1546–55.
2. Ott J, Stevens G, Groeger J, et al. Global epidemiology of hepatitis B virus infection: new estimates of age-specific HBsAg seroprevalence and endemicity. Vaccine 2012;30(12):2212–9.
3. James SL, Abate D, Abate KH, et al. Global, regional, and national incidence, prevalence, and years lived with disability for 354 diseases and injuries for 195 countries and territories, 1990–2017: a systematic analysis for the Global Burden of Disease Study 2017. Lancet 2018;392(10159):1789–858.
4. World Health Organization. Global health sector strategy on viral hepatitis 2016-2021. Towards ending viral hepatitis. Geneva (Switzerland): World Health Organization; 2016.
5. World Health Organization. Guidelines for the prevention care and treatment of persons with chronic hepatitis B infection. Geneva (Switzerland): World Health Organization; 2015.
6. Terrault NA, Lok AS, McMahon BJ, et al. Update on prevention, diagnosis, and treatment of chronic hepatitis B: AASLD 2018 hepatitis B guidance. Hepatology 2018;67(4):1560–99.
7. Terrault NA, Bzowej NH, Chang KM, et al. AASLD guidelines for treatment of chronic hepatitis B. Hepatology 2016;63(1):261–83.
8. Nelson NP, Jamieson DJ, Murphy TV. Prevention of perinatal hepatitis B virus transmission. J Pediatric Infect Dis Soc 2014;3(suppl_1):S7–12.
9. Chen D-S. Hepatitis B vaccination: the key towards elimination and eradication of hepatitis B. J Hepatol 2009;50(4):805–16.
10. Chang M-H, Chen C-J, Lai M-S, et al. Universal hepatitis B vaccination in Taiwan and the incidence of hepatocellular carcinoma in children. Taiwan Childhood Hepatoma Study Group. N Engl J Med 1997;336(26):1855–9.
11. Hepatitis B vaccines: WHO position paper—July 2017. Wkly Epidemiol Rec 2017; 92(27):369–92.
12. Holmberg SD, Suryaprasad A, Ward JWJM. Updated CDC recommendations for the management of hepatitis B virus-infected health-care providers and students. MMWR Recomm Rep 2012;61(3):1.
13. Cooper C, Mackie D. Hepatitis B surface antigen-1018 ISS adjuvant-containing vaccine: a review of HEPLISAV™ safety and efficacy. Expert Rev Vaccines 2011;10(4):417–27.

14. Sánchez-Fueyo A, Rimola A, Grande L, et al. Hepatitis B immunoglobulin discontinuation followed by hepatitis B virus vaccination: a new strategy in the prophylaxis of hepatitis B virus recurrence after liver transplantation. Hepatology 2000; 31(2):496–501.
15. Beasley RP, George C-YL, Roan C-H, et al. Prevention of perinatally transmitted hepatitis B virus infections with hepatitis B immune globulin and hepatitis B vaccine. Lancet 1983;322(8359):1099–102.
16. Ranger-Rogez S, Denis F. Hepatitis B mother-to-child transmission. Expert Rev Anti Infect Ther 2004;2(1):133–45.
17. Pan CQ, Duan Z, Dai E, et al. Tenofovir to prevent hepatitis B transmission in mothers with high viral load. N Engl J Med 2016;374(24):2324–34.
18. Chen HL, Lee CN, Chang CH, et al. Efficacy of maternal tenofovir disoproxil fumarate in interrupting mother-to-infant transmission of hepatitis B virus. Hepatology 2015;62(2):375–86.
19. Chang CY, Aziz N, Poongkunran M, et al. Serum aminotransferase flares in pregnant and postpartum women with current or prior treatment for chronic hepatitis B. J Clin Gastroenterol 2018;52(3):255–61.
20. Chang CY, Aziz N, Poongkunran M, et al. Serum alanine aminotransferase and hepatitis B DNA flares in pregnant and postpartum women with chronic hepatitis B. London: Nature Publishing Group; 2016.
21. Ganem D, Prince AM. Hepatitis B virus infection—natural history and clinical consequences. N Engl J Med 2004;350(11):1118–29.
22. Marcellin P, Gane E, Buti M, et al. Regression of cirrhosis during treatment with tenofovir disoproxil fumarate for chronic hepatitis B: a 5-year open-label follow-up study. Lancet 2013;381(9865):468–75.
23. Shimakawa Y, Njie R, Ndow G, et al. Development of a simple score based on HBeAg and ALT for selecting patients for HBV treatment in Africa. J Hepatol 2018;69(4):776–84.
24. Peeling RW, Boeras DI, Marinucci F, et al. The future of viral hepatitis testing: innovations in testing technologies and approaches. BMC Infect Dis 2017; 17(1):699.
25. Buti M, Gane E, Seto WK, et al. Tenofovir alafenamide versus tenofovir disoproxil fumarate for the treatment of patients with HBeAg-negative chronic hepatitis B virus infection: a randomised, double-blind, phase 3, non-inferiority trial. Lancet Gastroenterol Hepatol 2016;1(3):196–206.
26. Chan HL, Fung S, Seto WK, et al. Tenofovir alafenamide versus tenofovir disoproxil fumarate for the treatment of HBeAg-positive chronic hepatitis B virus infection: a randomised, double-blind, phase 3, non-inferiority trial. Lancet Gastroenterol Hepatol 2016;1(3):185–95.
27. Lim S, Wai C, Rajnakova A, et al. Fatal hepatitis B reactivation following discontinuation of nucleoside analogues for chronic hepatitis B. Gut 2002;51(4):597–9.
28. Chang ML, Liaw YF, Hadziyannis SJ. Systematic review: cessation of long-term nucleos(t)ide analogue therapy in patients with hepatitis B e antigen-negative chronic hepatitis B. Aliment Pharmacol Ther 2015;42(3):243–57.
29. Tenney DJ, Rose RE, Baldick CJ, et al. Long-term monitoring shows hepatitis B virus resistance to entecavir in nucleoside-naïve patients is rare through 5 years of therapy. Hepatology 2009;49(5):1503–14.
30. van Bömmel F, de Man RA, Wedemeyer H, et al. Long-term efficacy of tenofovir monotherapy for hepatitis B virus-monoinfected patients after failure of nucleoside/nucleotide analogues. Hepatology 2010;51(1):73–80.

31. Fung S, Kwan P, Fabri M, et al. Tenofovir disoproxil fumarate (TDF) vs. emtricitabine (FTC)/TDF in lamivudine resistant hepatitis B: a 5-year randomised study. J Hepatol 2017;66(1):11–8.

32. Shi Y-H, Shi C-H. Molecular characteristics and stages of chronic hepatitis B virus infection. World J Gastroenterol 2009;15(25):3099.

33. Chayanupatkul M, Omino R, Mittal S, et al. Hepatocellular carcinoma in the absence of cirrhosis in patients with chronic hepatitis B virus infection. J Hepatol 2017;66(2):355–62.

34. Aghoram R, Cai P, Dickinson JA. Alpha-foetoprotein and/or liver ultrasonography for screening of hepatocellular carcinoma in patients with chronic hepatitis B. Cochrane Database Syst Rev 2012;(9):CD002799.

35. Hann H-W, Fu X, Myers RE, et al. Predictive value of alpha-fetoprotein in the long-term risk of developing hepatocellular carcinoma in patients with hepatitis B virus infection–results from a clinic-based longitudinal cohort. Eur J Cancer 2012; 48(15):2319–27.

36. Heimbach JK, Kulik LM, Finn RS, et al. AASLD guidelines for the treatment of hepatocellular carcinoma. Hepatology 2018;67(1):358–80.

37. European Association for the Study of the Liver; European Association for the Study of the Liver. EASL 2017 clinical practice guidelines on the management of hepatitis B virus infection. J Hepatol 2017;67(2):370–98.

38. Sarin S, Kumar M, Lau G, et al. Asian-Pacific clinical practice guidelines on the management of hepatitis B: a 2015 update. Hepatol Int 2016;10(1):1–98.

39. Chou R, Easterbrook P, Hellard M. Methodological challenges in appraising evidence on diagnostic testing for WHO guidelines on hepatitis B and hepatitis C virus infection. BMC Infect Dis 2017;17(Suppl 1):694.

The Effects of Hepatic Steatosis on the Natural History of HBV Infection

Idrees Suliman, MD[a], Noha Abdelgelil, MBBCh[b],
Farah Kassamali, MD[c], Tarek I. Hassanein, MD[d],*

KEYWORDS

• Prevalence • Hepatitis B • NAFLD • NASH • Cirrhosis • HCC

KEY POINTS

• The prevalence of nonalcoholic fatty liver disease (NAFLD) is progressively increasing worldwide, especially with the increased incidence of metabolic syndrome and obesity.

• Chronic hepatitis B infection (CHB) patients with concomitant steatosis are at increased risk of hepatic fibrosis, cirrhosis, and hepatocellular carcinoma.

• Several studies have been conducted to better understand the interaction between CHB and NAFLD, both at the cellular level and clinically.

• Noninvasive diagnostic tests have been developed to predict fibrosis in CHB/NAFLD patients.

• Further research needs to be conducted to arrive at specific treatment guidelines in this patient population.

EPIDEMIOLOGY/PREVALENCE OF HEPATITIS B

Hepatitis B virus (HBV) infection affects millions of individuals worldwide, notably in Asia, Africa, and Pacific Islands.[1] Approximately 2 billion people have been affected by HBV worldwide.[2] After an acute infection, the progression to chronic hepatitis B infection (CHB) increases the risk for progression of fibrosis, cirrhosis, and hepatocellular carcinoma (HCC), contributing to increased global burden and mortality. The 2010 Global Burden of Disease study estimates HBV and outcome of chronic HBV to be the fifteenth leading cause of mortality worldwide.[3] The number of chronically

Disclosure Statement: The authors have nothing to disclose.
[a] Blake Medical Center Internal Medicine, 2020 59th St W, Bradenton, FL 34209, USA;
[b] Southern California Research Center, 131 Orange Avenue, Suite 101, Coronado, CA 92118, USA; [c] St. Mary's Medical Center, 450 Stanyan St, San Francisco, CA 94117, USA; [d] Southern California Liver Centers, 131 Orange Avenue, Suite 101, Coronado, CA 92118, USA
* Corresponding author.
E-mail address: thassanein@livercenters.com

Clin Liver Dis 23 (2019) 433–450
https://doi.org/10.1016/j.cld.2019.05.001
1089-3261/19/© 2019 Elsevier Inc. All rights reserved.

HBV-infected individuals ranges from 240 million to 350 million.[3] The prevalence of CHB varies around the world, with the highest prevalence occurring in Western sub-Saharan Africa (12%), followed by East Asia and Southeast Asia (5%–7%).[3] More than 20% of infected population live in South Sudan and Kiribati and as low as 0.01% in Norway and the United Kingdom.[4] Although the prevalence of CHB in the United States was estimated as 0.27%, more recent studies suggest that the prevalence might be higher, with as many as 2.2 million infected individuals, mostly (40%–70%) foreign born (**Fig. 1**).[1,5]

Hepatic steatosis, also known as fatty liver disease, consists of histopathologic spectrum of liver abnormalities, including nonalcoholic fatty liver disease (NAFLD), which has the potential to evolve into nonalcoholic steatohepatitis (NASH), fibrosis, cirrhosis, and HCC. The prevalence of NAFLD and NASH is increasing globally and believed due to Western dietary pattern and sedentary lifestyle.

NAFLD is known to be the most common liver disease in the world, notably in Asia, with an increasing prevalence in the United States, from 15% in 2005 to approximately 25% in 2017, and it correlates with the rise in obesity, dyslipidemia, and type 2 diabetes mellitus.[6,7] The prevalence of NAFLD in Europe and the Middle East ranges from 20% to 30% as well.[4] Other studies on the global impact of NAFLD suggest a similar prevalence in Japan, China, and Australia. In general, it is estimated that more than 1 billion people have NAFLD (**Fig. 2**).[8,9]

The increase in risk factors associated with metabolic syndrome, such as obesity, insulin resistance, and hyperlipidemia, have led to an increasing prevalence of NAFLD in developed and developing countries, along with the incidence of liver cirrhosis and HCC. Because liver fibrosis is a shared pathologic process in CHB-NAFLD patients, recent studies have been done to assess the interaction between HBV and fatty liver.[10,11] Approximately 5% to 7% of the world's population is a chronic carriers of HBV,[7] whereas 15% to 30% of the world's population has NAFLD.[12] According to EASL-EASD-EASO clinical practice guidelines, NAFLD is the most common liver disorder in Western countries, ranging from 17% to 46%, based on age, gender, ethnicity, and method of diagnosis.[13] On the other hand, multiple studies reported that approximately a quarter of CHB patients have concurrent steatosis, which is relative to that in the general population and may be lower when considering individuals with no alcohol consumption.[14]

In the United States, the prevalence of CHB is less than 0.5%, which is lower than in other countries, such as China (7%) and African countries (10%).[15] Individuals with CHB and coexisting NAFLD, however, are estimated to be more than 25% to 30%.[16,17]

INTERACTION BETWEEN HEPATITIS B VIRUS AND FATTY LIVER AT THE CELLULAR LEVEL

CHB and NAFLD are the focus of recent research efforts. Of particular importance is if NAFLD is associated with patients with CHB; and if so, what its effect is on the progression of chronic liver disease (CLD) to fibrosis and cirrhosis or the development of HCC.

Some studies reported an inverse relationship between CHB and steatosis whereas others showed a direct association between both diagnoses and suggested an increased risk of cirrhosis and HCC in CHB patients. The possible mechanisms behind the inverse relationship between steatosis and HBV infection are unclear, and available data are still not conclusive.

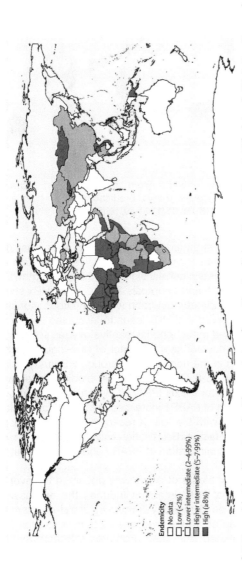

Fig. 1. Prevalence of CHB worldwide. (Reprinted with permission from Elsevier (Schweitzer A, Horn J, Mikolajczyk RT. Estimations of worldwide prevalence of chronic hepatitis B virus infection: a systematic review of data published between 1965 and 2013. Lancet. 2015 Oct 17;386:1546-55.)

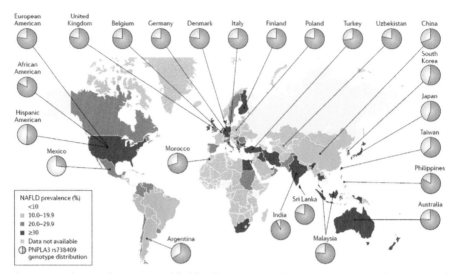

Fig. 2. Prevalence of NAFLD worldwide. (*From* Younossi Z, Anstee QM, Marietti M, et al. Global burden of NAFLD and NASH: trends, predictions, risk factors and prevention. Nat Rev Gastroenterol Hepatol. 2018 Jan;15(1):11-20, with permission.)

HBV is a partially double-stranded, circular DNA virus expressing codes for 4 proteins: C, X, P, and S. Hepatitis B protein X (HBx) has an important role in hepatitis B infection because it is involved in cellular signal transduction pathways and gene transcription affecting cell growth and apoptosis. Furthermore, HBx stimulates the mitrochondrial function through direct interaction with the mitochondrial respiratory chain complex subunit. It is believed that HBx leads to increased lipid accumulation in the liver as a result of increased mitochondrial reactive oxygen species levels and oxidative stress.[18] Thus, HBx may act as a promoter of viral-induced fatty liver. It also induces lipid accumulation in the hepatocytes through HBx/fatty acid–binding protein 1/hepatocyte nuclear factor 3-β, CCAAT/enhancer-binding protein α, and peroxisome proliferator-activated receptor α axis (PPARα), which consequently activates FABP1 promoter. Over-expression of FABP1 increases the rate of fatty acid uptake.[18] Direct interaction of HBx protein with the liver X receptor α or tumor necrosis factor (TNF) receptor 1 leads to nuclear factor κB activation and TNF production, inhibition of apolipoprotein B secretion, and stimulation of PPARγ and sterol-regulatory element-binding protein (SREBP)-1c.[19]

The effect of CHB on cholesterol levels was observed in several studies. Li and colleagues[20] reported that HBV infection induces the expression of cholesterol synthesis genes, such as 3-hydroxy-3-methylglutaryl-coenzyme A (HMG-CoA) reductase and LDL receptor, which predisposes to liver steatosis. Although Oehler and colleagues[21] suggested that HBV promotes bile acid synthesis and an increase in cholesterol level on binding to the Na taurocholate cotransporting polypeptide, a bile acid transporter, leading to induction of cholesterol 7-hydroxylase and up-regulation of SREBP-2 and HMG-CoA reductase. In contrast, Joo and colleagues[22] suggested that there is an inverse relationship between HBV infection and NAFLD. They showed that cholesterol levels significantly decrease in hepatitis B surface antigen (HBsAg)-positive patients whereas in the HBsAg-negative subjects, an increase in cholesterol levels was observed associated with elevation of alanine aminotransferase (ALT).

Pan and colleagues[23] reported that patatin-like phospholipase domain-containing protein 3 single-nucleotide pleomorphisms also predispose patients with CHB to hepatic steatosis but improve glucose metabolism by decreasing insulin resistance and glucose dysregulation. A recent study suggested that the gene of transmembrane 6 superfamily member 2 (TM6SF2) rs58542926 variant may help explain the relationship between CHB and hepatic steatosis. Kozlitina and colleagues[24] showed that when a nonsynonymous nucleotide pleomorphism occurs, a substitution of adenine for guanine encoding the nucleotide 499, the triglyceride (TG) content in the liver increases and the plasma levels of TG and low density lipoprotein cholesterol decrease. Another study by Eslam and colleagues,[25] including the International Liver Disease Genetics Consortium database of 507 CHB Chinese patients, confirmed the association between the rs58542926 T allele and steatosis in patients with CHB. No association between the severity of steatosis and the allele, however, was seen. Surprisingly, this variant also is associated with higher HBV DNA load. Oher studies suggested, however, that HBV may have more protective antisteatogenic effects than the steatogenic effects of HBx. In a study by Hui and colleagues,[16] an inverse association between steatosis and HBV DNA levels was observed in the treatment-naïve CHB patient group. Additionally, an obvious decrease in the median HBV DNA levels was seen as steatosis increases. In animal studies, accumulation of fat in the hepatocytes is believed to lessen viral replication directly or indirectly induce hepatocyte apoptosis, decreasing replication.[26,27] Zhang and colleagues[28] also showed an inverse association between HBV and steatosis. The Toll-like receptor (TLR) 4/myeloid differentiation factor 88 (MyD88) pathway was stimulated in NAFLD with stearic acid–induced steatosis in HBV-transgenic mice. This resulted in activation of the innate immune system and production of large amounts of proinflammatory cytokines, which contributed to HBV viral replication inhibition in patients with CHB/NAFLD. MyD88 is an adaptor for TLRs, leading to production of TNF-α and interleukin (IL)-6, which also have an important role in the development of NAFLD. Several other studies indicated that TLRs play a crucial role in the pathogenesis and progression of various CLDs, including HBV, HCV, NAFLD, fibrosis, and HCC.[29,30]

In human epidemiologic studies, Cheng and colleagues[31] showed an inverse relationship between the prevalence of fatty liver and positive HBsAg status in subjects older than 50 years whereas there was no significant association between HBV infection and fatty liver in subjects younger than 50 years. This may be due to the effects of serum Adiponectin on HBV infection, as showed by Wong and colleagues.[32] It is known that in animal studies, adiponectin suppresses fatty acid synthesis in the liver and opposes synthesis and release of TNF-α in adipose tissue.[33]

PREDICTION OF NONALCOHOLIC STEATOHEPATITIS IN HEPATITIS B VIRUS–INFECTED INDIVIDUALS

Thymosin beta-4 (Tb4) is a peptide produced by the thymus and is composed of 43 amino acids. It is believed that it has a protective role against liver cell damage and fibrosis. Levels of Tb4 in serum and tissues of patients with CHB/NAFLD have been studied. Results showed no statistical difference between the CHB/NAFLD group and the control group. Furthermore, no correlation with ALT, aspartate aminotransferase (AST), TGs, FGP, HBV DNA levels, and fat grading was seen; however, there was a negative correlation with inflammation and fibrosis score (P <.01). Tb4 may play a critical defense role in the disease progression and help regulate the chronic inflammation and fibrosis in CHB/NAFLD patients. Current studies reported lower Tb4 levels in patients with CHB/cirrhosis with significant decrease in acute-on-chronic liver failure and chronic liver failure. There were no significant differences in the transaminase level, hepatitis B e antigen ratio, and HBV-DNA load between the CHB/NAFLD group and control group, suggesting that steatosis is not directly caused by HBV infection. In contrast, there were differences in TGs and blood glucose in the CHB/NAFLD group, indicating that steatosis was related to the metabolic disorder of the host.[34] Kumar and Gupta[35] demonstrated that Tb4 has antioxidative stress effect through stimulation of antioxidase. Additionally, there was a negative correlation between Tb4 expression and that of the TNF-α in the serum and liver tissues. Moreover, Tb4 inhibited the activation of nuclear factor κB and expression of IL-8 induced by TNF-α.[36] Other studies confirmed that Tb4 could repair inflammation and protect the liver against fibrosis.[37,38]

Cytokeratin (CK) protein is essential to preserve normal liver structure and protect it from damage. CK18 is a filament protein characteristic of apoptosis in the liver. Liang and colleagues[39] investigated the CK18 fragments M30 and M65 in patients with CHB/NAFLD. Apoptosis is the most common physiologic manifestation in NASH and may be reflected by CK18 M30. It is believed that CK18 fragment M30 is closely related to hepatocyte inflammation and NASH. M30 levels were significantly higher in those patients compared with the non-NAFLD group, especially in patients with positive DNA and hepatitis B e antigen (HBeAg). M30 also correlated with ALT, AST, TGs, fasting plasma glucose, inflammation score, fibrosis score, and steatosis. This correlation indicates that inflammation and fibrosis are more severe in the combined group than without NAFLD. Consequently, CK18 M30 can be used to assess the level of inflammation in these patients. The sensitivities of CK18 M30, when compared with that of Controlled Attenuation Parameter (CAP), fasting plasma glucose, and log10 (HBV DNA), were 94.1%, 76.5%, 79.4%, and 67.6%, and the specificities were 67.7%, 87.1%, 64.5%, and 51.6%, respectively. Therefore, a new model combining CK18 M30, CAP, fasting plasma glucose, and HBV DNA level may be used as a simple and noninvasive method to predict NASH in patients with CHB/NAFLD, with sensitivity and specificity of the diagnosis of NASH of 100% and 80.6%, respectively. This will assist screening of patients for lifestyle modification, control of inflammation, and prevention of disease progression. M65 showed no significant difference between the 2 groups.[39]

Yang and colleagues[40] analyzed the lipid profiles in patients with NAFLD and CHB with and without NAFLD using ultraperformance liquid chromatography–tandem mass spectrometry. Results showed that monosaturated triacylglycerol (TAG_1) has similar diagnostic value as CK18 M30 and better diagnostic value than CK18 M65 and ALT. In the CHB group, TAG_1 showed better predictive value of NASH than CK18 M30, CK18 M65, and ALT. Plasmalogens are believed to protect polyunsaturated fatty acid from oxidative damage. Most of the serum plasmalogens were significantly decreased in both the NAFLD and CHB without NAFLD groups.[40] TAG_1 may serve as a specific biomarker for the diagnosis of NASH in NAFLD patients with or without HBV infection and may differentiate between different etiologies of abnormal ALT elevation and consequently identify the appropriate treatment in patients with concomitant CHB/NAFLD.[40]

CHRONIC HEPATITIS B INFECTION AND METABOLIC SYNDROME

A retrospective cohort showed that prevalence of metabolic syndrome in patients with CHB was significantly higher than in the control group.[41] The insulin resistance was not associated with HBsAg-positive patients in a study by Wang and colleagues.[42] Lee and colleagues[43] from Korea reported, however, that patients with CHB had higher levels of fasting insulin, homeostatic model assessment of insulin resistance (HOMA-IR) index, and lower quantitative insulin-sensitivity check index (QUICKI).

Shen and colleagues[44] tried to identify the risk factors for type 2 diabetes mellitus in patients infected with hepatitis B. His analysis demonstrated that besides general risk factors, 3 hepatitis B–related risk factors (high viral load, long duration of infection, and presence of cirrhosis) independently increased the risk of T2DM. A meta-analysis by Machado and colleagues[45] confirmed that the presence of NAFLD does not worsen the inflammation or the degree of fibrosis in patients with CHB. Although it is known that high HBV DNA load increases the risk of liver cirrhosis and HCC, this meta-analysis showed significant negative effect of HBV load on hepatic steatosis. On the other hand, Jarčuška and colleagues[46] reported that CHB patients with metabolic syndrome had significantly higher HBV DNA load compared with CHB patients with no metabolic syndrome. Similar results were observed regarding total cholesterol (TC) levels and apolipoprotein B100 levels. Patients with higher than normal levels of TC and apolipoprotein B100 had higher levels of HBV DNA compared with patients with normal values. Patients with low levels of TC often have advanced fibrosis that already impacts liver function. In the Risk Evaluation of Viral Load Elevation and Associated Liver Disease/Cancer-Hepatitis B Virus (REVEAL-HBV) study, HBV DNA load was inversely associated with extreme ($P = .004$) and central obesity ($P = .004$) in HBeAg-positive patients. In HBeAg-negative patients, inverse association with TGs was seen.[47]

Insulin resistance often plays a crucial role in the imbalance of hepatic lipids. Moreover, TAG deposition in the liver tissue aggravates hepatic insulin resistance and leads to an increase in the insulin-antagonizing cytokines. Also, increased levels of diacylglycerol (DAG) and ceramide cause insulin resistance, oxidative stress, apoptosis, and endoplasmic reticulum stress, which, in turn, are associated with lipotoxic liver injury in NASH.[48] Yang and colleagues[40] suggested that CHB may be protective against hyperlipidemia and insulin resistance because their results showed decreased serum total lipids, neutral lipids (TAG, diacylglycerol, and cholesteryl esters), and sphingolipids (ceramide and sphingomyelin) in the CHB without NAFLD group.

EFFECT OF NONALCOHOLIC FATTY LIVER DISEASE ON THE PROGRESSION OF CHRONIC HEPATITIS B (CLINICAL DATA)

The frequency of NAFLD encountered in CHB has been the subject of several research efforts. Multiple reports have found that CHB is associated with a lower frequency of metabolic syndrome and NAFLD (**Table 1**). Hazard ratios varied from 0.42 to 0.83 all were statistically significant.[22,49,50] These studies then suggest that CHB could be protective against the development of NAFLD. This was further demonstrated in a retrospective cross-sectional study in which 121 patients with HBV were compared with 263 volunteers. This research effort found that patients who were HBeAG positive and had elevated ALT levels also had a lower rate of metabolic syndrome compared with volunteers. The negative association between CHB and NAFLD is not uniformly present in the literature. One recent study found no association between CHB and NAFLD.[51]

With the conflicting data on the effect of CHB in the development of NAFLD, there have been several research efforts to determine whether it is viral or host metabolic factors that determine the development of NAFLD in patients with CHB. A vast majority of these studies have observed that host factors, such as body mass index (BMI), fasting plasma glucose, cholesterol levels, waist circumference, and fasting insulin, play a role in the development of NAFLD in the CHB population (**Table 2**).[11,31,52–56] In contrast, viral factors, such as viral load and antiviral treatment history, do not seem to contribute to the development of NAFLD. The data are conflicted in the role of HBeAg and the development of NAFLD, with studies showing that it either

Table 1
Publications on the association of nonalcoholic fatty liver disease and chronic hepatitis B infection

Authors, Year of Publication	Wong et al,[50] 2012	Joo et al,[22] 2017	Zhong et al,[49] 2018	Wang et al,[51] 2019
Country	China	South Korea	China	China
Total number of patients	1013	83,339	631	1866
Hazard ratio/OR of developing NAFLD in patients with CHB (95% CI)	0.42 (0.20–0.88)	0.83 (0.73–0.94)	0.64 (0.42–0.95)	0.656 (0.379–1.134)

has no effect on the development of NAFLD or possibly is protective. Although the factors that affect the development of NAFLD in the CHB remain to be fully elucidated, it seems that it is more the host factors rather than viral factors that determine the development of NAFLD. Of equal importance is the potential consequence of the development of NAFLD in CHB as it relates to active hepatitis, progression of CLD, and the development of HCC.

A recent study by Charatcharoenwitthaya and colleagues[57] in Thailand evaluated the prevalence of steatohepatitis and NAFLD in patients with CHB. The investigators suggested that steatohepatitis was associated with being overweight/obese (odds ratio [OR] 5.99) and hypertriglyceridemia (OR 2.95) without any association with viral factors. Additionally, steatohepatitis was an independent predictor of significant fibrosis (OR 10) and advanced fibrosis (OR 3.45) after adjusting for viremia and features of the metabolic syndrome. Another study by Zheng and colleagues[58] had similar results and was conducted in China. In this study, 106 patients with NAFLD and negative HBeAg were compared with those without NAFLD. Elevated fasting insulin and globulin levels were associated with more inflammation whereas elevated BMI and TC were associated with higher levels of fibrosis. Cai and colleageues,[59] in China evaluated and compared two cohorts of CHB patients, 149 patients with at least 1 component of metabolic syndrome with 1087 patients without any features of metabolic syndrome. A positive correlation with the number of features of metabolic syndrome and fibrosis was found. Also, elevated BMI, smoking, and alcohol intake all were associated with hepatic fibrosis in the NAFLD group. A randomized case-control study by Hui and colleagues[16] included 601 patients with CHB and NAFLD diagnosed by CAP, matched with 601 patients with CHB but without NAFLD. Patients in the severe steatosis group, compared with mild/moderate steatosis, had an increased percentage of severe fibrosis (23.2% vs 12.6%). Yen and colleagues[60] reported on 1513 patients with CHB, CHC, or NAFLD who were evaluated for the presence of cirrhosis. Across all 3 etiologies of CLD, elevated BMI was associated with the development of cirrhosis. Diabetes mellitus was associated only with cirrhosis in the CHC and NAFLD group.

Worsening fibrosis with concomitant NAFLD and CHB was not universally present in the literature. In a recent study by Pais and colleagues[61] that involved 110 patients with CHB, 111 patients with CHC, and 136 cases of NAFLD, metabolic factors and insulin resistance did not predict significant fibrosis. Similar results were obtained in another case-control study from China that involved 360 patients with CHB. In this study, there was no correlation between host metabolic factors and hepatic fibrosis. Instead, fibrosis was more prevalent in the non-NAFLD group.[62] In a third study that enrolled 1915 CHB patients, 260 of whom had concomitant NAFLD, steatosis did not correlate to hepatic fibrosis.[63] Rather, inflammatory grade, age, and viral load all

Table 2
Publications on the effect of viral and host factors in the development of alcoholic fatty liver disease in the chronic hepatitis B infection population

Authors, Year of Publication	Cheng et al,[31] 2013	Nau et al.[54] 2014	Poortahmasebi et al,[56] 2014	Yilmaz et al,[52] 2015	Pokorska-Śpiewak et al,[11] 2017	Chen et al,[53] 2018	Zhu et al,[55] 2019
Country	Taiwan	Brazil	Iran	Turkey	Poland	China	China
Total number of patients	33,439	83	160	88	78	144	2393
Factors positively associated	BMI, age, WC, SBP, fasting plasma glucose, TChole, LDL, TRI	Male, BMI, FI, PT, TChole, AST	Male, age, BMI, fasting plasma glucose, TChole	Age, BMI, TChole, HOMA-IR	BMI	FBSr, FI, TRI, TChole, LDL	BMI, DM, HTN
Factors negatively associated	None	None	HBeAg	None	None	None	None
Factors with no association with NAFLD	None	HTN, age, DM, HBeAg, VL, Rx	VL	VL, HBeAg, Rx	VL, ALT, AST, HBeAg	Age, gender	HBeAg, VL

Abbreviations: DM, diabetes mellitus; LDL, low-density lipoprotein; Rx, treatment of HBV; FI, fasting insulin; HTN, hypertension; Rx, Treatment; WC, waist circumference; PT, prothrombin activity; SBP, systolic blood pressure; TChole, total cholesterol; TRI, TG level; VL, HBV viral load.

were found contributing factors to the development of hepatic fibrosis. A smaller study in Indonesia that had 174 participants with CHB did not yield a significant difference in fibrosis, necroinflammation, or HBV DNA levels with regard to steatosis.[64]

CHRONIC HEPATITIS B, NONALCOHOLIC STEATOSIS, AND HEPATOCELLULAR CARCINOMA

CHB is a known risk factor for the development of HCC even in the absence of cirrhosis. Current research has evaluated if concomitant NAFLD with CHB would increase the risk of developing HCC. A retrospective study by Chan and colleagues[65] in Hong Kong evaluated a total of 270 patients with CHB, of whom 107 had concomitant NAFLD by biopsy. NAFLD in this patient population was associated with an increased risk of HCC with a hazard ratio of 7.27 (1.52–34.76). This finding was replicated by Lee and colleagues[66] in a recent study that enrolled 70 patients with NAFLD and CHB compared with 321 patients with CHB alone. Concomitant NAFLD with CHB was associated with a hazard ratio of 3.0; however, after adjusting for metabolic factors, it lost statistical significance. Diabetes mellitus, however, was found an independent risk factor for the development of HCC.

A study by Chan and colleagues[65] demonstrated increased risk of HCC among patients with concomitant CHB and steatosis. In 270 HBV patients, biopsy-proved hepatic steatosis increased the risk of developing HCC by 7.3-fold. They also reported an increased risk of HCC in patients with APOC3 gene polymorphism. Further work and more data are required, however, to confirm the higher risk of developing HCC in patients with CHB/NAFLD.

A particular area of interest is patients coinfected with CHB and CHC and its effect on the development of NAFLD. It is suggested that CHC, in particular genotype 3, increases the incidence of NAFLD independent of host factors.[11] The effect of hepatitis B on steatosis in hepatitis C virus co-infected subjects (BOSTIC) Study sought to evaluate this patient population and enrolled 85 patients with CHB/CHC, 112 with CHC, and 69 with CHB alone.[67] As is consistent with the literature, only BMI and not viral factors were associated with the development of NAFLD in the CHB population. In the CHC group, male gender, genotype 3, fasting plasma glucose, BMI, TGs, and age over 50 all were associated with steatosis. This finding also is consistent with previously published works. In the coinfected study population, only BMI and fasting plasma glucose were associated with the development of NAFLD. In subgroup analysis, even in patients with genotype 3, CHC and CHB together had less steatosis than in patients with genotype 3 CHC alone. This could suggest that there might be an underlying mechanism in CHB infection that is protective against the development of NAFLD.

DIAGNOSIS OF NONALCOHOLIC FATTY LIVER DISEASE IN HEPATITIS B VIRUS PATIENTS

The American Association for the Study of Liver Diseases (AASLD) updated their guidelines regarding the diagnosis and evaluation of NAFLD.[68] Although NAFLD and NASH should be considered in patients with obesity with or without type 2 diabetes mellitus, there currently are no screening guidelines. Laboratory values can be normal in patients with NAFLD; accordingly, liver ultrasound (US) and transient elastography are possible modalities that may complement in screening for NAFLD.

The gold standard for diagnosing NAFLD/NASH is liver biopsy, although it is associated with increased cost, subject to sampling error, and invasive. Other radiologic noninvasive evaluation for NAFLD includes magnetic resonance imaging/magnetic resonance enterography and estimated proton density fat fraction. There currently are no official guidelines for screening for NAFLD in the CHB patient population; however, a significant number of these individuals undergo US every 6 months for HCC screening.

In evaluating NAFLD in patients with CHB, it may be desirable to detect NASH because this has treatment implications regarding the appropriateness of initiating antiviral therapy and the progression of CLD.

There are several laboratory, biometric, elastographic, and imaging modalities available for detecting NAFLD in patients with CHB. Laboratory values include fasting plasma glucose, TC, TGs, and CK18 M30. Transient elastography measures include acoustic radiation force impulse by shear wave velocity (ARFI) and CAP by FibroScan®. The most commonly used imaging modality for the detection of NAFLD in CHB is still US with its known limitations.

The FibroScan®-based CAP was compared with liver biopsy in a recent study performed in Taiwan by Wang and colleagues[69]; 88 patients underwent CAP measurements to detect steatosis in a blinded manner and subsequently underwent biopsy to determine the area under the receiver operating curves (AUROCs), sensitivity, and specificity to detect steatosis. The sensitivities of detecting stage 1 (11%–33%), stage 2 (34%–66%), and stage 3 (>66%) were 69.0%, 83.3%, and 100.0%, respectively. This corresponded to specificities of 71.8%, 78.1%, and 96.9% for stage 1, stage 2, and stage 3, respectively. The AUROCs for CAP for stage 1, stage 2, and stage 3 were 0.711, 0.868, and 0.974, respectively. Active inflammation and fibrosis did not alter CAP measurements in this study.

US detection of NAFLD was evaluated in a recent study in Canada by Kelly and colleagues,[70] who involved 109 patients; 44% of research participants had steatosis on biopsy. The sensitivity of detecting steatosis by US was 60%, and 75% of patients without steatosis by biopsy were correctly identified by US. A semiquantitative ultrasound score, called the ultrasonographic fatty liver indicator (US-FLI), recently was developed in Italy.[71] Using this tool, a score between 2 and 8 is determined by allotting points for various US appearances that range from liver-kidney contrast, vessel blurring, and areas of focal sparing. This study included various diagnosis of CLD, including CHB, chronic hepatitis C, NAFLD, and others. Mild steatosis (at least 10% steatosis by biopsy) with a cutoff of greater than 2 on the score was associated with a sensitivity of 90.1% and specificity of 90.0%. Moderate steatosis (>30% by biopsy) using a cutoff value of greater than 3 yielded a sensitivity of 88.5% and specificity of 87%. Severe steatosis was detected with a cutoff value of greater than 5 and had a sensitivity of 88.5% and specificity of 87%.[71]

US and CAP both have potential utility in detecting NAFLD in patients with CHB, and a recent study compared CAP, US, and a laboratory-based hepatic steatosis index (HSI) using liver biopsy as the gold standard.[72] In this study, 366 nonobese patients with CHB, of whom 137 had biopsy-proved hepatic steatosis. AUROCs for detecting more than 5% steatosis were 0.780 for CAP and 0.655 for the HSI. In detecting patients with 5% to 33% steatosis, the detection rates were 65.3% for CAP, 56.5% for HSI, and 17.7% for US. In detecting group stages 2–3 (>33%), the detection rate for CAP was 92.3%, 100% for HSI, and 53.8% for US. This study suggests that CAP and HSI may be superior to regular US.[72] There currently are no established data comparing CAP to the US-FLI.

Several laboratory parameters and screening tools have been proposed to screen for NAFLD in the CHB patient population. One such measure, the steatosis index of patients with HBV infection, was proposed and validated recently in China.[17] It consists of measuring BMI, hemoglobin, TGs, and serum uric acid. For detecting steatosis greater than 33%, the AUROCs were 0.823 and 0.839 using a steatosis threshold greater than 22% on biopsy. Another research group in China developed and evaluated a fatty liver test in patients with CHB.[2] In this research effort of 1312 patients, 618 had steatosis by CAP, and were included. The fatty liver test consisted of a formula from the measurements of diastolic blood pressure, weight, and waistline. The AUROCs for detecting steatosis were 0.79 during the training phase and 0.82 during the validation phase. One possible limitation, however, is that CAP rather than liver biopsy was used; however, being able to predict NAFLD from typical measurements obtained in a routine office visit is appealing.

ARFI is yet another elastography measure and it was recently compared with FibroScan® and the laboratory-based Forns index in a research effort conducted in China.[73] Sensitivity of ARFI was greater than FibroScan® at all stages of steatosis except greater than stage 4. The Forns index had comparable sensitivities and specificities to FibroScan® and ARFI.

NONINVASIVE TESTS TO PREDICT FIBROSIS IN CHRONIC HEPATITIS B INFECTION/ NONALCOHOLIC FATTY LIVER DISEASE

Gamma-glutamyl transpeptidase–to–platelet ratio (GPR), a novel fibrosis model, could be used as a noninvasive test to predict liver fibrosis and cirrhosis in CHB/ NAFLD patients early on, allowing prompt and appropriate treatment to decrease the disease burden. It was proposed by Lemoine and colleagues[74] and showed a better diagnostic performance in significant and severe fibrosis compared with other previously used models (APRI [aspartate aminotransferase–to–eplatelet ratio index] and FIB-4 [fibrosis-4 index]) in CHB/NAFLD patients. In a study by Li and colleagues,[15] no statistical significance was seen between GPR and APRI in diagnosing cirrhosis ($P = .104$). GPR had good negative predictive value for excluding significant fibrosis (91%), severe fibrosis (98%), and cirrhosis (100%) but low positive predictive value for diagnosing significant fibrosis (65%), severe fibrosis (39%), and cirrhosis (30%). Similarly, APRI and FIB-4 had low positive predictive values for diagnosing significant fibrosis (47% and 37%, respectively), severe fibrosis (25% and 23%, respectively), and cirrhosis (21% and 14%, respectively). GPR showed a relatively higher positive predictive values, however, compared with APRI and FIB-4.

A recent study compared 31 patients with NAFLD and CHB to 34 patients with NASH and CHB by biopsy to determine which factors were associated with NASH.[39] In this study, elevations of serum marker CK18 M30, higher CAP measurements, and elevated fasting plasma glucose were all independent risk factors for NASH. The AUROCs for CK18 M30, CAP, and elevated fasting plasma glucose were 0.94, 0.77, and 0.79,respectively. Specificity for CK18 M30 was 67% whereas CAP was 87% and fasting plasma glucose was 64%. When these 3 measures were combined, the AUROC was 1 with a specificity of 80%.

Evaluation of NAFLD and NASH in CHB is an emerging management strategy given the increasing prevalence of NAFLD in this population with the current obesity epidemic. In this treatment population, elevated ALT levels could be the result of NAFLD, HBV immune active phase, or a combination of both. Noninvasive measures to detect NAFLD and possibly NASH are attractive because they avoid the invasiveness of liver biopsy and can be used to make treatment decisions regarding the appropriateness of initiating antiviral therapy. Additionally, these measures can be repeated over the course of treatment to gauge treatment response to measures aimed at CHB and NAFLD.

The AASLD updated their guidelines regarding the treatment of CHB in 2018.[75] The recommendation is to treat all patients with HBeAg-positive immune active and HBeAg-negative immune active patients with antiviral therapy. The 6 approved antiviral therapies for CHB in the United States are pegylated interferon, lamivudine, telbivudine, entecavir, adefovir, and tenofovir. The AASLD, however, recommends monotherapy with pegylated interferon, entecavir, or tenofovir as first-line agents in light of the fact that these agents are associated with less long-term resistance.

There also exist guidelines from the AASLD regarding the treatment of NAFLD. Lifestyle modifications, such as weight loss, avoidance of alcohol, and aggressive treatment of hypertension, hyperlipidemia, and diabetes, remain a cornerstone of treatment.[68] Medical therapies specific for NAFLD include thiazolidinediones and vitamin E. Glucagon-like peptide-1 analogs are a potential specific treatment of NAFLD; however, they currently are not recommended for this indication alone. There currently are sparse recommendations regarding the treatment of CHB in patients with concomitant NAFLD.

The data regarding the selection, efficacy, and outcomes of treating patients with NAFLD and CHB infection are conflicting.[76]

Two recently conducted studies in patients with CHB on antivirals found that there was less ALT normalization in patients with CHB with concomitant NAFLD compared with CHB alone (**Table 3**).[76,77] Two other studies also found that NAFLD had no impact on viral response to treatment with entecavir or tenofovir.[78,79]

Given both the paucity and conflicting nature of the data regarding treatment response to antiviral therapy and outcome data in patients with concomitant NAFLD and CHB, it is difficult to make specific recommendations regarding treatment approaches in this patient population. Given that the risk factors associated with NAFLD are harbingers of other medical illnesses, such as atherosclerotic cardiovascular disease, these should be addressed with both medical and lifestyle interventions. Whether their control gains extra significance or alters liver-related morbidity, mortality, and transplant rates remains to be determined. Further research efforts in the areas of treatment response, natural history, and outcome data regarding patients with concomitant NAFLD and CHB are required before more specific recommendations can be made.

Table 3
Publications on the treatment response in chronic hepatitis B infection and nonalcoholic fatty liver disease

Author, Year of Publication	Jin et al,[81] 2012	Dogan et al,[78] 2015	Gong et al,[80] 2015	Ceylan et al,[79] 2016	Chen et al,[77] 2017
Country	China	Turkey	China	Turkey	China
Total number of patients	65	63	89	132	153
Antiviral	Entecavir	Entecavir or tenofovir	Pegylated interferon	Entecavir or tenofovir	Entecavir
ALT normalization	Less in NAFLD[a]	No difference	No difference	Not reported	Less in NAFLD[a]
Hepatitis B e seroconversion	Less in NAFLD[a]	Not reported	No difference	Not reported	No difference
Viremic response	No difference	No difference	Less in NAFLD[a]	No difference	Less in NAFLD[a]

[a] Statistically significant.

REFERENCES

1. Kowdley KV, Wang CC, Welch S, et al. Prevalence of chronic hepatitis B among foreign-born persons living in the United States by country of origin. Hepatology 2012;56(2):422–33.
2. Ou H, Cai S, Liu Y, et al. A noninvasive diagnostic model to assess nonalcoholic hepatic steatosis in patients with chronic hepatitis B. Therap Adv Gastroenterol 2017;10(2):207–17.
3. MacLachlan JH, Cowie BC. Hepatitis B virus epidemiology. Cold Spring Harb Perspect Med 2015;5(5):a021410.
4. Schweitzer A, Horn J, Mikolajczyk RT, et al. Estimations of worldwide prevalence of chronic hepatitis B virus infection: a systematic review of data published between 1965 and 2013. Lancet 2015;386(10003):1546–55.
5. Jefferies M, Rauff B, Rashid H, et al. Update on global epidemiology of viral hepatitis and preventive strategies. World J Clin Cases 2018;6(13):589–99.
6. Perumpail BJ, Khan MA, Yoo ER, et al. Clinical epidemiology and disease burden of nonalcoholic fatty liver disease. World J Gastroenterol 2017;23(47):8263–76.
7. Xiong J, Zhang H, Wang Y, et al. Hepatitis B virus infection and the risk of nonalcoholic fatty liver disease: a meta-analysis. Oncotarget 2017;8(63):107295–302.
8. Loomba R, Sanyal AJ. The global NAFLD epidemic. Nat Rev Gastroenterol Hepatol 2013;10(11):686–90.
9. Younossi Z, Anstee QM, Marietti M, et al. Global burden of NAFLD and NASH: trends, predictions, risk factors and prevention. Nat Rev Gastroenterol Hepatol 2018;15(1):11–20.
10. Morales MR, Sendra C, Romero-Gomez M. Hepatitis B and NAFLD: lives crossed. Ann Hepatol 2017;16(2):185–7.
11. Pokorska-Śpiewak M, Kowalik-Mikołajewska B, Aniszewska M, et al. Liver steatosis in children with chronic hepatitis B and C: prevalence, predictors, and impact on disease progression. Medicine (Baltimore) 2017;96(3):e5832.
12. Kanto T, Yoshio S. Hepatitis action plan and changing trend of liver disease in Japan: viral hepatitis and nonalcoholic fatty liver disease. Euroasian J Hepatogastroenterol 2017;7(1):60–4.
13. European Association for the Study of The Liver (EASL), European Association for the Study of Diabetes (EASD), European Association for the Study of Obesity (EASO). EASL-EASD-EASO clinical practice guidelines for the management of non-alcoholic fatty liver disease. J Hepatol 2016;64(6):1388–402.
14. Pais R, Rusu E, Ratziu V. The impact of obesity and metabolic syndrome on chronic hepatitis B and drug-induced liver disease. Clin Liver Dis 2014;18(1):165–78.
15. Li Q, Lu C, Li W, et al. The gamma-glutamyl transpeptidase to platelet ratio for non-invasive assessment of liver fibrosis in patients with chronic hepatitis B and non-alcoholic fatty liver disease. Oncotarget 2017;8(17):28641–9.
16. Hui RWH, Seto WK, Cheung KS, et al. Inverse relationship between hepatic steatosis and hepatitis B viremia: results of a large case-control study. J Viral Hepat 2018;25(1):97–104.
17. Zhang Z, Wang G, Kang K, et al. Diagnostic accuracy and clinical utility of a new noninvasive index for hepatic steatosis in patients with hepatitis B virus infection. Sci Rep 2016;6:32875.
18. Wu YL, Peng XE, Zhu YB, et al. Hepatitis B virus X protein induces hepatic steatosis by enhancing the expression of liver fatty acid binding protein. J Virol 2015;90(4):1729–40.

19. Haga Y, Kanda T, Sasaki R, et al. Nonalcoholic fatty liver disease and hepatic cirrhosis: comparison with viral hepatitis-associated steatosis. World J Gastroenterol 2015;21(46):12989–95.
20. Li YJ, Zhu P, Liang Y, et al. Hepatitis B virus induces expression of cholesterol metabolism-related genes via TLR2 in HepG2 cells. World J Gastroenterol 2013;19(14):2262–9.
21. Oehler N, Volz T, Bhadra OD, et al. Binding of hepatitis B virus to its cellular receptor alters the expression profile of genes of bile acid metabolism. Hepatology 2014;60(5):1483–93.
22. Joo EJ, Chang Y, Yeom JS, et al. Hepatitis B virus infection and decreased risk of nonalcoholic fatty liver disease: a cohort study. Hepatology 2017;65(3):828–35.
23. Pan Q, Chen MM, Zhang RN, et al. PNPLA3 rs1010023 predisposes chronic hepatitis B to hepatic steatosis but improves insulin resistance and glucose metabolism. J Diabetes Res 2017;2017:4740124.
24. Kozlitina J, Smagris E, Stender S, et al. Exome-wide association study identifies a TM6SF2 variant that confers susceptibility to nonalcoholic fatty liver disease. Nat Genet 2014;46(4):352–6.
25. Eslam M, Mangia A, Berg T, et al. Diverse impacts of the rs58542926 E167K variant in TM6SF2 on viral and metabolic liver disease phenotypes. Hepatology 2016;64(1):34–46.
26. Zhang Z, Pan Q, Duan XY, et al. Fatty liver reduces hepatitis B virus replication in a genotype B hepatitis B virus transgenic mice model. J Gastroenterol Hepatol 2012;27(12):1858–64.
27. Chu CM, Lin DY, Liaw YF. Does increased body mass index with hepatic steatosis contribute to seroclearance of hepatitis B virus (HBV) surface antigen in chronic HBV infection? Int J Obes (Lond) 2007;31(5):871–5.
28. Zhang RN, Pan Q, Zhang Z, et al. Saturated Fatty Acid inhibits viral replication in chronic hepatitis B virus infection with nonalcoholic Fatty liver disease by toll-like receptor 4-mediated innate immune response. Hepat Mon 2015;15(5):e27909.
29. Seki E, Brenner DA. Toll-like receptors and adaptor molecules in liver disease: update. Hepatology 2008;48(1):322–35.
30. Broering R, Lu M, Schlaak JF. Role of Toll-like receptors in liver health and disease. Clin Sci (Lond) 2011;121(10):415–26.
31. Cheng YL, Wang YJ, Kao WY, et al. Inverse association between hepatitis B virus infection and fatty liver disease: a large-scale study in populations seeking for check-up. PLoS One 2013;8(8):e72049.
32. Wong VW, Wong GL, Yu J, et al. Interaction of adipokines and hepatitis B virus on histological liver injury in the Chinese. Am J Gastroenterol 2010;105(1):132–8.
33. Masaki T, Chiba S, Tatsukawa H, et al. Adiponectin protects LPS-induced liver injury through modulation of TNF-alpha in KK-Ay obese mice. Hepatology 2004;40(1):177–84.
34. Liang J, Cai W, Han T, et al. The expression of thymosin β4 in chronic hepatitis B combined nonalcoholic fatty liver disease. Medicine (Baltimore) 2016;95(52): e5763.
35. Kumar S, Gupta S. Thymosin beta 4 prevents oxidative stress by targeting antioxidant and anti-apoptotic genes in cardiac fibroblasts. PLoS One 2011;6(10): e26912.
36. Qiu P, Wheater MK, Qiu Y, et al. Thymosin beta4 inhibits TNF-alpha-induced NF-kappaB activation, IL-8 expression, and the sensitizing effects by its partners PINCH-1 and ILK. FASEB J 2011;25(6):1815–26.

37. Xiao Y, Qu C, Ge W, et al. Depletion of thymosin β4 promotes the proliferation, migration, and activation of human hepatic stellate cells. Cell Physiol Biochem 2014;34(2):356–67.

38. Barnaeva E, Nadezhda A, Hannappel E, et al. Thymosin beta4 upregulates the expression of hepatocyte growth factor and downregulates the expression of PDGF-beta receptor in human hepatic stellate cells. Ann N Y Acad Sci 2007; 1112:154–60.

39. Liang J, Liu F, Wang F, et al. A noninvasive score model for prediction of NASH in patients with chronic hepatitis B and nonalcoholic fatty liver disease. Biomed Res Int 2017;2017:8793278.

40. Yang RX, Hu CX, Sun WL, et al. Serum monounsaturated triacylglycerol predicts steatohepatitis in patients with non-alcoholic fatty liver disease and chronic hepatitis B. Sci Rep 2017;7(1):10517.

41. Jarcuska P, Drazilova S, Fedacko J, et al. Association between hepatitis B and metabolic syndrome: current state of the art. World J Gastroenterol 2016;22(1): 155–64.

42. Wang CC, Hsu CS, Liu CJ, et al. Association of chronic hepatitis B virus infection with insulin resistance and hepatic steatosis. J Gastroenterol Hepatol 2008;23(5): 779–82.

43. Lee JG, Lee S, Kim YJ, et al. Association of chronic viral hepatitis B with insulin resistance. World J Gastroenterol 2012;18(42):6120–6.

44. Shen Y, Zhang J, Cai H, et al. Identifying patients with chronic hepatitis B at high risk of type 2 diabetes mellitus: a cross-sectional study with pair-matched controls. BMC Gastroenterol 2015;15:32.

45. Machado MV, Oliveira AG, Cortez-Pinto H. Hepatic steatosis in hepatitis B virus infected patients: meta-analysis of risk factors and comparison with hepatitis C infected patients. J Gastroenterol Hepatol 2011;26(9):1361–7.

46. Jarčuška P, Janičko M, Kružliak P, et al. Hepatitis B virus infection in patients with metabolic syndrome: a complicated relationship. Results of a population based study. Eur J Intern Med 2014;25(3):286–91.

47. Chiang CH, Yang HI, Jen CL, et al. REVEAL-HBV Study Group. Association between obesity, hypertriglyceridemia and low hepatitis B viral load. Int J Obes (Lond) 2013;37(3):410–5.

48. Pagadala M, Kasumov T, McCullough AJ, et al. Role of ceramides in nonalcoholic fatty liver disease. Trends Endocrinol Metab 2012;23(8):365–71.

49. Zhong GC, Wu YL, Hao FB, et al. Current but not past hepatitis B virus infection is associated with a decreased risk of nonalcoholic fatty liver disease in the Chinese population: a case-control study with propensity score analysis. J Viral Hepat 2018;25(7):842–52.

50. Wong VW, Wong GL, Chu WC, et al. Hepatitis B virus infection and fatty liver in the general population. J Hepatol 2012;56(3):533–40.

51. Wang B, Li W, Fang H, et al. Hepatitis B virus infection is not associated with fatty liver disease: evidence from a cohort study and functional analysis. Mol Med Rep 2019;19(1):320–6.

52. Yilmaz B, Koklu S, Buyukbayram H, et al. Chronic hepatitis B associated with hepatic steatosis, insulin resistance, necroinflammation and fibrosis. Afr Health Sci 2015;15(3):714–8.

53. Chen XL, Han YD, Wang H. Relations of hepatic steatosis with liver functions, inflammations, glucolipid metabolism in chronic hepatitis B patients. Eur Rev Med Pharmacol Sci 2018;22(17):5640–6.

54. Nau AL, Soares JC, Shiozawa MB, et al. Clinical and laboratory characteristics associated with dyslipidemia and liver steatosis in chronic HBV carriers. Rev Soc Bras Med Trop 2014;47(2):158–64.

55. Zhu L, Jiang J, Zhai X, et al. Hepatitis B virus infection and risk of non-alcoholic fatty liver disease: a population-based cohort study. Liver Int 2019;39(1):70–80.

56. Poortahmasebi V, Alavian SM, Keyvani H, et al. Hepatic steatosis: prevalence and host/viral risk factors in Iranian patients with chronic hepatitis B infection. Asian Pac J Cancer Prev 2014;15(9):3879–84.

57. Charatcharoenwitthaya P, Pongpaibul A, Kaosombatwattana U, et al. The prevalence of steatohepatitis in chronic hepatitis B patients and its impact on disease severity and treatment response. Liver Int 2017;37(4):542–51.

58. Zheng RD, Xu CR, Jiang L, et al. Predictors of hepatic steatosis in HBeAg-negative chronic hepatitis B patients and their diagnostic values in hepatic fibrosis. Int J Med Sci 2010;7(5):272–7.

59. Cai S, Ou Z, Liu D, et al. Risk factors associated with liver steatosis and fibrosis in chronic hepatitis B patient with component of metabolic syndrome. United European Gastroenterol J 2018;6(4):558–66.

60. Yen YH, Chang KC, Tsai MC, et al. Elevated body mass index is a risk factor associated with possible liver cirrhosis across different etiologies of chronic liver disease. J Formos Med Assoc 2018;117(4):268–75.

61. Pais R, Rusu E, Zilisteanu D, et al. Prevalence of steatosis and insulin resistance in patients with chronic hepatitis B compared with chronic hepatitis C and non-alcoholic fatty liver disease. Eur J Intern Med 2015;26(1):30–6.

62. Zheng RD, Chen JN, Zhuang QY, et al. Clinical and virological characteristics of chronic hepatitis B patients with hepatic steatosis. Int J Med Sci 2013;10(5):641–6.

63. Shi JP, Fan JG, Wu R, et al. Prevalence and risk factors of hepatic steatosis and its impact on liver injury in Chinese patients with chronic hepatitis B infection. J Gastroenterol Hepatol 2008;23(9):1419–25.

64. Lesmana LA, Lesmana CR, Pakasi LS, et al. Prevalence of hepatic steatosis in chronic hepatitis B patients and its association with disease severity. Acta Med Indones 2012;44(1):35–9.

65. Chan AW, Wong GL, Chan HY, et al. Concurrent fatty liver increases risk of hepatocellular carcinoma among patients with chronic hepatitis B. J Gastroenterol Hepatol 2017;32(3):667–76.

66. Lee YB, Ha Y, Chon YE, et al. Association between hepatic steatosis and the development of hepatocellular carcinoma in patients with chronic hepatitis B. Clin Mol Hepatol 2019;25(1):52–64.

67. Goossens N, de Vito C, Mangia A, et al. Effect of hepatitis B virus on steatosis in hepatitis C virus co-infected subjects: a multi-centre study and systematic review. J Viral Hepat 2018;25(8):920–9.

68. Chalasani N, Younossi Z, Lavine JE, et al. The diagnosis and management of nonalcoholic fatty liver disease: practice guidance from the American Association for the Study of Liver Diseases. Hepatology 2018;67(1):328–57.

69. Wang CY, Lu W, Hu DS, et al. Diagnostic value of controlled attenuation parameter for liver steatosis in patients with chronic hepatitis B. World J Gastroenterol 2014;20(30):10585–90.

70. Kelly EM, Feldstein VA, Etheridge D, et al. Sonography predicts liver steatosis in patients with chronic hepatitis B. J Ultrasound Med 2017;36(5):925–32.

71. Ballestri S, Nascimbeni F, Baldelli E, et al. Ultrasonographic fatty liver indicator detects mild steatosis and correlates with metabolic/histological parameters in various liver diseases. Metabolism 2017;72:57–65.

72. Xu L, Lu W, Li P, et al. A comparison of hepatic steatosis index, controlled attenuation parameter and ultrasound as noninvasive diagnostic tools for steatosis in chronic hepatitis B. Dig Liver Dis 2017;49(8):910–7.

73. Dong DR, Hao MN, Li C, et al. Acoustic radiation force impulse elastography, FibroScan®, Forns' index and their combination in the assessment of liver fibrosis in patients with chronic hepatitis B, and the impact of inflammatory activity and steatosis on these diagnostic methods. Mol Med Rep 2015;11(6):4174–82.

74. Lemoine M, Shimakawa Y, Nayagam S, et al. The gamma-glutamyl transpeptidase to platelet ratio (GPR) predicts significant liver fibrosis and cirrhosis in patients with chronic HBV infection in West Africa. Gut 2016;65(8):1369–76.

75. Terrault NA, Lok ASF, McMahon BJ, et al. Update on prevention, diagnosis, and treatment of chronic hepatitis B: AASLD 2018 hepatitis B guidance. Hepatology 2018;67(4):1560–99.

76. Laho T, Clarke JD, Dzierlenga AL, et al. Effect of nonalcoholic steatohepatitis on renal filtration and secretion of adefovir. Biochem Pharmacol 2016;115:144–51.

77. Chen J, Wang ML, Long Q, et al. High value of controlled attenuation parameter predicts a poor antiviral response in patients with chronic hepatits B. Hepatobiliary Pancreat Dis Int 2017;16(4):370–4.

78. Dogan Z, Filik L, Ergül B, et al. Comparison of first-year results of tenofovir and entecavir treatments of nucleos(t)ide-naive chronic hepatitis B patients with hepatosteatosis. Saudi J Gastroenterol 2015;21(6):396–9.

79. Ceylan B, Arslan F, Batırel A, et al. Impact of fatty liver on hepatitis B virus replication and virologic response to tenofovir and entecavir. Turk J Gastroenterol 2016;27(1):42–6.

80. Gong L, Liu J, Wang J, et al. Hepatic steatosis as a predictive factor of antiviral effect of Pegylated Interferon therapy in patients with hepatitis B. Transplant Proc 2015;47(10):2886–91.

81. Jin X, Chen YP, Yang YD, et al. Association between hepatic steatosis and entecavir treatment failure in Chinese patients with chronic hepatitis B. PLoS One 2012;7(3):e34198.

Hepatitis B in Pregnant Women and their Infants

Alicia M. Cryer, DO[a,1], Joanne C. Imperial, MD[b,*]

KEYWORDS

- Pregnancy • Chronic hepatitis B • Mother-to-child transmission • Antiviral therapy
- Postexposure prophylaxis • Postpartum hepatitis flares

KEY POINTS

- Mother to child transmission (MTCT) is the major risk factor for development of chronic hepatitis B (CHB).
- All pregnant women should be screened for CHB.
- Hepatitis B virus (HBV) vaccination is safe and effective in pregnant women not infected with, or not immune to, HBV.
- Antiviral therapy for highly viremic hepatitis B surface antigen–positive (HBsAg+) mothers (HBV DNA >200,000 IU/mL) can significantly reduce MTCT, is recommended in the third trimester, and can be discontinued within a few weeks postpartum.
- All infants born from HBsAg+ mothers should receive hepatitis B immunoglobulin plus HBV vaccine within 12 hours to 24 hours after birth.

HEPATITIS B VIRUS TRANSMISSION DURING PREGNANCY

It is generally accepted that mother-to-child transmission (MTCT) occurs around the birth of the infant, it is believed to be due to exposure to maternal blood and cervical secretions, and is dependent on maternal HBV DNA levels. Although hepatitis B can present as an acute infection during pregnancy, and previously was a more common reason for abnormal maternal liver enzymes, vaccination programs have significantly reduced this risk.[1] If acute HBV is contracted, the likelihood of transmission to the infant is dependent on the timing of the infection and highest when mothers acquire HBV in the third trimester. It is recommended that all pregnant women undergo screening for HBV, and, although these recommendations are likely to be upheld for those with health insurance, there are definite gaps in screening and linkage to care, evident predominantly in underinsured populations.[2]

Disclosures: The authors have nothing to disclose.
[a] Department of Gynecology and Obstetrics, Loma Linda Medical Center, Loma Linda, CA, USA;
[b] Southern California Liver Center, San Diego, CA, USA
[1] Present address: 23683 Sonata Drive, Murieta, CA 92562.
* Corresponding author. 442 Littlefield Avenue South, San Francisco, CA 94080.
E-mail addresses: joanne.imperial@gmail.com; jimperial@blademed.com

The American College of Obstetricians and Gynecologists (ACOG) and Centers for Disease Control and Prevention (CDC) agree—all pregnant women should undergo screening for HBsAg to assess active hepatitis B infection (**Table 1**).[3] Women who report never receiving HBV vaccination may be tested for hepatitis B surface antibody (anti-HBs) and, if negative, should receive HBV vaccination. This is especially important for those women at high risk for acquisition of HBV (**Box 1**).[4] Women with established immunity (anti-HBs >10 IU/mL) need no further work-up. Those with low or nonexistent anti-HBs may lack immunity or may have declining antibody titers.[5] If the seroprotection is a result of hepatitis B vaccination, the anti-HBs titer can wane over time, resulting in levels that may be confused with nonimmunity. To adequately assess these patients, a 1-time challenge dose of hepatitis B vaccine may be administered.[5] If seroprotected, there should be a rapid and appropriate immunologic response, resulting in an increase in anti-HBs. If anti-HBs is again documented to be negative, completion of a second vaccine series with 2 additional doses is recommended. Vaccine nonresponders are defined as those individuals who remain anti-HBs negative, despite 2 complete vaccination series. It is important to counsel mothers that completion of another hepatitis B vaccination series is not indicated.[5]

For women with no previous hepatitis B immunization and no evidence of prior infection, an HBV vaccination series should be initiated. A proposed accelerated protocol should establish a high level of immunity early in the pregnancy.[6] All women with negative HBsAg, and who qualify as having a high-risk lifestyle, should be retested at 28 weeks and again at time of delivery admission.[7] A high-risk lifestyle is defined as one that increases the likelihood of HBV exposure and includes use of intravenous drugs, close contact with someone who has chronic HBV, or history of multiple sexual partners. For unvaccinated pregnant women with known hepatitis B exposure presenting for the first time at delivery, standard postexposure prophylaxis protocol for the newborn should be initiated and is discussed in detail later.

Table 1
Hepatitis B serology interpretation for determination of need for hepatitis B virus vaccination

Test	Result	Interpretation
HBsAg	Negative	Nonimmune, susceptible
HBcAb	Negative	
HBsAb	Negative	
HBsAg	Negative	Resolved HBV infection
HBcAb	Positive	
HBsAb	Positive	
HBsAg	Positive	Chronically infected
HBcAb IgM	Negative	
HBcAb IgG	Positive	
HBsAb	Negative	
HBsAg	Negative	Immunity due to HBV vaccination
HBcAb	Negative	
HBsAb	Positive	
HBsAg	Positive	Acutely infected
HBcAb IgM	Positive	
HBsAb	Negative	

Abbreviations: HBsAg, Hepatitis B surface antigen; HBcAb, Hepatitis B core antibody; HBeAg, Hepatitis B e antigen; HBeAb, Hepatitis B e antibody; HBsAb, Hepatitis B surface antibody; HBcAb, Hepatitis B core antibody (igM and IgG).

From Centers for Disease Control and Prevention. Interpretation of Hepatitis B Serologic Test Results. Available at: https://www.cdc.gov/hepatitis/hbv/pdfs/serologicchartv8.pdf.

> **Box 1**
> **Examples of individuals at high risk for chronic hepatitis B**
>
> Those born in areas where HBV is of high or intermediate endemicity (prevalence >2%)
>
> Travelers to countries with intermediate or high prevalence of HBV infection
>
> Those with sexual contact with individuals infected with HBV
>
> Persons living in a household with an HBV-infected individual
>
> Intravenous drug users
>
> Heterosexuals with multiple sexual partners
>
> Persons receiving blood transfusions using infected blood
>
> Health care workers exposed to infected blood or body fluids through contact with needles or medical devices
>
> *Adapted from*: Hepatitis B Questions and Answers for Health Professionals | CDC. Centers for Disease Control and Prevention. https://www.cdc.gov/hepatitis/hbv/hbvfaq.htm. Revised October 31, 2018.

NATURAL HISTORY OF HEPATITIS B IN PREGNANCY

The course of chronic hepatitis B (CHB) in the pregnant woman is generally mild; however, because there are many phases of infection (**Fig. 1**), close follow-up of all chronically HBV-infected women is recommended during the entire pregnancy. For those women who are HBsAg+ and hepatitis B e antigen negative (HBeAg−), with low-level viremia, the risk of transmission to the infant is approximately 10% without immune prophylaxis given at birth. Infants born to HBsAg+, HBeAg+, and mothers

Diagnosis of Chronic HBV

- **HBsAg-positive**
- **Immune-tolerant phase**
  - Normal liver enzymes
  - Very high HBV DNA level
  - HBeAg+: marker of infectivity
  - Children, teens, young adults
- **Inactive HBV carrier**
  - Normal liver enzymes
  - HBeAg-, HBeAb+
  - Undetectable or low HBV DNA (<1000 IU/mL)
- **Chronic active HBV**
  - Abnormal liver enzymes (ALT >1.5 x normal, ALT >30)
  - HBeAg+
  - HBV DNA >20,000 IU/mL

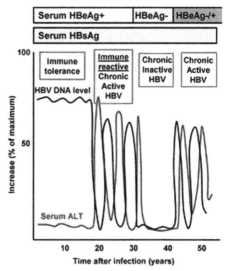

Fig. 1. Phases of chronic HBV infection. (*From* Dunkelberg, JC; Thiel, KW; Leslie, KK. Hepatitis B and C in pregnancy: a review and recommendations for care. Journal of Perinatology 2014;34(12):882–891; with permission.)

with high viral loads, have a 90% chance of developing chronic HBV if not given immune prophylaxis. Approximately 25% of are at risk for development of cirrhosis, liver failure, and/or hepatocellular carcinoma during their lifetimes. The MTCT rates of CHB are highest for those chronic HBsAg+ carriers who are foreign-born, particularly in Asian countries and areas where HBV genotype C is endemic,[8] but the recent opioid epidemic has brought with it a resurgence of acute hepatitis B in non–foreign-born mothers, with approximately 1000 new cases of CHB in infants born of HBV-infected mothers identified annually in the United States.[9] Many high-risk women (see **Box 1**) who present to obstetrics clinics are either immune tolerant and have high levels of HBV DNA (HBeAg+ CHB) or have circulating levels of HBV DNA and normal or near-normal alanine aminotransferase (ALT) levels (HBeAg− CHB). The highly viremic HBV-infected mothers present the greatest risk for MTCT, even when their newborns are given postexposure prophylaxis.[10,11] Regardless of stage, pregnancy usually does not result in significant changes in the clinical course of HBV infection.

There have been rare case reports, however, of fulminant liver failure or severe hepatic flares occurring during pregnancy or in the postpartum period (discussed later).[12–14]

IMPACT OF PREGNANCY ON HEPATITIS B VIRUS INFECTION

Pregnancy results in many physiologic changes, has multiorgan effects, and is an immunotolerant state. It is associated with significant hormonal changes, including an increase in adrenocorticoids, progesterone, and estrogen. Consideration of these immunologic changes is paramount to treating a pregnant woman with active HBV. During pregnancy, the maternal immune system adapts to tolerate external antigens and allow for the development of the semiallogenic fetus. Overall, proinflammatory processes have been found to decrease whereas anti-inflammatory processes increase.[15] These changes are required for proper implantation and growth of the placenta, allow for the development of maternal-fetal interface, and help avoid rejection of the developing fetus. The natural course of HBV infection, however, may be impacted due to these immunologic changes. The increase in steroid hormones seen early in pregnancy results in depressed cell-mediated immunity. Animal studies have demonstrated that estrogen and progesterone have a detrimental effect on T-cell development, both in number and activity.[15–17] This may explain why loss of HBsAg in pregnant women acutely infected with HBV is less likely than that observed in nonpregnant women. Pregnancy is believed a risk factor for the development of CHB if an acute exposure to HBV occurs.[18]

IMPACT OF HEPATITIS B VIRUS INFECTION ON PREGNANCY

If found during screening of a pregnant woman, a positive HBsAg warrants further investigation. Additional tests should include an HBeAg, hepatitis B e antibody (HBeAb), HBV DNA, complete blood cell count, comprehensive metabolic panel, international normalized ratio (INR), and liver ultrasound. For diagnosis of acute HBV infection, HBV IgM anti–core antibody (anti-HBc) must be obtained; if positive, acute HBV infection is confirmed. As discussed previously, pregnant women who become infected with acute HBV may be more likely to develop CHB due to the immunologic changes that occur during pregnancy.

Acute HBV infection commonly is managed with supportive care, and antiviral therapy has not been shown to have an impact on the course of the disease.[19] Patients should be monitored frequently with liver function tests and prothrombin time/INR.

In addition, they should be assessed for mental status changes that could signal the development of a fulminant or subacute HBV, both of which would necessitate referral for urgent liver transplantation. Depending on the timing of development of fulminant or subacute disease, there very well may be compromise the health or life of the fetus.

Development of an acute HBV infection during pregnancy has been associated with gestational diabetes, increased postpartum hemorrhage, preterm delivery, and low birthweights.[20–22] The risk of MTCT of HBV is dependent on the timing of the exposure and highest in the third trimester of pregnancy. Although there is a 10% likelihood of transmission to the newborn if maternal infection occurs in the first trimester, the risk of HBV transmission is as high as 60% if exposure occurs in the third trimester.[23]

INDICATIONS FOR USE OF ANTIVIRAL THERAPY FOR HEPATITIS B VIRUS IN PREGNANCY

Women in their childbearing years already may require antiviral therapy for active CHB infection, especially if diagnosed with HBV cirrhosis. **Table 2** lists the HBV antiviral therapies as pregnancy category B (tenofovir and telbivudine) and category C (lamivudine, adefovir, and entecavir).

Table 2
Food and Drug Administration pregnancy categories and hepatitis B virus antiviral therapy

Category	Food and Drug Administration Description	Hepatitis B Virus Therapy
A	Adequate and well-controlled studies have failed to demonstrate a risk to the fetus in the first trimester of pregnancy (and there is no evidence of risk in later trimesters).	
B	Animal reproduction studies have failed to demonstrate a risk to the fetus and there are no adequate and well-controlled studies in pregnant women or animal studies, which have shown an adverse effect, but adequate and well-controlled studies in pregnant women have failed to demonstrate a risk to the fetus in any trimester.	Telbivudine Tenofovir
C	Animal reproduction studies have shown an adverse effect on the fetus, and there are no adequate and well-controlled studies in humans, but potential benefits may warrant use of the drug in pregnant women despite potential risks.	Lamivudine Entecavir Adefovir
D	There is positive evidence of human fetal risk based on adverse-reaction data from investigational or marketing experience or studies in humans, but potential benefits may warrant use of the drug in pregnant women despite potential risks.	
x	Studies in animals or humans have demonstrated fetal abnormalities and/or there is positive evidence of human fetal risk based on adverse-reaction data from investigational or marketing experience, and the risks involved in use of the drug in pregnant women clearly outweigh potential benefits.	Interferon

From Pan CQ, Lee HM. Antiviral Therapy for Chronic Hepatitis B in Pregnancy. Semin Liver Dis. 2013;33(2):138–46; with permission.

Although all pregnant women with HBV cirrhosis should be maintained on chronic antiviral therapy to avoid potential HBV flares and hepatic decompensation, it may be possible in certain cases to delay or discontinue treatment in those nonfibrotic/cirrhotic mothers until after the pregnancy is completed (**Fig. 2**). Recent data have shown that the newer antiviral nucleoside and nucleotide analogs are effective in maintaining durable suppression of HBV viral DNA, with very low levels of break-through resistance (<1%) and significant reversal of fibrosis/cirrhosis in patients with advanced liver disease,[24–26] but comprehensive data on use and safety in pregnancy are lacking, with the exception of cohort studies done in small numbers of patients[27–29] as well as numerous meta-analyses.[30] Tenofovir, due to the experience in those pregnant HIV+ mothers on antiretroviral therapy, along with its high barrier to breakthrough resistance, is the recommended antiviral treatment of HBsAg+ pregnant women, when indicated.[7]

Balancing the benefits versus the risks of medications given to pregnant women is always of utmost importance, and, if it were not for the significant rate of postexposure prophylaxis failure (9%) in highly viremic HBeAg+ mothers (>200,000 IU/mL HBV DNA),[30] it would be unlikely that studies would be done in this group of patients. Large randomized controlled trials are needed, but, in their absence, evidence thus far indicates that when antiviral therapy should be given in the third trimester of pregnancy to highly viremic HBeAg+ mothers (**Box 2**).

The Antiretroviral Pregnancy Registry was established in 1989 to evaluate potential teratogenic effects of HIV agents. This registry confirmed that lamivudine and tenofovir

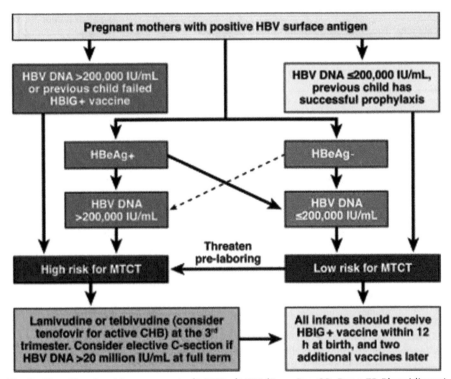

Fig. 2. Algorithm for risk assessment of MTCT of HBV. (*From* Pan CQ, Duan ZP, Bhamidimarri KR, et al. An algorithm for risk assessment and intervention of mother to child transmission of hepatitis B virus. Clin Gastroenterol Hepatol 2012;10(5):452–9; with permission.)

Box 2
Results of giving antiviral therapy in the third trimester of pregnancy

- Antiviral therapy results in significant maternal HBV DNA reduction.

- No significant changes in ALT, creatinine, or creatine kinase levels are noted between treated and control group mothers.

- The limited safety data suggest no increased risk of maternal or fetal serious adverse events.

- Infants of mothers treated with antiviral therapy have significantly less HBsAg, HBeAg, and HBV DNA positivity compared with controls.

- Rates of immune prophylaxis failure and MTCT are significantly lower in infants when highly viremic mothers received antiviral therapy during last trimester compared with controls.[31]

---

used in pregnant women for the treatment of HIV was not associated with an increased risk of birth defects or fetal deaths compared with those seen in the general population.[32] The most serious adverse event reported with use of nucleos(t)ide analogs includes the development of lactic acidosis, which can result in fetal death, and has been reported rarely in infants of HIV-infected mothers but not observed in infants born to HBV-infected mothers taking antiviral therapy. Although limited safety data are not available, the use of antiviral agents in highly viremic pregnant women (HBV DNA >200,000 IU/mL) currently is accepted.[30]

An additional indication for the use of antiviral therapy during pregnancy is for treatment of HBsAg+ mothers with acute exacerbation of ALT (>5 × upper limit of normal) due to reactivation of CHB, especially if advanced fibrosis is present. Antiviral treatment can be initiated at any time point during the pregnancy as necessary, and, although use throughout pregnancy in the HIV-infected mothers has not been shown associated with increased rates of fetal birth defects compared with controls, there are few data available regarding its usage during the entire pregnancy for HBV-infected mothers.

MANAGEMENT OF PREGNANT WOMEN WITH HEPATITIS B VIRUS CIRRHOSIS

As discussed previously, for those HBV-infected pregnant women with advanced fibrosis, initiation and or continuation of antiviral therapy is mandatory to prevent episodes of acute exacerbation of HBV and/or decompensated liver disease.[7] Pregnancy in patients with cirrhosis occurs rarely, because advanced liver disease frequently occurs later in life, after the end of reproductive years. Although for pregnant women with compensated cirrhosis there may not be significant increased risks, however for those women with decompensated HBV cirrhosis, unique risks exist throughout their pregnancy and include higher rates of spontaneous abortion, fetal prematurity, life-threatening variceal bleeding, liver failure and decompensation, and postpartum hemorrhage.[33] In addition, should hepatocellular carcinoma develop during pregnancy, the course is much more aggressive, with poor outcomes likely.

These HBV-infected mothers could be on multiple medications, some of which also could have an impact on the outcome of their pregnancy. Therefore, balancing of benefits and risks is of utmost importance in the management of this patient population. As facility with taking care of cirrhotic patients increases and outcomes continue to improve, seeing more pregnant women presenting with cirrhosis is likely. Pregnancy worsens portal hypertensive hemodynamics and the most dreaded complications occur in patients with clinically significant portal hypertension (hepatic venous pressure >10 mm Hg), who can develop esophageal variceal bleeding and liver failure, which carries a mortality rate as high as 50%. Variceal bleeding is most likely to occur in the second trimester or third trimester of pregnancy, when maternal blood flow is maximally expanded and increased fetal growth may cause venacaval compression.

Esophageal band ligation is likely the treatment of choice for HBV cirrhotic mothers with known varices (medium or large varices) that have not bled and for treatment of acute variceal hemorrhage in pregnancy, because it is preferable to the use of chronic nonselective β-blockers in this group of patients.[34] Transjugular intrahepatic portosystemic shunt has been successfully done in pregnant women, although few cases have been reported in the literature.[35] Upper gastrointestinal endoscopy should be performed in all pregnant cirrhotic HBV women, early in the course of pregnancy. Screening for hepatocellular carcinoma with ultrasound is safe and recommended in all cirrhotic patients, including pregnant women. There are few reports of hepatocellular carcinoma developing during pregnancy, and, in most cases, the prognosis is poor, because the tumor growth may be accelerated due to increased estrogen levels as well as the associated gestational immune suppression seen in pregnancy.[36,37]

PERFORMANCE OF OTHER PROCEDURES IN THE PREGNANT WOMEN

When considering invasive procedures during pregnancy and labor course, the risks and benefits must be assessed and discussed with the mother. Procedures likely to be performed on pregnant women include the following:

- Amniocentesis
  - Amniocentesis should be performed with caution in pregnant women with high HBV DNA greater than 10^7 IU/mL.
  - The transmission risk of HBV is low with pregnant women receiving amniocentesis when viral loads are low, and the procedure is performed with a 22-gauge needle under ultrasound guidance.[38,39]
- Cesarean section
  - There is controversy surrounding the preferred delivery for pregnant women with cirrhosis secondary to HBV.
  - ACOG and CDC recommend vaginal as the preferred delivery mode.
  - Cesarean section does not need to be performed to decrease MTCT although a slight decrease in MTCT may occur if cesarean section is completed prior to the onset of labor contractions in pregnant women with high HBV DNA levels.[38,39]
  - This minimal decrease in transmission does not normally outweigh the risks associated with undergoing abdominal surgery.
  - However there is controversy surrounding the preferred delivery for pregnant women with cirrhosis secondary to HBV.
- Internal monitoring with intrauterine pressure catheter or fetal scalp electrodes
  - These intrapartum devices have not well studied in HBV-infected women
  - There is no reported contraindication to their use, but they should be used judiciously.[39]

POSTPARTUM MANAGEMENT OF HEPATITIS B VIRUS–INFECTED MOTHERS AND THEIR INFANTS

The postpartum period for HBV-infected mothers provides its own set of challenges regarding management of both the newborn infant as well as the mother. The most significant obstacle is overcoming the rate of MTCT.[40] Postexposure prophylaxis has become the standard of care and has significantly reduced MTCT of HBV. Hepatitis B immunoglobulin (HBIG) and HBV vaccination should be provided within 12

Table 3			
Doses for immune prophylaxis of infants born of hepatitis B virus–infected mothers			
Infants Weight at Birth	**Hepatitis B Surface Antigen Positive**	**Hepatitis B Surface Antigen Unknown**	**Hepatitis B Surface Antigen Negative**
<2000 g	HBV vaccine <12 h after birth. This is not included in the 3-shot vaccine series. HBIG <12 h after birth	Test HBsAg on admission HBV vaccine <12 h HBIG <12 h unless HBsAg is found negative	Administer HBV vaccination at 1 month of age or on hospital discharge (whichever comes first)
>2000 g	HBV vaccine <12 h after birth HBIG <12 h after birth	Test HBsAg on admission HBV vaccine <12 h HBIG within 7 d or on hospital discharge if HBsAg is positive or remains unknown	HBV vaccination <24 h after birth

Adapted from Lee C, Gong Y, Brok J, et al. Hepatitis B immunisation for newborn infants of hepatitis B surface antigen-positive mothers. Cochrane Database Syst Rev 2006;(2):CD004790; with permission.

hours to 24 hours after birth, regardless of an infant's weight (**Table 3**). Serologic testing for the newborn child should be performed 1 month to 2 months after completion of vaccination series, the ideal testing time 9 months to 12 months of age.[23,41]

It is important to continue close follow-up of HBV-infected mothers in the postpartum period because transaminase flares are common. A transaminase flare is defined as an ALT greater than 3-times to 5-times the upper limit of normal. Approximately 25% of HBsAg+ women may develop ALT flares postpartum, more commonly in women who are HBeAg+.[42,43] It is hypothesized that these flares are due to immune reconstitution and they have been associated with a higher level of HBsAg seroconversion in the postpartum period (up to 17%).[7] Hepatic flares usually are mild and resolve with no sequelae. Associated risk factors have not been well characterized, but studies have shown that risk of hepatic flare is increased when mothers are HBeAg+, have markedly elevated HBV DNA levels, and are of younger age.[44] There are no data to support a specified duration of antiviral therapy, initiated in the third trimester, to decrease the incidence of postpartum HBV flares.[42,43] It is important that HBV-infected mothers establish ongoing care with providers who specialize in the treatment of HBV, to continually monitor the course of HBV infection after pregnancy, to determine if/when initiation of antiviral therapy is appropriate, and to monitor for hepatocellular carcinoma for HBV cirrhotic women.

RECOMMENDATIONS ON BREAST FEEDING

Discontinuation of antiviral therapy should occur soon after delivery for those mothers planning to breastfeed and within 4 weeks to 12 weeks for women who are not breast feeding.[7] The ACOG, CDC, and World Health Organization agree that breastfeeding is safe in infants who have received postexposure prophylaxis for HBV.[3] A large meta-analysis has shown that breastfeeding does not increase the risk of MTCT.[11,45,46] Special care is needed, however, to avoid cracked or dry nipples or mastitis, because these may be a source of MTCT.[47,48] For women who need to continue antiviral therapy, controversy still exists around continuation of breastfeeding. Much of the literature available is focused on the safety of breastfeeding in HIV+ mothers on antiretroviral therapy. The American Association for the Study of Liver Diseases recommends that HBsAg+ mothers should consider breastfeeding, even if on antiviral therapy for HBV, as long as there are no specific contraindications.[7,49,50]

SUMMARY

Postexposure prophylaxis of infants born to HBsAg+ mothers is proven to reduce MTCT. There is still room for improvement in identification of hepatitis B in pregnant women and continued efforts should be made for this purpose. Although large randomized controlled trials are not available, use of antiviral therapy in the third trimester of pregnancy for those highly viremic HBeAg+ mothers seems safe and effective.

REFERENCES

1. Gupta I, Ratho RK. Immunogenicity and safety of two schedules of hepatitis B vaccination during pregnancy. J Obstet Gynaecol Res 2003;29:84–6.
2. Harris AM, Isenhour C, Schillie S, et al. Hepatitis B virus testing and care among pregnant women using commercial claims data, United States, 2011-2014. Infect Dis Obstet Gynecol 2018;2018:4107329.
3. Practice advisory: hepatitis B prevention. The American College of Obstetricians and Gynecologists; 2018. Available at: https://www.acog.org/Clinical-guidance-and-publications. Accessed November 19, 2018.
4. Castillo E, Murphy K, Schalkwyk J. No. 342-Hepatitis B and pregnancy. J Obstet Gynaecol Can 2017;39(3):181–90.
5. Centers for Disease Control and Prevention. Division of Viral Hepatitis. Hepatitis B questions and answers for health professionals. Center for Disease Control and Prevention website; 2018. Available at: https://www.cdc.gov/hepatitis/hbv/hbvfaq.htm. Accessed November 20, 2018.
6. Rac MWF, Sheffield JS. Prevention and management of viral hepatitis in pregnancy. Obstet Gynecol Clin North Am 2014;41(4):573–92.
7. Terrault NA, Lok ASF, Mcmahon BJ, et al. Update on prevention, diagnosis, and treatment of chronic hepatitis B: AASLD 2018 hepatitis B guidance. Hepatology 2018;67(4):1560–99.
8. Livingstone SE, Simonetti JP, Bulkow LR, et al. Clearance of hepatitis B e antigen in patients with chronic hepatitis B and genotypes A, B, C,D, and F. Gastroenterology 2007;133:452–7.
9. Centers for Disease Control and Prevention. Division of viral hepatitis. Surveillance for viral hepatitis-United States 2014. Center for Disease Control and Prevention website; 2016. Available at: https://www.cdc.gov/hepatitis/statistics/2014surveillance/index.htm. Accessed March 23, 2017.
10. Pan CQ, Duan ZP, Bhamidimarri KR, et al. An algorithm for risk assessment and intervention of mother to child transmission of hepatitis B virus. Clin Gastroenterol Hepatol 2012;10:452–9.
11. Yi P, Chen R, Huang Y, et al. Management of mother-to-child transmission of hepatitis B virus: propositions and challenges. J Clin Virol 2016;77:32–9.
12. Yang M, Qin Q, Fang Q, et al. Cesarean section to prevent mother-to-child transmission of hepatitis B virus in China: a meta-analysis. BMC Pregnancy Childbirth 2017;17(1):303.
13. Liu J, Wang J, Qi C, et al. Baseline Hepatitis B virus titer predicts initial postpartum hepatic flare: a multicenter prospective study. J Clin Gastroenterol 2018;52(10):902–7.

14. Chen HL, Wen WH, Chang MH. Management of pregnant women and children: focusing on preventing mother-to-infant transmission. J Infect Dis 2017; 216(suppl_8):S785–91.
15. Navaneethan U, Al Mohajer M, Shata MT. Hepatitis B and pregnancy: understanding the pathogenesis. Liver Int 2008;28(9):1190–9.
16. Chamroonkul N, Piratvisuth T. Hepatitis B during pregnancy in endemic areas: screening, treatment, and prevention of mother-to-child transmission. Paediatr Drugs 2017;19(3):173–81.
17. Rijhsinghani AG, Thompson K, Bhatia SK, et al. Estrogen blocks early t cell development in the thymus. Am J Reprod Immunol 1996;36(5):269–77.
18. Han YT, Sun C, Liu CX, et al. Clinical features and outcome of acute hepatitis B in pregnancy. BMC Infect Dis 2014;14:368.
19. Tillman HL, Zachou k, Dalekos GN. Management of severe acute to fulminant hepatitis B: to treat or not to treat or when to treat? Liver Int 2012;32(4):544–53.
20. Tan J, Liu X, Mao X, et al. HBsAg positivity during pregnancy and adverse maternal outcomes: a retrospective cohort analysis. J Viral Hepat 2016;23(10): 812–9.
21. Sirilert S, Traisrisilp K, Sirivatanapa P, et al. Pregnancy outcomes among chronic carriers of hepatitis B virus. Int J Gynaecol Obstet 2014;126(2):106–10.
22. Liu J, Zhang S, Liu M, et al. Maternal pre-pregnancy infection with hepatitis B virus and the risk of preterm birth: a population-based cohort study. Lancet Glob Health 2017;5(6):e624–32.
23. Whittaker G, Herrera JL. Hepatitis B in pregnancy. South Med J 2014;107(3): 195–200.
24. Tenney DJ, Rose RE, Baldick CJ, et al. Long-term monitoring shows hepatitis B resistance to entecavir in nucleoside-naïve patients is rare through 5 years of therapy. Hepatology 2009;49(5):1503–14.
25. Hadziyannis SJ, Tassopoulos NC, Heathcote EJ, et al. Long-term therapy with adefovir dipovoxil for HBeAg- chronic hepatitis B for up to 5 years. Gastroenterology 2006;131(6):1743–51.
26. Chang TT, Liau YF, Wu SS, et al. Long term entecavir therapy results in reversal of fibrosis/cirrhosis in patients with chronic hepatitis B. Hepatology 2010;52(3): 886–93.
27. Xu WM, Cui YT, Wang L, et al. Lamivudine in late pregnancy to prevent perinatal transmission of hepatitis B virus infection: a multicenter, randomized, double-blind, placebo-controlled study. J Viral Hepat 2009;16(2):94–103.
28. Pan CQ, Han GR, Jiang HX, et al. Telbivudine prevents vertical transmission from HBeAg-positive women with chronic hepatitis B. Clin Gastroenterol Hepatol 2012; 10(5):520–6.
29. Pan CQ, Lee HM. Antiviral therapy for chronic hepatitis B in pregnancy. Semin Liver Dis 2013;33(2):138–46.
30. Brown RS Jr, McMahon BJ, Lok AS, et al. Antiviral therapy in chronic hepatitis B viral infection during pregnancy: a systemic review and meta-analysis. Hepatology 2016;63(1):319–33.
31. Jonas M. Hepatitis B and pregnancy: an underestimated issue. Liver Int 2009; 29(s1):133–9.
32. Liu M, Cai H, Yi W. Safety of telbivudine treatment for chronic hepatitis B for the entire pregnancy. J Viral Hepat 2013;20(Suppl 1):65-70.
33. Tan J, Surti B, Saab S. Pregnancy and cirrhosis. Liver Transpl 2008;14(8): 1081–91.

34. Starkel P, Horsmans Y, Geubel A. Endoscopic band ligation: a safe technique to control bleeding esophageal varices in pregnancy. Gastrointest Endosc 1998; 48(2):212–4.

35. Lodato F, Cappelli A, Montagnani M, et al. Transjugular intrahepatic portosystemicshunt: a case report of rescue management of unrestrainable variceal bleeding in a pregnant woman. Dig Liver Dis 2008;40:387–90.

36. Lau WY, Leung WT, Ho S, et al. Hepatocellular carcinoma during pregnancy and its comparison with other pregnancy-associated malignancies. Cancer 1995; 75(11):2669–76.

37. Alverez de la Rosa M, Nicolás-Pérez D, Muñiz-Montes JR, et al. Evolution and management of a hepatocellular carcinoma during pregnancy. J Obstet Gynaecol Res 2006;32(4):437–9.

38. Dionne-Odom J, Tita ATN, Silverman NS. Hepatitis B in pregnancy: screening, treatment, and prevention of vertical transmission. Am J Obstet Gynecol 2016; 214(1):6–14.

39. Dunkelberg JC, Berkley EMF, Thiel KW, et al. Hepatitis B and C in pregnancy: a review and recommendations for care. J Perinatol 2014;34(12):882–91.

40. Zhang L, Gui X, Wang B, et al. A study of immunoprophylaxis failure and risk factors of hepatitis B virus mother-to-infant transmission. Eur J Pediatr 2014;173(9): 1161–8.

41. Committee on Infectious Diseases. Committee on Fetus and Newborn. Elimination of perinatal hepatitis B: providing the first vaccine dose within 24 hours of birth. Pediatrics 2017;140(3):1–5.

42. Chang CY, Aziz N, Poongkunran M, et al. Serum aminotransferase flares in pregnant and postpartum women with current or prior treatment for chronic hepatitis B. J Clin Gastroenterol 2018;52(3):255–61.

43. Chang ML, Liaw YF. Hepatitis B flares in chronic hepatitis B: pathogenesis, natural course, and management. J Hepatol 2014;61(6):1407–17.

44. Schillie S, Walker T, Veselsky S, et al. Outcomes of infants born to women infected with hepatitis B. Pediatrics 2015;135(5):1141–7.

45. Zheng Y, Lu Y, Ye Q, et al. Should chronic hepatitis B mothers breastfeed? A meta analysis. BMC Public Health 2011;11:502.

46. Shi Z, Yang Y, Wang H, et al. Breastfeeding of newborns by mothers carrying hepatitis B virus; a meta analysis and systemic review. Arch Pediatr Adolesc Med 2011;165(9):837–46.

47. Ayoub W, Cohen E. Hepatitis B management in the pregnant patient: an update. J Clin Transl Hepatol 2016;4(3):241–7.

48. Breastfeeding: hepatitis B or C infections. Center for Disease Control and Prevention website; 2018. Available at: https://www.cdc.gov/breastfeeding/breast feeding-special-circumstances/maternal-or-infant-illnesses/hepatitis.html. Accessed November 20, 2018.

49. Petrova M, Kamburov V. Breastfeeding and chronic HBV infection: clinical and social implications. World J Gastroenterol 2010;16(40):5042–6.

50. Ehrhardt S, Xie C, Guo N, et al. Breastfeeding while taking lamivudine or tenofovir disoproxil fumarate: a review of the evidence. Clin Infect Dis 2015;60(2):275–8.

HBV/HCV Coinfection in the Era of HCV-DAAs

Rashed Abdelaal, BS[a,b], Beshoy Yanny, MD[a,b,c], Mohamed El Kabany, MD[a,b,c],*

KEYWORDS

- Hepatitis B and C coinfection • Sustained viral response • Hepatitis B reactivation

KEY POINTS

- The interaction between HBV and HCV in coinfected individuals and the mechanism of HBV reactivation remain poorly understood.
- Because of lack of large multicenter studies, the data regarding screening, risk factors for coinfection, and treatment remain scattered and conflicting.
- Based on the most recent review of the literature, patients undergoing HCV treatment with newly developed DAAs should undergo screening for hepatitis B and receive careful monitoring or prophylaxis treatment, specially individuals with HBsAg positivity or HBV DNA positivity.
- More studies are needed to evaluate the possibility of genotype interaction, different types of DAAs, and geographic distribution given that many of the previously described cases were in Chinese, Japanese, and US studies.
- More prospective multicenter studies are needed to further elucidate the duration of prophylaxis treatment after discontinuation of DAA therapy.

INTRODUCTION

Coinfection with hepatitis B virus (HBV) and hepatitis C virus (HCV) is not uncommon. Epidemiologic studies suggest that approximately 10% to 15% of patients with hepatitis C infection are coinfected with HBV.[1,2] Because of the lack of large-scale studies, these numbers may underestimate the true number of patients coinfected

Role in the Study: Study concept and design (M.E. Kabany, R. Abdelaal); acquisition of data (R. Abdelaal); analysis and interpretation of data (M.E. Kabany, R. Abdelaal, B. Yanny); drafting of the article (R. Abdelaal, B. Yanny, M.E. Kabany); critical revision of the article for important intellectual content (M.E. Kabany, B. Yanny); statistical analysis (B. Yanny, M.E. Kabany); administrative, technical, or material support; study supervision (M.E. Kabany, B. Yanny).
The authors have nothing to disclose.
[a] Department of Surgery, University of California at Los Angeles, 200 Medical Plaza, Suite 214, Los Angeles, CA 90095, USA; [b] Department of Transplant Hepatology, University of California at Los Angeles, Los Angeles, CA, USA; [c] Department of Medicine, University of California at Los Angeles, Los Angeles, CA, USA
* Corresponding author. University of California Los Angeles, 200 Medical Plaza, Suite 214, Los Angeles, CA 90095.
E-mail address: melkabany@mednet.ucla.edu

with HCV/HBV. Coinfection has been reported up to 30% of cases in certain geographic areas. Patients who are coinfected with HCV/HBV have faster progression to cirrhosis and complications of liver disease compared with monoinfected patients.[1] The host's immune system plays an important role in controlling viral replication for both viruses, usually leading to predominance of one over the other. Hepatitis C is usually more predominant in coinfected individuals. Immunosuppression of the host or eradication of hepatitis C can change this paradigm, causing hepatitis B reactivation.[3-5] Hepatitis B reactivation can have a wide clinical spectrum from minimal hepatitis up to devastating acute or acute on chronic liver failure. Hepatitis B reactivation has been reported recently in patients being treated with direct-acting antiviral (DAA) therapy for HCV.[1-8] The United States Food and Drug Administration (FDA) issued a warning to that extent in October 2016 as a result of cases of hepatitis B reactivation.[8] This raised the awareness of practitioners to check for active or occult HBV coinfection in patients being treated for hepatitis C and patients undergoing immunosuppression therapy.

Accordingly, patients coinfected HBV/HCV have heterogeneous clinical manifestations. There is either HCV predominance, with high HCV RNA levels and low HBV DNA levels, or rarely HBV predominance, with high HBV DNA levels and low HCV RNA levels. This highlights the importance of practitioner awareness to screen high-risk populations and start treatment or prophylaxis appropriately. because of the lack of large multicenter studies, the data regarding screening, risk factors for coinfection, and treatment remain scattered and conflicting. This review discusses viral interactions between HCV and HBV, risk factors for coinfection, screening, mechanism, and risk of hepatitis B reactivation in patients undergoing HCV treatment with DAAs, treatment of HCV/HBV coinfection, prevention of reactivation, and major society guidelines for screening and prevention.

VIRAL INTERACTIONS BETWEEN HEPATITIS C VIRUS AND HEPATITIS B VIRUS

Hepatitis C is usually the dominant infection in individuals chronically infected with hepatitis B and C.[9-13] On rare occasions, HBV dominates; this is believed to be secondary to the time of infection. This relationship between the 2 viruses has previously been explained by 3 theories. The interjection between the 2 viruses and how one can flare after eradication of the other is still poorly understood. However, previously accepted explanations remarked on (1) direct inhibition of HCV to HBV replication; (2) an increase in the available replication space after eradication of one virus; (3) loss of host immune responses to one of the viruses, usually hepatitis B, or production of an immune inhibitory signal of one virus to improve replication over the other.[12]

First, direct inhibition of HCV to HBV viral replication is discussed. In a human hepatocyte, HCV core protein was shown to interfere with HBV gene expression and replication by directly interacting with HBV proteins. More recently, it has been shown that in a mouse model, coexpression of HCV core protein did not interfere with HBV replication or gene expression. The limitation of these models is that overexpression of HCV proteins rather than replicating virus was used.[12-16] A more recent study demonstrated that both viruses can replicate in the same hepatocyte in vitro. Similarly, fluorescent in situ hybridization on patient samples recently showed that HCV and HBV can infect the same hepatocyte at similar replication rates.[12] Thus, the more recent literature does not support direct viral interference between HBV and HCV.

Second, we review how an increase in the available replication space after eradication of one virus affects the replication of the other virus. Hepatitis B generally reactivates after eradication of hepatitis C. It is possible that fast eradication of hepatitis C produces an uninhibited space for HBV to replicate in the liver cell. Previous evidence suggests that HBV replication space is not limited in HBV/HCV coinfection. In chronic HCV, 21%–45% of hepatocytes contained HCV RNA. Similarly, in chronic HBV, 21%–27% of hepatocytes were found to have covalently closed circular DNA or to be infected with HBV.[8,12–18] This means that both viruses occupy a minority of hepatocytes, and there are ample available hepatocytes to support coinfection. Previous evidence also shows that 1 hepatocyte is capable of accommodating both viruses, including successful replication. Lastly, the turnover rate of HCV-infected hepatocytes is believed to be short even in the absence of therapy (estimated at between 4 and 29 days), so enough new hepatocytes that are susceptible to infection should be available at any given time.[12] This makes the theory of increased space of replication after eradication of 1 virus possible but unlikely overall.

Third, hepatitis C can induce an interferon-abundant state that inhibits HBV replication versus directly activating the host lymphocytes against HBV.[12–16] HCV infection stimulates production of interferon-stimulated genes (ISGs) in the liver, which are highly expressed during chronic infection. Many ISGs have antiviral effects. These high intrahepatic ISGs are insufficient to suppress HCV replication and may suppress HBV replication in some cases. Circulating interferon gamma-induced protein 10 (IP-10), an intrahepatic ISG that is strongly associated with intrahepatic ISG expression, was significantly higher in patients coinfected with HBV/HCV when HCV was the dominant virus and correlated with HCV RNA levels.[8,12] In vitro studies are scarce in this area; however, 1 study supports the theory that in the chronically HCV-infected liver, the HCV-induced interferon (IFN)-α/β response creates an antiviral state that limits both the initiation and the replication of HBV in cells whose type I interferon-stimulated gene expression profile does not preclude HBV infection.[8,12–25] Direct stimulation by HCV to host lymphocytes was previously accepted as a possible mechanism for limiting HBV replication; however, there are not enough data to support this theory and hence it is highly unlikely.

RISK FACTORS FOR COINFECTION

Modes of transmission of HCV and HBV are similar and coinfection is not unlikely. Both hepatitis B and C are transmitted by way of contact with infected bodily fluids or blood. Well-known modes of transmission include sharing needles with infected blood during intravenous drug use or for medications such as insulin in the same household of an infected individual, tattoos with unclean equipment, blood transfusions before 1992, unprotected sexual intercourse with an infected individual, work-related exposure to infected fluids or blood, babies born to infected mothers during the birthing process, and in countries that lack sanitation equipment in the medical field due to shortage of resources with re-use of dental and medical equipment in endemic countries.[25–27] Patients in these groups should be considered high-risk individuals and should be screened for coinfection.

SCREENING

There are no current guidelines for screening patients for coinfection with HCV/HBV. Previous reports and expert opinion recommendations do exist. Generally, individuals with a first episode of acute hepatitis should be screened for all viral causes, including hepatitis B and C. Some patients may be inoculated with both viruses at once and present with acute hepatitis as a result of simultaneous coinfection. Patients with known chronic hepatitis B or C infection who present with a new acute hepatitis picture should also be screened, especially those who continue to exhibit high-risk behavior such as injecting drugs or having multiple sex partners. Patients who are undergoing hepatitis C treatment should also be screened for hepatitis B before treatment (see the section on major society guidelines).

HEPATITIS B REACTIVATION

Hepatitis B reactivation has been commonly described in patients exposed to HBV who are undergoing immunosuppressive and cytotoxic therapy.[3–5] HBV reactivation is characterized by an increase in serum HBV DNA in patients with previously low or undetected serum HBV DNA, because of inactive or resolved HBV infection.[6,7,28] Reactivation is usually followed by the reappearance of HBV activity (HBV DNA detectability or increase >1 log) or a flare of hepatitis in previously minimal or inactive disease characterized by an increase in serum alanine aminotransferase level 3 to 10 times the upper level of normal.[6,7,9] Antiviral prophylaxis is recommended in patients considered at high risk for HBV reactivation.[4,5] Hepatitis B reactivation has also been described in patients who undergoing treatment with the earlier interferon-based hepatitis C regimens.[1] With the emergence of HBV reactivation reported in coinfected patients undergoing DAA therapy, the need for prophylactic antiviral therapy to prevent HBV reactivation has more recently become a concern for these patients.

Patients at the highest risk for reactivation are those with hepatitis B surface antigen (HBsAg) and core antibody (HBcAb) positivity. It is recommended that patients in this cohort undergo prophylaxis with hepatitis B antiviral therapy. Patients undergoing anti-CD20 antibody therapy (eg, rituximab) or undergoing stem cell transplantation, have a high risk for reactivation and must be on prophylaxis with antiviral therapy during and for a longer duration after discontinuation of the immunosuppressive medications (for specifics on duration and drug of choice for prophylaxis, see the section on major society guidelines). Patients with HBcAb-positive and HBsAg-negative serology are at a lower risk for reactivation, however because of poor outcomes with reactivation, prophylaxis is still indicated in patients undergoing anti-CD-20 therapy. In this lower risk population undergoing immunosuppressive or cytotoxic therapy other than anti-CD-20 agents, on-demand antiviral therapy may be an option if reactivation occurs during treatment. The risk of HBV reactivation during DAA treatment remains unclear. Some studies show the risk of reactivation of HBV is about 1% to 2% of patients treated with DAAs for hepatitis C with concurrent HBV serologic markers, whereas other studies show no concern for reactivation.[28] Nevertheless, the FDA issued a black-boxed warning in 2016 indicating the risk of HBV reactivation, leading to increased awareness and better monitoring of individuals coinfected with HCV/HBV or those previously exposed to HBV with serologies consistent with HBcAb positivity.

HEPATITIS B REACTIVATION IN PATIENTS UNDERGOING HEPATITIS C VIRUS TREATMENT WITH DIRECT-ACTING ANTIVIRALS

Interaction between hepatitis B and C as described here is altered by treatment of HCV. The introduction of DAA therapy changed the paradigm for hepatitis C treatment. DAAs have proven to be safe and effective thus far. Recent case reports and studies suggest a risk of HBV reactivation during treatment of HCV with the DAA drug class (**Table 1**). Prospective and retrospective cohort studies looking at the risk of HBV reactivation, in general, are listed in **Table 2**. In these studies, HBV reactivation occurred in patients with "occult" HBV (HBcAb positivity, HBsAg negativity) and patients who were actively infected with HBsAg positive and have a detectable viral load.[8,27–36]

Table 1
Previously reported hepatitis B reactivation case reports

Reference	Gender	Age	HIV Coinfection	HCV Genotype	Previous Treatment	DAA Regimen	Profile Before DAAs	HBV DNA (IU/mL) Before/After DAAs
Collins et al,[23] 2015	M	55	No	1a	IFN/ribavirin	Sofosbuvir/simeprevir	Inactive carrier	2300/22 million
Collins et al,[23] 2015	M	57	No	1a	IFN/ribavirin	Sofosbuvir/simeprevir	Occult infection	20/11,255
Ende et al,[22] 2015	F	59	No	1b	IFN/ribavirin	Sofosbuvir/simeprevir/ribavirin	Resolved infection	Undetectable/29 million
Takayama et al,[19] 2016	M	69	No	1b	No treatment	Daclatasvir/asunaprevir	Inactive carrier	310/10 million
De Monte et al,[21] 2016	M	53	Yes	4d	IFN/ribavirin	Sofosbuvir/ledipasvir	Resolved infection	Undetectable/960 million
Hayashi et al,[20] 2016	F	83	No	1b	No treatment	Daclatasvir/asunaprevir	Unclear	Undetectable/1,000,000
Madonia et al,[24] 2016	F	62	No	2	No treatment	Sofosbuvir/ribavirin	Resolved infection	Undetectable/2,080,000

Abbreviations: F, female; M, male.

Table 2
The risk of hepatitis B reactivation

Reference	Study Type	Conclusion and Recommendations	Number and Characteristics of Patients Reported
Loggi et al,[25] 2017	Retrospective cohort	No evidence of reactivation	44 patients HBcAb-positive
Mücke et al,[26] 2017	Retrospective cohort	No evidence of reactivation in patients treated with various DAAs	272 patients HBcAb-positive (HBsAg-positive, n = 9; HBsAg-negative, n = 263)
Ogawa et al,[27] 2017	Retrospective cohort	No evidence of reactivation in patients treated with various DAAs	63 patients with resolved HBV infection
Belperio et al,[29] 2017	Retrospective cohort	Reactivation of varying severity, even in the setting of isolated HBcAb	62,290 VA patients treated with DAAs (allcomers). 0.7% (377 patients) HBsAg-positive. No individual chart review performed
Yeh et al,[30] 2017	Retrospective cohort	There was minimal impact of anti-HBc seropositivity on HCV efficacy and safety. For patients with current HBV infection, the risk of HBV reactivation was present and monitoring the HBV DNA level during therapy is warranted	64 patients, 57 HBcAb-positive and 7 patients HBsAg-positive
Yanny et al,[34] 2018	Retrospective cohort	No reactivation was noted in patients treated with ledipasvir-sofosbuvir	283 patients, a total of 45% of patients were HBcAb-positive and HBsAg-negative
Tamori et al,[8] 2018	Retrospective cohort	Minimal risk of reactivation in patients with isolated HBcAb	Among 765 patients, there was 0.1% risk of reactivation, which was not clinically significant
Liu et al,[35] 2018	Prospective cohort	The combination of ledipasvir and sofosbuvir for 12 wk produced a sustained virologic response in 100% of patients with HCV infection who were coinfected with HBV. Most patients had an increased level of HBV DNA not associated with signs or symptoms	111 patients did not have clinically significant reactivation
Butt et al,[36] 2018	Retrospective cohort	HBV reactivation is relatively uncommon after DAA therapy and not higher than among those treated with a PEG/RBV regimen. The small numbers of persons treated with a DAA regimen who do develop HBV reactivation have a shortened survival compared with those without HBV reactivation	>23,000 patients retrospectively reported no significant reactivation

Abbreviation: PEG/RBV, peginterferon plus ribavirin.

Most studies to date suggest minimal risk for HBV reactivation with DAA treatment versus a nonclinically significant risk. Most of the studies looking at the risk of reactivation are retrospective cohort studies. Previous reactivations have been reported mainly in retrospective case reports or case series. The largest study to date was a prospective study by Wang and colleagues in a Chinese population.[16,28–34] Data are scarce for areas with diverse populations such as large metropolitan areas. This also poses the question of possible genetic predisposition or possibly interactions between only certain HCV/HBV genotypes. It is also unclear whether the risk for reactivation is linked to a certain DAA or HCV genotype because subgroup analyses are lacking in recent studies. **Table 1** shows the major studies published thus far with the risk of reactivation.[34]

Overall, the risk of HBV reactivation with DAA therapy in patients with isolated HBcAb positivity seems to be a rare event. The risk of a flare in patients with HBsAg positivity and low-titer positive polymerase chain reaction remains unclear.[34] Patients coinfected with hepatitis B and C should not be denied DAA therapy, however they should be closely monitored as described in the guidelines (see next section). Generally, HBV reactivation can be devastating and life threatening in patients receiving immune suppression or chemotherapy. HBV reactivation with DAA use can present clinically without any symptoms and has a silent course, but could present as severe as fulminant liver failure requiring liver transplantation. Existing data are not sufficient to support preemptive therapy in all patients previously exposed to or actively infected with HBV undergoing DAA therapy.[25–27,29] Current evidence is also not sufficient to support not checking HBV status while on DAA therapy. More studies are needed to further evaluate the risk of HBV reactivation in different patient demographics, the influence of both HBV and HCV genotypes, the mechanism of HBV reactivation, and the association with different regimens of DAA.

MAJOR SOCIETY GUIDELINES FOR HEPATITIS B VIRUS REACTIVATION: SCREENING, TREATMENT, AND PREVENTION

The American Association for the Study of Liver Diseases (AASLD) suggests that all patients with HCV who are about to initiate DAA therapy should be assessed for HBV coinfection by checking the presence of HBsAg, anti-HBs, and anti-HBc. In addition, patients with positive HBsAg should be tested for HBV DNA viral load before the initiation of DAA therapy.[27–34] For patients who meet the criteria for HBV treatment because of active HBV infection, HBV treatment should be administered before or during the HCV treatment. Patients with low or undetectable HBV DNA levels should be monitored at regular intervals (usually no more than once every 4 weeks) for HBV reactivation, and patients with HBV DNA levels that meet treatment criteria should begin HBV therapy. For those patients with positive anti-HBc or anti-HBs and anti-HBc, there are no sufficient recommendations for HBV therapy; however, if patients present with increased liver enzyme levels during or after DAA therapy, the possibility of HBV reactivation should be excluded. European Association for the Study of the Liver (EASL) guidelines suggest that patients should be tested for HBs antigen, anti-HBc, and anti-HBs antibodies before the initiation of DAA therapy. If HBs antigen is present, or if HBV DNA is detectable in HBs antigen-negative, anti-HBc antibody-positive patients ("occult" hepatitis B), then concurrent HBV therapy is indicated. However, more studies are needed to elucidate the cost effectiveness and safety of long-term use versus discontinuation of hepatitis B therapy initiated during DAA treatment versus its discontinuation after HCV cure.[27–36] Starting HBV therapy during DAA treatment poses the question whether discontinuation is appropriate after HCV cure in patients

Table 3
HBV/HCV coinfection: AASLD and EASL recommendations

Criteria	AASLD	EASL
Test HCV patients for HBsAg	Yes	Yes
HCV patients with positive HBsAg	• At risk of flares during HCV DAA therapy • During DAA therapy, monitor HBV DNA and ALT every 4–8 weeks and for 3 months post treatment	• Monitor closely • Recommend concomitant nucleos(t)ide analogue prophylaxis until week 12 post DAA therapy
HCV patients with negative HBsAg and anti-HBc positive	• At low risk of flares during HCV DAA therapy • During DAA therapy: monitor ALT at baseline, at end of treatment, and during follow-up • If ALT increases or does not normalize during treatment or post treatment then monitor HBV DNA and HBsAg	• Monitor closely • Test for HBV reactivation in case of increased level of ALT
HBV treatment	• Based on HBV-DNA and ALT levels • Treat per AASLD guidelines	• Treat per AASLD guidelines

Abbreviation: ALT, alanine aminotransferase.
Data from Terrault N, Lok ASF, McMahon BJ, et al. Update on prevention, diagnosis and treatment of chronic hepatitis B: AASLD 2018 hepatitis B guidance. Hepatology 2018;67(4):1560–99; EASL 2017 clinical practice guidelines on the management of hepatitis B virus infection. J Hepatol 2017;67:370–98.

who otherwise would only need to be monitored periodically.[34] **Table 3** summarizes key points from each of the two major societies: AASLD and EASL.

SUMMARY

The interaction between HBV and HCV in coinfected individuals and the mechanism of HBV reactivation remain poorly understood. Because of the lack of large multicenter studies, the data regarding screening, risk factors for coinfection, and treatment remain scattered and conflicting. Based on the most recent review of the literature, patients undergoing HCV treatment with newly developed DAAs should undergo screening for hepatitis B and receive careful monitoring or prophylaxis treatment, specially individuals with HBsAg or HBV DNA positivity. More studies are needed to evaluate the possibility of genotype interaction, different types of DAAs, and geographic distribution given that many of the cases described previously were in Chinese and Japanese studies. More prospective multicenter studies are also needed to further elucidate the duration of prophylaxis treatment after discontinuation of DAA therapy.

REFERENCES

1. Kawagishi N, Suda G, Onozawa M, et al. Comparing the risk of hepatitis B virus reactivation between direct-acting antiviral therapies and interferon-based therapies for hepatitis C. J Viral Hepat 2017;24(12):1098–106.
2. Serper M, Forde KA, Kaplan DE. Rare clinically significant hepatic events and hepatitis B reactivation occur more frequently following rather than during direct-acting antiviral therapy for chronic hepatitis C: data from a national US cohort. J Viral Hepat 2017;25(2):187–97.

3. Gupta S, Govindarajan S, Fong TL, et al. Spontaneous reactivation in chronic hepatitis B: patterns and natural history. J Clin Gastroenterol 1990;12:562.
4. Reddy KR, Beavers KL, Hammond SP, et al. American Gastroenterological Association Institute guideline on the prevention and treatment of hepatitis B virus reactivation during immunosuppressive drug therapy. Gastroenterology 2015; 148:215.
5. Lok AS, McMahon BJ. Chronic hepatitis B: update 2009. Hepatology 2009; 50:661.
6. Bessone F, Dirchwolf M. Management of hepatitis B reactivation in immunosuppressed patients: an update on current recommendations. World J Hepatol 2016;8:385–94.
7. Hoofnagle JH. Reactivation of hepatitis B. Hepatology 2009;49:S156–65.
8. Tamori A, Abiru S, Enomoto H, et al. Low incidence of hepatitis B virus reactivation and subsequent hepatitis in patients with chronic hepatitis C receiving direct-acting antiviral therapy. J Viral Hepat 2018;25(5):608–11.
9. Huang YW, Chung RT. Management of hepatitis B reactivation in patients receiving cancer chemotherapy. Therap Adv Gastroenterol 2012;5:359–70.
10. Bersoff-Matcha SJ, Cao K, Jason M, et al. Hepatitis B virus reactivation associated with direct-acting antiviral therapy for chronic hepatitis C virus: a review of cases reported to the U.S. Food and drug administration adverse event reporting system. Ann Intern Med 2017;166:792–8.
11. Konstantinou D, Deutsch M. The spectrum of HBV/HCV coinfection: epidemiology, clinical characteristics, viral interactions and management. Ann Gastroenterol 2015;28:221–8.
12. Balagopal A, Thio CL. Editorial commentary: another call to cure hepatitis B. Clin Infect Dis 2015;61(8):1307–9.
13. Coffin CS, Mulrooney-Cousins PM, Lee SS, et al. Profound suppression of chronic hepatitis C following superinfection with hepatitis B virus. Liver Int 2007;27:722–6.
14. Dai CY, Yu ML, Chuang WL, et al. Influence of hepatitis C virus on the profiles of patients with chronic hepatitis B virus infection. J Gastroenterol Hepatol 2001;16: 636–40.
15. Hamzaoui L, El Bouchtili S, Siai K, et al. Hepatitis B virus and hepatitis C virus coinfection: a therapeutic challenge. Clin Res Hepatol Gastroenterol 2013;37: e16–20.
16. Potthoff A, Wedemeyer H, Boecher WO, et al. The HEP-NET B/C co-infection trial: a prospective multicenter study to investigate the efficacy of pegylated interferon-alpha2b and ribavirin in patients with HBV/HCV co-infection. J Hepatol 2008;49:688–94.
17. Nakamura M, Kanda T, Nakamoto S, et al. Reappearance of serum hepatitis B viral DNA in patients with hepatitis B surface antigen seroclearance. Hepatology 2015;62:1329.
18. Wang C, Ji D, Chen J, et al. Hepatitis due to reactivation of hepatitis B virus in endemic areas among patients with hepatitis C treated with direct-acting antiviral agents. Clin Gastroenterol Hepatol 2016;5:30370–6.
19. Takayama H, Sato T, Ikeda F, et al. Reactivation of hepatitis B virus during interferon-free therapy with daclatasvir and asunaprevir in patient with hepatitis B virus/hepatitis C virus co-infection. Hepatol Res 2016;46:489–91.
20. Hayashi K, Ishigami M, Ishizu Y, et al. A case of acute hepatitis B in a chronic hepatitis C patient after daclatasvir and asunaprevir combination therapy: hepatitis B virus reactivation or acute self-limited hepatitis. Clin J Gastroenterol 2016;9: 252–6.

21. De Monte A, Courjon J, Anty R, et al. Direct-acting antiviral treatment in adults infected with hepatitis C virus: reactivation of hepatitis B virus coinfection as a further challenge. J Clin Virol 2016;78:27–30.

22. Ende AR, Kim NH, Yeh MM, et al. Fulminant hepatitis B reactivation leading to liver transplantation in a patient with chronic hepatitis C treated with simeprevir and sofosbuvir: a case report. J Med Case Rep 2015;9:164.

23. Collins JM, Raphael KL, Terry C, et al. Hepatitis B virus reactivation during successful treatment of hepatitis C virus with sofosbuvir and simeprevir. Clin Infect Dis 2015;61:1304–6.

24. Madonia S, Orlando E, Madonia G, et al. HCV/HBV coinfection: the dark side of DAAs treatment. Liver Int 2016;37(7):1086–7.

25. Loggi E, Gitto S, Galli S, et al. Hepatitis B virus reactivation among hepatitis C patients treated with direct-acting antiviral therapies in routine clinical practice. J Clin Virol 2017;93:66–70.

26. Mücke VT, Mücke MM, Peiffer KH, et al. No evidence of hepatitis B virus reactivation in patients with resolved infection treated with direct-acting antivirals for hepatitis C in a large real-world cohort. Aliment 25. Pharmacol Ther 2017;46(4):432–9.

27. Ogawa E, Furusyo N, Murata M, et al. Potential risk of HBV reactivation in patients with resolved HBV infection undergoing direct-acting antiviral treatment for HCV. Liver Int 2017;38(1):76–83.

28. Terrault NA, Bzowej NH, Chang K-M, et al. AASLD guidelines for treatment of chronic hepatitis B. Hepatology 2016;63:261–83.

29. Belperio PS, Shahoumian TA, Mole LA, et al. Evaluation of hepatitis B reactivation among 62,920 veterans treated with oral hepatitis C antivirals. Hepatology 2017;66(1):27–36.

30. Yeh ML, Huang CF, Hsieh MH, et al. Reactivation of hepatitis B in patients of chronic hepatitis C with hepatitis B virus infection treated with direct acting antivirals. J Gastroenterol Hepatol 2017;32(10):1754–62.

31. Lin ZH, Xin YN, Dong QJ, et al. Performance of the aspartate aminotransferase-to-platelet ratio index for the staging of hepatitis C-related fibrosis: an updated meta-analysis. Hepatology 2011;53:726–36.

32. AASLD-IDSA recommendations for testing, managing, and treating adults infected with hepatitis C virus. Hepatology 2015;62:932–54.

33. Aggeletopoulou I, Konstantakis C, Manolakopoulos S, et al. Risk of hepatitis B reactivation in patients treated with direct-acting antivirals for hepatitis C. World J Gastroenterol 2017;23(24):4317–23.

34. Yanny BT, Latt NL, Saab S, et al. Risk of hepatitis B virus reactivation among patients treated with ledipasvir-sofosbuvir for hepatitis C virus infection. J Clin Gastroenterol 2018;52(10):908–12.

35. Liu CJ, Chuang WL, Sheen IS, et al. Efficacy of ledipasvir and sofosbuvir treatment of HCV infection in patients coinfected with HBV. Gastroenterology 2018;154(4):989–97.

36. Butt AA, Yan P, Shaikh OS, et al. Hepatitis B reactivation and outcomes in persons treated with directly acting antiviral agents against hepatitis C virus: results from ERCHIVES. Aliment Pharmacol Ther 2018;47(3):412–20.

Antiretroviral Effects on HBV/HIV Co-infection and the Natural History of Liver Disease

David L. Wyles, MD[a,b],*

KEYWORDS

- HIV • HBV • Antiretrovirals • Natural history • HAART

KEY POINTS

- Hepatitis B virus (HBV) coinfection is prevalent (~10%) in those with human immunodeficiency virus (HIV) infection.
- Many HIV antiretrovirals also possess potent anti-HBV activity.
- HBV coinfection increases all cause and liver-related mortality in persons with HBV-HIV coinfection.
- HBV active antiretroviral therapy is associated with high rates of HBV DNA suppression.
- Long-term studies have not definitively shown decreased rates liver-related outcomes related to HBV treatment in HBV-HIV–infected persons.

The presence of chronic hepatitis B virus (HBV) infection in persons living with human immunodeficiency virus (PLWH) is a key consideration in selecting and maintaining antiretroviral therapy (ART). Fortunately, modern ART regimens commonly include agents with potent and durable anti-HBV activity. The benefits of long-term HBV suppression in the setting of HIV coinfection, in which a more aggressive HBV disease course is seen, are just now being appreciated. In the future, persons with HBV-HIV coinfection will be a key population in which to evaluate the safety and efficacy of novel HBV therapeutics.

EPIDEMIOLOGY OF HEPATITIS B VIRUS IN THOSE WITH HUMAN IMMUNODEFICIENCY VIRUS

Several factors contribute to the increased prevalence of chronic HBV (CHB) infection in persons with HIV infection. Overlapping transmission risks, including percutaneous

Disclosures: Research funds paid to author's institution from Gilead Sciences.
[a] Division of Infectious Diseases, Denver Health Medical Center, 601 Broadway Street, MC 4000, Denver, CO 80204, USA; [b] Division of Infectious Diseases, University of Colorado School of Medicine, Aurora, CO, USA
* 601 Broadway Street, MC 4000, Denver, CO 80204, USA.
E-mail address: David.Wyles@dhha.org

exposures to contaminated blood or body fluid (eg, injection drug use or unsafe medical practices) and high-risk sexual exposures, are most common for HIV and may also lead to HBV acquisition later in life. Globally, vertical transmission was a major source of current prevalent HBV infections. However, outside of areas endemic for HBV infection, vertical transmission is unlikely to play a major role in HIV-HBV coinfection. In addition to common routes of exposure, preexisting HIV infection contributes to an increased rate of transition from acute to CHB coinfection.

Numerous cohort studies of HIV-infected persons from North America, Europe, and Australia have found an HBV coinfection prevalence of 5% to 10% based on hepatitis B surface antigen (HBsAg) positivity.[1–5] Initial reports from the Multicenter AIDS Cohort Study (MACS) of men who have sex with men (MSM) recruited during the pre-ART era found a prevalence of CHB infection of 8.3% (213 per 2559) in HIV-positive (+) MSM.[1] A similar CHB prevalence of 8.7% was found in the EuroSIDA cohort encompassing sites in Europe and South America.[4] The prominent role that presumed HBV sexual transmission plays in development of HIV-HBV coinfection was highlighted by the significant increase in MSM as the HIV transmission risk factor in those with HBV coinfection in the EuroSIDA cohort (50% with HBsAg vs 45% without, $P<.0001$).

More recent analyses suggest a stable to slightly decreased prevalence of HIV-HBV coinfection. A recent analysis from the North American Cohort Collaboration on Research and Design (NA-ACCORD), collected from 12 clinical sites from 1996 to 2010, found a CHB prevalence of 7% (2229 per 34,119) using a combined definition for CHB of a positive HBsAg, hepatitis e antigen (HBeAg), or DNA.[6] A more stringent definition of CHB infection (2 HBsAg+ >6 months apart) was used within the US Military HIV Natural History Study and an overall prevalence of 4.3% (117 per 2769) was found.[5] Because this is a dynamic cohort with patients moving in and out, cross-sectional prevalence by year was also evaluated. The peak CHB prevalence was found in 1995 (9.6%) with significant decrease through 2008 (2.3%; $P<.001$ for trend). When examining an epidemiologic data set with reported cases of HBV, hepatitis C virus (HCV), and HIV in 15 states and 2 cities, only 2% of more than 500,000 PLWH were found to have HBV infection using probabilistic matching.[7] For comparison, the most recent estimates of CHB infection prevalence in the general US population is 0.3%.[8–10]

Finally, in areas where HBV infection remains endemic, a higher prevalence of HIV-HBV coinfection is found. For example, in Ghana 17% of PLWH were HBsAg+.[11] Similarly, in China data suggest a HIV-HBV coinfection prevalence of 10% to 15%.[12,13]

COMPARATIVE VIROLOGY AND ANTIVIRAL TARGETS

Before a discussion of the impact of antiviral therapy on the natural history of HBV in the setting of HIV coinfection, it is illustrative to examine the viral basis for why many HIV nucleoside or nucleotide reverse transcriptase inhibitors (NRTIs) also possess anti-HBV activity (**Table 1**). Shortly after full sequences of HBV, and other animal-associated hepadnaviruses, were available, it became clear that they were evolutionarily related to retroviruses, including HIV-1.[14] In particular, it was noted that the putative HBV polymerase (P protein) had a high degree of homology with key conserved domains with the reverse transcriptase (RT) of retroviruses. Subsequently, in vitro and early clinical studies confirmed the anti-HBV activity of several antiretroviral (ARV) drugs, including zalcitabine (ddC) and lamivudine (3TC).[15,16]

Table 1			
Activity of human immunodeficiency virus nucleosides or nucleotides against hepatitis B virus			
HIV Nucleosides or Nucleotides	**HBV Activity**	**HBV Resistance**	**FDA Approval for HBV**
Abacavir	No	No	N/A
Didanosine	No	No	N/A
Lamivudine	Yes	M204V	Yes (1998)
Emtricitabine	Yes	M204V	No
Stavudine	No	No	N/A
Tenofovir Disoproxil fumarate	Yes	A194T, N236T[a]	Yes (2008)
Tenofovir alafenamide	Yes	A194T, N236T[a]	Yes (2016)
Zidovudine	No	No	N/A

Abbreviations: FDA, US Food and Drug Administration; HBV, hepatitis B virus; HIV, human immunodeficiency virus; N/A, not applicable.
 [a] Clinical impact of these variants remains inconclusive.

Although a high-resolution crystal structure of the HBV P protein has not been solved, contemporary studies have extended the understanding of structural homologies between the HBV P protein and HIV RT using mutational analysis and computer modeling. Most notably, HBV P protein possesses a conserved YMDD motif in the polymerase active site, similar to HIV RT.[17] Deoxyribonucleotide specificity seems to be conferred by a conserved aromatic amino acid (F423 in the case of HBV) within the deoxynucleoside triphosphate binding pocket, analogous to the conserved Y115 in HIV RT.[18] These examples of sequence-conserved sites, along with their presumed functional or structural similarities, underlie the activity of many approved HIV NRTIs on HBV P protein. An extension of these analyses offers possibility concerning why select HIV NRTIs do not possess anti-HBV activity. Drawing inference from sequence analogies between drug-resistant HIV RT and wild-type HBV P protein sequences, it seems nucleotide or amino acids changes that confer resistance NRTIs, such as zidovudine (AZT), didanosine (ddI), and stavudine (D4T) in HIV-1 (eg, Q151M or T69S insertion complex), are consensus sequences in the HBV P protein.[17]

Most first-line and second-line nucleoside or nucleotide inhibitors currently approved for use in CHB infection were initially developed as ARVs, including 3TC, adefovir (ADV), tenofovir disoproxil fumarate (TDF) and tenofovir alafenamide (TAF) (**Table 2**). All of these medications, except ADV, are currently approved for treatment of HIV and commonly used in modern highly active ART (HAART) regimens. Although ADV was developed as a potential ARV, the doses required to attain anti-HIV activity (60–120 mg) resulted in significant nephrotoxicity and thus it was abandoned as an HIV-1 therapy.[19–21] At the lower dose used for HBV (10 mg), ADV does not have any appreciable anti-HIV activity.[22,23] Emtricitabine (FTC) is another approved HIV NRTI that also has potent anti-HBV activity; however it is not approved for treatment of CHB.[24]

Despite the recognized similarities between P protein and HIV RT and cross-activity of several antivirals, not all anti-HBV nucleotides were immediately recognized to have anti-HIV activity. Entecavir (ETV) is a potent guanosine-analog inhibitor of HBV replication that was not found to have anti-HIV-1 activity in initial studies using cell lines and a cell death readout as a surrogate for HIV replication inhibition (50% effective

Table 2
Activity of hepatitis B virus nucleosides or nucleotides against human immunodeficiency virus-1

HBV Nucleosides or Nucleotides	HIV Activity	HIV Resistance	FDA Approval for HIV
Adefovir	No[a]	No[a]	No
Lamivudine	Yes	M184V	Yes (1995)
Entecavir	Yes	M184V	No
Telbivudine	No	No	No
TDF	Yes	K65R	Yes (2001)
TAF	Yes	K65R	Yes (2015)

[a] HIV activity and resistance selection not seen at doses used for HBV.

concentration >10 μM).[25] Based on this initial characterization, ETV was recommended for treatment of HBV in those with HIV who did not also require HIV treatment. In 2007, 3 cases were reported of HIV-HBV coinfected patients who were not on HIV therapy and were treated with ETV monotherapy for HBV. All also showed decreases in HIV RNA with selection of the M184V resistance mutation in HIV in 1 of the 2 patients assessed.[26] Companion in vitro studies using sensitive single round infection assays (capable of detecting infections at the single cell level) demonstrated potent low nM anti-HIV activity of ETV. Interesting, the anti-HIV activity plateaued at modest levels despite being detected at low ETV concentration and may account for how it was missed by less sensitive assays. Subsequent studies showed ETV-triphosphate was a substrate for HIV RT and could inhibit replication in vitro by acting as a nonobligate chain terminator.[27] Furthermore, it was shown that the M184V mutation resulted in less efficient incorporation of ETV-TP.

Telbivudine (LdT) was approved for CHB infection in 2006 and is currently considered a second-line option for CHB infection (American Association for the Study of Liver Diseases, 2018).[28] Initial in vitro characterization demonstrated potent HBV inhibition without HIV-1 activity[29]; however, 2 case reports suggested it may have anti-HIV-1 activity.[30,31] Interestingly, the patients in both case reports were on dual HBV therapy with ADV plus LdT. Despite these reports, convincing follow-up in vitro studies demonstrate a lack of anti-HIV activity and inability of LdT-TP to be incorporated by HIV RT.[32,33] On balance, it seems unlikely that LdT has significant anti-HIV activity. Regardless, the need for HBV therapy in the absence of HIV therapy for coinfected patients is now almost nonexistent given the strong recommendations for treatment of all PLWH as soon as HIV infection is recognized.[34]

PRE–HIGHLY ACTIVE ANTIRETROVIRAL THERAPY NATURAL HISTORY OF HEPATITIS B VIRUS INFECTION

Multiple factors affect the natural history of CHB infection and the resultant risk of cirrhosis and hepatocellular carcinoma. Chief among these factors are duration of infection, HBV DNA levels, HBeAg status, and concomitant liver disease or toxins (eg, nonalcoholic fatty liver disease or excessive alcohol). The understanding of a potential bidirectional impact of coinfection with HIV and HBV has evolved as treatment approaches for both of these chronic infections have changed.

Before the advent of HAART, morbidity and mortality in PLWH, whether coinfected with HBV or not, were dominated by the progression to AIDS and death related to advanced immunosuppression or untreated HIV.[35,36] For instance, in a cohort of more than 470 patients with HIV followed in Los Angeles from 1993 to 2001, the overall mortality rate was 28% with no significant difference between HIV ($n = 126$, 33% mortality) and HIV-HBV ($n = 72$, 26% mortality).[36] Interestingly, some early studies suggested the degree of liver inflammation based on transaminases and thus HBV liver disease progression may be slowed owing to immunosuppression in the setting of HIV coinfection.[37,38]

One of the few studies to include liver biopsy found higher rates of cirrhosis in HIV-HBV compared with HBV monoinfected MSM in France.[39] In a cross-sectional analysis of 132 MSM with CHB infection (65 HIV coinfected), liver biopsy was performed in all subjects and combined with HBV DNA, ALT, and albumin measurements to characterize subjects both biochemically and histologically. HIV-HBV coinfected subjects had higher HBV DNA levels and lower alanine aminotransferase (ALT), in agreement with other studies. Pathologically, no difference in median histologic activity index was seen between the 2 groups yet cirrhosis was present in 13% (9 per 67) of those with HBV and 28% (18 per 65) of those with HIV-HBV ($P = .04$). Multivariate analysis, which accounted for duration of HBV infection, alcohol use, and HBeAg status, demonstrated a significant association between HIV coinfection and cirrhosis with a relative risk (RR) of 4.2 (1.3–13.8, $P = .03$). This is a better appreciated, yet still obscure, concept.

Larger prospective cohort studies were the first to demonstrate increased all-cause and liver mortality in the setting of HIV-HBV coinfection before the introduction of HAART. In the Los Angeles cohort, although all-cause mortality was similar between HIV and HIV-HBV infected groups, liver-related mortality was significantly higher in those with HBV coinfection (6% vs 15%, $P = .04$).[36] In a multivariate analysis, viral hepatitis coinfection (HCV and HBV combined) was associated with an RR for liver death of 5.9 (CI 1.7–20, $P = .003$). Not surprisingly, alcohol use greater than 50gm/d and a CD4 nadir less than 200 were also associated with liver-related death, although the RR was lower at about 2. Although time period (pre-HAART vs post-HAART) was not specifically evaluated, receipt of 0 to 2 ARVs (suggested by the investigators as a surrogate for pre-HAART outcomes) was also significantly associated with liver-related death in those with viral hepatitis coinfection (RR 2.9 [1.3–6.7], $P = .01$).

Some of the most robust data on outcomes in HIV-HBV–coinfected persons (HBsAg+) comes from the prospective MACS cohort, which enrolled MSM in 4 major metropolitan areas across the United States starting in 1987.[1] The cohort included 213 HIV+-HBV+, 139 HIV-HBV+, 2346 HIV+-HBV−, and 3093 HIV−-HBV−. Across the entire study period (1987–2000), liver-related mortality was significantly higher in HIV-HBV participants (14.2 per 1000 person-years [p-y]) than those with HIV alone (1.7 per 1000 p-y) or HBV alone (0.8 per 1000 p-y). In an analysis restricted to outcomes before 1996, the advent of HAART, all-cause mortality was significantly higher in PLWH who were coinfected with HBV (12.3 per 1000 p-y vs 1.6 per 1000 p-y; RR 7.6) than those with HIV alone. Before the introduction of HAART, liver-related mortality was relatively low in HIV+ participants (2.5 per 1000 p-y).

TREATMENT OF HEPATITIS B VIRUS IN THOSE WITH HUMAN IMMUNODEFICIENCY VIRUS

Antiviral treatment of HBV in the setting of HIV coinfection is simplified (compared with HBV alone) because (1) immediate initiation of HAART is recommend for all persons with HIV infection and (2) multiple first-line HIV regimens also deliver complete HBV therapy. These conditions remove the need for assessments of HBV DNA levels, HBeAg status, and hepatic transaminases or fibrosis stage to determine candidacy for HBV antiviral therapy. However, these assessments remain critical for proper management of patients with HIV-HBV coinfection. Of the currently recommended initial regimens for HIV by the US Department of Health & Human Services or International Antiviral Society–USA panels, only abacavir-3TC-dolutegravir is not recommended for use in HIV-HBV coinfection due to 3TC monotherapy for HBV.[34,40]

Suboptimal rates of HBV DNA suppression combined with high rates of resistance selection underlie the recommendations against the use of 3TC monotherapy to treat CHB, regardless of coinfection status. Studies of 3TC HBV monotherapy given in the setting of HIV ART have demonstrated high rates of resistance development. After 1 year, 20% to 25% demonstrate 3TC resistance, which progressively increases such that resistance is detectable in greater than 50% at 2 years and greater than 90% after 4 years.[41–43] These are somewhat higher than those found in HBV monoinfection studies.[44] Although the M204V/I variant is invariably present, the rate of selection of double (M204V/I + L180M) or triple mutants (+V173L) was found to increase with longer 3TC exposure.[43]

Tenofovir-based therapies (either TDF or TAF) are first-line for management of HBV in the setting of HIV coinfection. Regardless of prior 3TC exposure and/or resistance, rates of HBV DNA suppression in HBeAg+ patients are 30% to 50% at 1 year, 70% to 80% at 2 years, and greater than 90% after 4 to 5 years on therapy.[45,46] As in HBV monoinfection, HBV DNA suppression rates are even higher in HBeAg− patients. Despite high rates of viral suppression, HBsAg loss is relatively infrequent (10%–15%) at 5 years.[45] Because tenofovir (administered as TDF or TAF) is often given with 3TC or FTC, HIV-HBV coinfection was a logical place to study whether combination therapy provides any virologic or clinical benefit compared with tenofovir alone in the context of a suppressive HIV ARV regimen. Although data are mixed, the preponderance of evidence does not suggest a significant benefit to combination therapy in terms of HBV DNA viral load decrease or suppression, biochemical normalization, or serologic response.[47–50] A recent meta-analysis conducted in HBV-HIV coinfection came to the same conclusion.[46]

Despite the potent anti-HBV activity of tenofovir, during long-term follow-up, a minority of patients fail to completely suppress HBV DNA or have periods of viral breakthrough or rebound. Poor or intermittent compliance seems to be the predominant reason for suboptimal response.[51–53] Two important concepts related to this are that (1) HIV suppression can be maintained despite HBV nonresponse or breakthrough related to poor adherence and (2) genotypic resistance to tenofovir in HBV is not encountered.[54]

Although limited data suggest entecavir intensification is successful in improving rates of HBV viremia suppression in those with HIV coinfection already on a tenofovir-based regimen[55]; whether this approach results in any clinical benefit over the long-term remains an unanswered clinical question and may depend on factors such as magnitude of the viremia and underlying fibrosis stage.

IMPACT OF ANTIRETROVIRAL THERAPY ON THE NATURAL HISTORY OF HEPATITIS B VIRUS IN HUMAN IMMUNODEFICIENCY VIRUS
Incident Hepatitis B Virus Infection

Fully active HBV therapy (containing at least 1 first-line HBV agent) given in the setting of HAART has the potential to alter the natural history of CHB infection but may also modulate the risk of HBV acquisition and/or the risk of chronic infection development after acute infection. Consistent with an increased HBV prevalence in those with HIV infection, incident HBV infection is also recognized more frequently. Incident HBV infection after HIV infection has been evaluated in multiple studies with a 50% to 90% decrease in incident infections being consistently found after the introduction of HAART.[2,5,56–58] Although multiple studies have shown a decrease in incident HBV infection while on ART, data are mixed on whether ART regimens containing HBV-specific agents (3TC-FTC or TDF) confer additional protection against incident infection. In one of the first studies to report on this phenomenon, Kellerman and colleagues[2] found a 50% decrease in incident HBV infection in the Spectrum of HIV Disease project; however, the risk reduction was the same regardless of whether 3TC was a component of the ART regimen. This study predated use of tenofovir prodrugs.

In a prospective Japanese cohort, the incidence rate of HBV for HIV+ MSM not on ART was 6.72 per 100 p-y.[57] Receipt of ART containing at least 1 HBV active agent reduced this rate by 90% (hazard ratio 0.11, $P<.001$). ART with no HBV active agents was not found to be protective in this study, although the observation period was short (114 p-y). Intriguingly, no HBV infections were found in those on TDF-containing ART, although this was not statistically significant given the small numbers. Similarly, a cohort from Amsterdam only found a significant decrease in incident HBV infection in HIV+ MSM who were on HBV-active HAART. Furthermore, this study showed an additional benefit of TDF-containing ART compared with 3TC-containing ART (95% reduction vs 53% reduction).[56]

The largest study conducted to date of incident HBV infection in MSM comes from the MACS cohort with more than 9 years of follow-up (25,000 p-y).[58] This study is also unique in that it enrolled HIV− MSM and could compare HBV incidence between HIV+ (n = 591) and HIV− (n = 1784) MSM, as well as assess the impact of HAART. HBV incidence was higher in HIV-infected MSM compared with HIV− (1.49 per 100 p-y vs 0.78 per 100 p-y, respectively). However, HBV incidence decreased significantly in both groups during the HAART era (incidence rate ratio [IRR] 0.2, CI 0.1–0.4, and 0.3, CI 0.2–0.4, respectively). Other suggested factors, such as increased HBV vaccination rates in MSM, are likely also contributing to decreasing incidence. Despite this overall effect, a benefit of HAART on decreasing HBV incidence was seen within the HIV+ MSM group. HIV-infected MSM on HAART with a suppressed HIV RNA level demonstrated an 80% reduction in incident HBV infection. Being prescribed HAART but not having a suppressed HIV viral load offered no protection. Because nearly all HAART regimens in the cohort contained 3TC, no comparison could be made between HAART regimens with and without HBV-active agents. In contrast to other studies, no additional benefit of TDF-containing ART was found. Taken together, studies suggest a large effect of HAART-containing HBV-active agents on reducing HBV incidence in at-risk HIV+ MSM. Whether these benefits are directly conferred to the individual taking HBV-active HAART or are realized through reductions in HBV DNA levels in persons with chronic infection who are potential transmitters is unclear.

Development of Chronic Hepatitis B Virus Infection

Acquisition of HBV later in life (late teens, adults) is associated with a low rate of transition to chronic infection that is less than 5%.[59,60] Established HIV infection at the time of HBV infection increases the rate of transition from acute to CHB infection. In pre-HAART era, rates of transition to CHB infection were found to range from 20% to 25%.[61,62] Contemporary studies suggest a decrease in the risk for development of chronic infection with effective HIV therapy. For instance, in the Spectrum of HIV Disease Project, approximately 7% of 316 incident HBV infections became chronic when 80% of the study population was on some form of ART.[2] In a Department of Defense study, which spanned the HAART era, 20.4% (37 per 181) of incident HBV infection went on to chronic infection.[5] However, when analyzed by time periods, the rate of chronic infection decreased from 1.2 cases per 100 p-y in the pre-HAART era to 0.12 cases per 100 p-y in the HAART era (P<.001). Although effective treatment with ARVs seems to decrease the risk of development of chronic infection, whether ART that contains HBV-specific antivirals further decreases that risk is unclear.

Natural History of Chronic Hepatitis B Virus Infection

There are limited long-term data on the impact of HBV antiviral therapy on the natural history of CHB in PLWH, particularly in the HAART era (after 1996) and with the use of tenofovir-based therapies (after 2001). As noted previously, early studies of HBV-HIV coinfection in the pre-HAART or early-HAART eras were dominated by mortality related to HIV disease combined with relatively less effective 3TC-based monotherapy for HBV. In the MACS cohort, mortality rate in HBsAg+ PLWH was seen to increase from 1996 to 2000 compared with before 1996 (24.7 per 1000 p-y vs 12.7 per 1000 p-y, respectively).[1] Among potential explanations for lack of a clear impact of HBV-active therapy posited by the investigators was ART-related hepatotoxicity, viral rebound or intermittent therapy, enhanced immune response after HIV control, and improved survival leading to longer cumulative HBV exposure. A later analysis from the MACS cohort reexamined mortality rates by HBV status with a longer follow-up period on HAART (median 6.6 years in CHB group).[63] Despite the longer time on therapy, AIDS-related mortality (17 per 1000 p-y) and liver-related mortality (22 per 1000 p-y) remained higher in the CHB group and was not substantially different from the earlier analysis. Although AIDS-related mortality remained higher, it was not statistically significantly higher than HIV-monoinfected groups when accounting for baseline CD4 and HIV RNA suppression. This analysis was limited by relatively small numbers with CHB (n = 45) and because only about 50% were on tenofovir-based HAART.

Additional cohort studies from Europe and a meta-analysis also found increased rates of all-cause mortality and/or liver-related mortality in HBV-HIV coinfected persons.[4,64] Also similar to the MACS cohort, the EuroSIDA cohort did not demonstrate that time on HBV-active HAART was associated with any significant decrease in the liver-related outcomes. Again, this is limited because nearly all HBV-active medication exposure was to 3TC and numbers and time on follow-up for this group was limited. In the meta-analysis, there was a 32% increased risk of mortality in the HBV-HIV coinfected group.[64] Mortality rate remained significantly elevated in both the pre-HAART and HAART eras (IRR 1.60; 1.07–2.39 and 1.30; 1.03–1.60, respectively).

An analysis from the NA-ACCORD cohort represents the largest evaluation to date on the impact of HAART on the development of endstage liver disease (ESLD) in HBV-HIV coinfection. Data collected from 12 clinical sites over 14 years, including over 2200 persons infected with HBV and HIV (with or without HCV), were analyzed according to 3 ART periods: early ART (1996–2000), mid-ART (2001–2005), and modern ART (2006–2010).[6] As expected, the proportion of HBV coinfected persons receiving ART containing HBV-active agents (3TC, FTC, or TDF) and tenofovir-based regimens, respectively, increased significantly over time (64%/0% early ART period to 78%/65% modern ART period). Consistent with nearly all other cohorts, the rates of ESLD were higher in those coinfected with HBV compared with HIV alone, regardless of the ART time period (incidence rate per 1000 p-y: early 8.23 versus 1.18, middle 9.75 versus 1.31, modern 7.50 versus 1.26). Within the HBV coinfected group, a trend in decreased rates of development of ESLD was seen in going from mid-ART to modern-ART period. The adjusted IRR was 0.69 (95% CI 0.38–1.26). Although not statistically significant, this was the only group for which a decrease in incidence of ESLD was seen. A competing risk analysis, which took into account time on study, found a further reduction in the risk of ESLD in those with HBV-HIV in the modern ART era compared with the middle ART era with longer time on study. This suggests that a longer time on a highly potent anti-HBV and HIV regimen confers continued benefits in terms of prevention of ESLD development.

In addition to looking at liver-related mortality, several recent studies have looked the impact of HBV-active ART on liver fibrosis as assessed by transient elastography (TE). In 2 cohorts from Africa, after 1 year of TDF-based therapy, significant decreases in liver stiffness were noted.[65,66] A study from Ghana performed TE 1 year apart in 76 HBV-HIV infected participants, of which 88% had been on 3TC-containing ART for a median of 45 months and 49% achieved HBV DNA suppression.[65] Initial TE suggested advanced fibrosis in 20% (Fibrosis stage 3: 7.6–9.4 kPa; Fibrosis stage 4 >9.4 kPa) and 16% after 1 year. HBeAg positivity and HBV DNA levels greater than 2000 IU/mL were associated a higher prevalence of advanced fibrosis. A second study from Zambia included 61 HBV-HIV coinfected participants; however, in this study, ART was started at the initial visit and 98% were on TDF-based ART.[66] TE was performed at baseline and 1 year later. HBV viral suppression was achieved in 65% at 1 year. A mean decrease of 0.7 kPa was seen in the cohort, with the proportion having greater than or equal to F2 fibrosis ($\geq$5.9 kPa) going from 46% to 21%. The proportion assessed as having cirrhosis by TE ($\geq$9.4 kPa) went from 8.2% to 1.6%. When compared with HBV− HIV-infected participants in the same cohort, HBV coinfection was associated with an odds ratio of 7.7 for significant fibrosis at 1 year (CI 2.89–20.57). Among those with HBV-HIV, there was no association with HBV DNA level and change in fibrosis over 1 year. Although intriguing, these data require additional follow-up and, ideally, validation with other means of fibrosis staging (eg, liver biopsy); early or rapid improvement in liver stiffness is likely due to decrease in liver inflammation and may not correlate with actual fibrosis regression.

Finally, one small study demonstrated improvements in the clinical parameters of ESLD in a small cohort of HBV-HIV infected subjects.[67] Among 7 subjects with cirrhosis and HBV coinfection treated with TDF-containing ART for a median of 28 months, significant improvements in albumin and prothrombin time were noted. In addition, all 3 subjects with Child-Pugh stage B or C cirrhosis had improvement to stage A at the end of follow-up. These data are similar to what has been previously described in HBV monoinfected patients with advanced liver disease.[68,69]

SUMMARY AND FUTURE DIRECTIONS

HIV coinfection affects the natural history of HBV infection across all stages of disease, from initial exposure and the development of chronic infection to fibrosis progression and death due to liver disease. Before the advent of HAART, morbidity and mortality related to AIDS dominated, although cohort studies clearly identified an adverse impact of HBV coinfection on mortality in persons living with HIV. As effective therapies for HIV arrived, HBV-related liver disease emerged as a major cause of death. HIV cohorts were instrumental in highlighting the shortcomings of 3TC-based HBV treatment and were among the first to demonstrate high levels of 3TC genotypic resistance in HBV over short periods of time.

Currently, nearly all recommended first-line HIV ART regimens provide potent HBV therapy, in the form of tenofovir prodrugs, as a component. Furthermore, all patients with HBV-HIV are recommended to initiate treatment with an ART regimen containing tenofovir, often in combination with a second nucleoside with anti-HBV activity (3TC or

FTC). Tenofovir-based HIV therapy achieves high rates of HBV DNA suppression with essentially no risk of genotypic HBV resistance. Despite this, a dramatic benefit in terms of amelioration of HBV-related disease impact has yet to be clearly documented in cohort studies. This likely stems from multiple factors, including incomplete uptake and adherence; persistent impact of other factors, such as alcohol or HIV itself, on liver disease in coinfected subjects; and relatively short time periods of follow-up since the widespread introduction of tenofovir.

Future research goals should include continued follow-up of cohorts and more widespread inclusion of longitudinal fibrosis assessment (eg, TE). Because TAF has only recently been introduced and has demonstrated more rapid and higher rates of biochemical normalization in registrational studies, it will be interesting to see whether wide spread use of TAF in HBV-HIV may be associated with more dramatic long-term benefits.[70] Finally, as novel therapies for CHB infection are developed, studies in HBV-HIV coinfected subjects should be prioritized given the more aggressive disease phenotype.

REFERENCES

1. Thio CL, Seaberg EC, Skolasky R Jr, et al. HIV-1, hepatitis B virus, and risk of liver-related mortality in the Multicenter Cohort Study (MACS). Lancet 2002;360: 1921–6.

2. Kellerman SE, Hanson DL, McNaghten AD, et al. Prevalence of chronic hepatitis B and incidence of acute hepatitis B infection in human immunodeficiency virus-infected subjects. J Infect Dis 2003;188:571–7.

3. Dore GJ, Cooper DA, Barrett C, et al. Dual efficacy of lamivudine treatment in human immunodeficiency virus/hepatitis B virus-coinfected persons in a randomized, controlled study (CAESAR). The CAESAR Coordinating Committee. J Infect Dis 1999;180:607–13.

4. Konopnicki D, Mocroft A, de Wit S, et al. Hepatitis B and HIV: prevalence, AIDS progression, response to highly active antiretroviral therapy and increased mortality in the EuroSIDA cohort. AIDS 2005;19:593–601.

5. Chun HM, Fieberg AM, Hullsiek KH, et al. Epidemiology of Hepatitis B virus infection in a US cohort of HIV-infected individuals during the past 20 years. Clin Infect Dis 2010;50:426–36.

6. Klein MB, Althoff KN, Jing Y, et al. Risk of end-stage liver disease in HIV-viral hepatitis coinfected persons in North America from the early to modern antiretroviral therapy eras. Clin Infect Dis 2016;63:1160–7.

7. Bosh KA, Coyle JR, Hansen V, et al. HIV and viral hepatitis coinfection analysis using surveillance data from 15 US states and two cities. Epidemiol Infect 2018;146:920–30.

8. Ioannou GN. Hepatitis B virus in the United States: infection, exposure, and immunity rates in a nationally representative survey. Ann Intern Med 2011;154: 319–28.

9. Roberts H, Kruszon-Moran D, Ly KN, et al. Prevalence of chronic hepatitis B virus (HBV) infection in U.S. Households: National Health and Nutrition Examination Survey (NHANES), 1988-2012. Hepatology 2016;63:388–97.

10. Polaris Observatory Collaborators. Global prevalence, treatment, and prevention of hepatitis B virus infection in 2016: a modelling study. Lancet Gastroenterol Hepatol 2018;3:383–403.

11. Geretti AM, Patel M, Sarfo FS, et al. Detection of highly prevalent hepatitis B virus coinfection among HIV-seropositive persons in Ghana. J Clin Microbiol 2010;48: 3223–30.
12. Xie J, Han Y, Qiu Z, et al. Prevalence of hepatitis B and C viruses in HIV-positive patients in China: a cross-sectional study. J Int AIDS Soc 2016;19:20659.
13. Wu S, Yan P, Yang T, et al. Epidemiological profile and risk factors of HIV and HBV/HCV co-infection in Fujian Province, southeastern China. J Med Virol 2017;89:443–9.
14. Miller RH, Robinson WS. Common evolutionary origin of hepatitis B virus and retroviruses. Proc Natl Acad Sci U S A 1986;83:2531–5.
15. Doong SL, Tsai CH, Schinazi RF, et al. Inhibition of the replication of hepatitis B virus in vitro by 2',3'-dideoxy-3'-thiacytidine and related analogues. Proc Natl Acad Sci U S A 1991;88:8495–9.
16. Benhamou Y, Katlama C, Lunel F, et al. Effects of lamivudine on replication of hepatitis B virus in HIV-infected men. Ann Intern Med 1996;125:705–12.
17. Das K, Xiong X, Yang H, et al. Molecular modeling and biochemical characterization reveal the mechanism of hepatitis B virus polymerase resistance to lamivudine (3TC) and emtricitabine (FTC). J Virol 2001;75:4771–9.
18. Beck J, Vogel M, Nassal M. dNTP versus NTP discrimination by phenylalanine 451 in duck hepatitis B virus P protein indicates a common structure of the dNTP-binding pocket with other reverse transcriptases. Nucleic Acids Res 2002;30:1679–87.
19. Deeks SG, Collier A, Lalezari J, et al. The safety and efficacy of adefovir dipivoxil, a novel anti-human immunodeficiency virus (HIV) therapy, in HIV-infected adults: a randomized, double-blind, placebo-controlled trial. J Infect Dis 1997;176: 1517–23.
20. Barditch-Crovo P, Toole J, Hendrix CW, et al. Anti-human immunodeficiency virus (HIV) activity, safety, and pharmacokinetics of adefovir dipivoxil (9-[2-(bis-pivaloyloxymethyl)-phosphonylmethoxyethyl]adenine) in HIV-infected patients. J Infect Dis 1997;176:406–13.
21. Fisher EJ, Chaloner K, Cohn DL, et al. The safety and efficacy of adefovir dipivoxil in patients with advanced HIV disease: a randomized, placebo-controlled trial. AIDS 2001;15:1695–700.
22. Delaugerre C, Marcelin AG, Thibault V, et al. Human immunodeficiency virus (HIV) Type 1 reverse transcriptase resistance mutations in hepatitis B virus (HBV)-HIV-coinfected patients treated for HBV chronic infection once daily with 10 milligrams of adefovir dipivoxil combined with lamivudine. Antimicrob Agents Chemother 2002;46:1586–8.
23. Sheldon JA, Corral A, Rodés B, et al. Risk of selecting K65R in antiretroviral-naive HIV-infected individuals with chronic hepatitis B treated with adefovir. AIDS 2005; 19:2036–8.
24. Saag MS. Emtricitabine, a new antiretroviral agent with activity against HIV and hepatitis B virus. Clin Infect Dis 2006;42:126–31.
25. Innaimo SF, Seifer M, Bisacchi GS, et al. Identification of BMS-200475 as a potent and selective inhibitor of hepatitis B virus. Antimicrob Agents Chemother 1997; 41:1444–8.
26. McMahon MA, Jilek BL, Brennan TP, et al. The HBV drug entecavir - effects on HIV-1 replication and resistance. N Engl J Med 2007;356:2614–21.
27. Domaoal RA, McMahon M, Thio CL, et al. Pre-steady-state kinetic studies establish entecavir 5'-triphosphate as a substrate for HIV-1 reverse transcriptase. J Biol Chem 2008;283:5452–9.

28. Update on prevention, diagnosis, and treatment of chronic hepatitis B: AASLD 2018 hepatitis B guidance - Terrault - 2018 - Hepatology - Wiley Online Library. Available at: https://aasldpubs.onlinelibrary.wiley.com/doi/10.1002/hep.29800. Accessed December 10, 2018.

29. Standring DN, Bridges EG, Placidi L, et al. Antiviral beta-L-nucleosides specific for hepatitis B virus infection. Antivir Chem Chemother 2001;12(Suppl 1):119–29.

30. Gentile I, Bonadies G, Carleo MA, et al. In vivo antiviral activity of telbivudine against HIV-1: a case report. Infez Med 2013;21:216–9.

31. Low E, Cox A, Atkins M, et al. Telbivudine has activity against HIV-1. AIDS 2009; 23:546–7.

32. Lin K, Karwowska S, Lam E, et al. Telbivudine exhibits no inhibitory activity against HIV-1 clinical isolates in vitro. Antimicrob Agents Chemother 2010;54: 2670–3.

33. van Maarseveen NM, Wensing AM, de Jong D, et al. Telbivudine exerts no antiviral activity against HIV-1 in vitro and in humans. Antivir Ther 2011;16:1123–30.

34. What to start adult and adolescent ARV. AIDSinfo. Available at: https://aidsinfo. nih.gov/guidelines/html/1/adult-and-adolescent-arv/11/what-to-start.   Accessed November 16, 2018.

35. Mai AL, Yim C, O'Rourke K, et al. The interaction of human immunodeficiency virus infection and hepatitis B virus infection in infected homosexual men. J Clin Gastroenterol 1996;22:299–304.

36. Bonacini M, Louie S, Bzowej N, et al. Survival in patients with HIV infection and viral hepatitis B or C: a cohort study. AIDS 2004;18:2039–45.

37. Rustgi VK, Hoofnagle JH, Gerin JL, et al. Hepatitis B virus infection in the acquired immunodeficiency syndrome. Ann Intern Med 1984;101:795–7.

38. Gilson RJ, Hawkins AE, Beecham MR, et al. Interactions between HIV and hepatitis B virus in homosexual men: effects on the natural history of infection. AIDS 1997;11:597–606.

39. Colin JF, Cazals-Hatem D, Loriot MA, et al. Influence of human immunodeficiency virus infection on chronic hepatitis B in homosexual men. Hepatology 1999;29: 1306–10.

40. Saag MS, Benson CA, Gandhi RT, et al. Antiretroviral drugs for treatment and prevention of HIV infection in adults: 2018 recommendations of the International Antiviral Society-USA panel. JAMA 2018;320:379–96.

41. Benhamou Y, Bochet M, Thibault V, et al. Long-term incidence of hepatitis B virus resistance to lamivudine in human immunodeficiency virus-infected patients. Hepatology 1999;30:1302–6.

42. Wolters LMM, Niesters HG, Hansen BE, et al. Development of hepatitis B virus resistance for lamivudine in chronic hepatitis B patients co-infected with the human immunodeficiency virus in a Dutch cohort. J Clin Virol 2002;24:173–81.

43. Matthews GV, Bartholomeusz A, Locarnini S, et al. Characteristics of drug resistant HBV in an international collaborative study of HIV-HBV-infected individuals on extended lamivudine therapy. AIDS 2006;20:863–70.

44. Chang T-T, Lai CL, Chien RN, et al. Four years of lamivudine treatment in Chinese patients with chronic hepatitis B. J Gastroenterol Hepatol 2004;19:1276–82.

45. de Vries–Sluijs TEMS, Reijnders JG, Hansen BE, et al. Long-term therapy with tenofovir is effective for patients Co-infected with human immunodeficiency virus and hepatitis B virus. Gastroenterology 2010;139:1934–41.

46. Price H, Dunn D, Pillay D, et al. Suppression of HBV by tenofovir in HBV/HIV co-infected patients: a systematic review and meta-analysis. PLoS One 2013;8: e68152.

47. Schmutz G, Nelson M, Lutz T, et al. Combination of tenofovir and lamivudine versus tenofovir after lamivudine failure for therapy of hepatitis B in HIV-coinfection. AIDS 2006;20:1951–4.

48. Matthews GV, Seaberg E, Dore GJ, et al. Combination HBV therapy is linked to greater HBV DNA suppression in a cohort of lamivudine-experienced HIV/HBV coinfected individuals. AIDS 2009;23:1707–15.

49. Lee YB, Jung EU, Kim BH, et al. Tenofovir monotherapy versus tenofovir plus lamivudine or telbivudine combination therapy in treatment of lamivudine-resistant chronic hepatitis B. Antimicrob Agents Chemother 2015;59:972–8.

50. Alvarez-Uria G, Ratcliffe L, Vilar J. Long-term outcome of tenofovir disoproxil fumarate use against hepatitis B in an HIV-coinfected cohort. HIV Med 2009; 10:269–73.

51. Matthews GV, Seaberg EC, Avihingsanon A, et al. Patterns and causes of suboptimal response to tenofovir-based therapy in individuals coinfected with HIV and hepatitis B virus. Clin Infect Dis 2013;56:e87–94.

52. Boyd A, Gozlan J, Maylin S, et al. Persistent viremia in human immunodeficiency virus/hepatitis B coinfected patients undergoing long-term tenofovir: virological and clinical implications. Hepatology 2014;60:497–507.

53. Wong TC, Lan A, Kiser JJ, et al. Novel quantification of tenofovir disoproxil fumarate adherence in human immunodeficiency virus/hepatitis B coinfected patients with incomplete hepatitis B virus viral suppression. Hepatology 2016;64: 999–1000.

54. Audsley J, Arrifin N, Yuen LK, et al. Prolonged use of tenofovir in HIV/hepatitis B virus (HBV)-coinfected individuals does not lead to HBV polymerase mutations and is associated with persistence of lamivudine HBV polymerase mutations. HIV Med 2009;10:229–35.

55. Luetkemeyer AF, Charlebois ED, Hare CB, et al. Resistance patterns and response to entecavir intensification among HIV-HBV-coinfected adults with persistent HBV viremia. J Acquir Immune Defic Syndr 2011;58:e96–9.

56. Heuft MM, Houba SM, van den Berk GE, et al. Protective effect of hepatitis B virus-active antiretroviral therapy against primary hepatitis B virus infection. AIDS 2014;28:999–1005.

57. Gatanaga H, Hayashida T, Tanuma J, et al. Prophylactic effect of antiretroviral therapy on hepatitis B virus infection. Clin Infect Dis 2013;56:1812–9.

58. Falade-Nwulia O, Seaberg EC, Snider AE, et al. Incident hepatitis B virus infection in HIV-infected and HIV-uninfected men who have sex with men from pre-HAART to HAART periods: a cohort study. Ann Intern Med 2015;163:673–80.

59. Wright TL, Lau JY. Clinical aspects of hepatitis B virus infection. Lancet 1993;342: 1340–4.

60. Hyams KC. Risks of chronicity following acute hepatitis B virus infection: a review. Clin Infect Dis 1995;20:992–1000.

61. Hadler SC, Judson FN, O'Malley P, et al. Outcome of hepatitis B virus infection in homosexual men and its relation to prior human immunodeficiency virus infection. J Infect Dis 1991;163:454–7.

62. Bodsworth NJ, Cooper DA, Donovan B. The influence of human immunodeficiency virus type 1 infection on the development of the hepatitis B virus carrier state. J Infect Dis 1991;163:1138–40.

63. Hoffmann CJ, Seaberg EC, Young S, et al. Hepatitis B and long-term HIV outcomes in coinfected HAART recipients. AIDS 2009;23:1881–9.

64. Nikolopoulos GK, Paraskevis D, Hatzitheodorou E, et al. Impact of hepatitis B virus infection on the progression of AIDS and mortality in HIV-infected individuals: a cohort study and meta-analysis. Clin Infect Dis 2009;48:1763–71.

65. Stockdale AJ, Phillips RO, Beloukas A, et al. Liver fibrosis by transient elastography and virologic outcomes after introduction of tenofovir in lamivudine-experienced adults with HIV and hepatitis B virus coinfection in Ghana. Clin Infect Dis 2015;61:883–91.

66. Vinikoor MJ, Sinkala E, Chilengi R, et al. Impact of antiretroviral therapy on liver fibrosis among human immunodeficiency virus-infected adults with and without HBV coinfection in Zambia. Clin Infect Dis 2017;64:1343–9.

67. Matthews GV, Cooper DA, Dore GJ. Improvements in parameters of end-stage liver disease in patients with HIV/HBV-related cirrhosis treated with tenofovir. Antivir Ther 2007;12:119–22.

68. Yao FY, Terrault NA, Freise C, et al. Lamivudine treatment is beneficial in patients with severely decompensated cirrhosis and actively replicating hepatitis B infection awaiting liver transplantation: a comparative study using a matched, untreated cohort. Hepatology 2001;34:411–6.

69. Kapoor D, Guptan RC, Wakil SM, et al. Beneficial effects of lamivudine in hepatitis B virus-related decompensated cirrhosis. J Hepatol 2000;33:308–12.

70. Agarwal K, Brunetto M, Seto WK, et al. 96 weeks treatment of tenofovir alafenamide vs. tenofovir disoproxil fumarate for hepatitis B virus infection. J Hepatol 2018;68:672–81.

Screening and Prophylaxis to Prevent Hepatitis B Reactivation

Introduction and Immunology

Joe Sasadeusz, MBBS, PhD, FRACP[a,b,*], Andrew Grigg, MBBS, FRACP, FRCPA, MD[c],
Peter D. Hughes, MBBS, PhD, FRACP[b,d], Seng Lee Lim, MBBS, FRACP, FRCP, MD[e],
Michaela Lucas, MD, Dr Med, FRACP, FRCPA[f],
Geoff McColl, MBBS, BMedSc, MEd, PhD, FRACP[g],
Sue Anne McLachlan, MBBS, MSc, FRACP[h], Marion G. Peters, MD, MBBS[i],
Nicholas Shackel, MB, FRACP, PhD[j], Monica Slavin, MBBS, FRACP, MD[d,k],
Vijaya Sundararajan, MD, MPH[b,h,l], Alexander Thompson, PhD, FRACP[b,h],
Joseph Doyle, MBBS, MPH, PhD, FRACP, FAFPHM[m,n], James Rickard, PhD[c],
Peter De Cruz, MBBS, PhD, FRACP[b], Robert G. Gish, MD[o,1],
Kumar Visvanathan, MBBS, PhD, FRACP[b,h,1]

KEYWORDS

- Hepatitis B virus • Hepatitis B immunology • Innate • Adaptive • Reactivation
- Prophylaxis

[a] Peter Doherty Institute for Infection and Immunity, Elizabeth Street, Melbourne, Victoria 3000, Australia; [b] University of Melbourne, Grattan Street, Parkville, Victoria 3010, Australia; [c] Olivia Newton John Cancer Research Institute, Austin Hospital, 145 Studley Road, Heidelberg, Victoria 3084, Australia; [d] Royal Melbourne Hospital, 300 Grattan Street, Parkville, Victoria 3050, Australia; [e] National University of Singapore, 21 Lower Kent Ridge Road, Singapore 119077, Singapore; [f] University of Western Australia, 35 Stirling Highway, Crawley, Western Australia 6009, Australia; [g] University of Queensland Oral Health Centre, 288 Herston Road, Queensland 4006, Australia; [h] St Vincent's Hospital, 41 Victoria Street, Fitzroy, Victoria 3065, Australia; [i] University of California, San Francisco, S357 Parnassus Avenue, San Francisco, CA 94143, USA; [j] Ingham Institute, 1 Campbell Street, Liverpool, Sydney, New South Wales 2170, Australia; [k] Victorian Comprehensive Cancer Centre, 305 Grattan Street, Melbourne, Victoria 3000, Australia; [l] Department of Public Health, La Trobe University, Plenty Road, Bundoora, Victoria 3086, Australia; [m] The Alfred and Monash University, 85 Commercial Road, Melbourne, Victoria 3004, Australia; [n] Burnet Institute, 85 Commercial Road, Melbourne, Victoria 3004, Australia; [o] Division of Gastroenterology and Hepatology, Department of Medicine, Stanford University, Stanford University Medical Center, 300 Pasteur Drive, Stanford, CA 94305, USA

[1] Co-Senior Authors.
* Corresponding author. Peter Doherty Institute for Infection and Immunity, 792 Elizabeth Street, Melbourne, Victoria 3000, Australia.
E-mail address: j.sasadeusz@mh.org.au

Clin Liver Dis 23 (2019) 487–492
https://doi.org/10.1016/j.cld.2019.04.009
1089-3261/19/© 2019 Elsevier Inc. All rights reserved.

KEY POINTS

- Because of the persistence of covalently closed circular DNA (cccDNA) in hepatocytes, HBV is never eradicated, even in patients who lose HBsAg and seroconvert to anti-HBs, and reactivation can occur.
- The presence of anti-HBc+ is the best current marker of the cccDNA persistence.
- HBV-specific T cells are the most important effector mechanism of viral clearance in acute hepatitis B.
- HBV is an active repressor of innate immune pathways in NK cells, monocytes, and hepatocytes.
- The risk of reactivation following treatment with many different drug classes can be divided into low-, moderate-, and high-risk based on the expected likelihood of reactivation.

BACKGROUND

In 4 articles in this issue, we present a consensus statement that was conceived in response to the large unmet need for guidelines for the management of hepatitis B virus (HBV) infection in the setting of immunosuppression. Current recommendations are limited, with nearly all guidelines focused on hematological malignancies and, to a lesser extent, some solid tumors. Few of the guidelines address the wider range of other immunosuppressive states in which reactivation may occur, including those that occur in organ transplantation or in those receiving treatment with any of the many immunosuppressive agents, including biological response modifiers, in current use for treatment of multiple diseases. They also do not address the reactivation that can occur in those receiving the direct-acting antivirals (DAAs) used in the treatment of hepatitis C virus (HCV). Furthermore, none of the guidelines address the potential of new emerging biological agents to cause reactivation of HBV. This leads to great uncertainty in how to manage these patients by individual clinicians. There is great need for medical guidance in managing these issues. In the 4 articles we focus on the treatment of patients with HBV infection, chronic hepatitis B (CHB) infection, and occult hepatitis B infection (OBI), in an extensive range of immunosuppressive scenarios. The aim is to focus on screening and prophylaxis in patients who would not normally require treatment of CHB and does not directly address management of patients who do need ongoing treatment. Well-developed guidelines for this clinical scenario are available elsewhere.[1]

The consensus statement group was specifically formed to consist of specialist infectious disease physicians, hepatologists, and gastroenterologists with expert knowledge in the management of hepatitis B, but also included specialist physicians from therapeutic areas who work with immunosuppressive agents. Individuals met face to face at a 2-day meeting that was held in Melbourne on September 28 to 29, 2016. Each individual was given the responsibility to review the data in a particular area of immunosuppression and present it as an oral presentation to the wider group. After this, a group discussion ensued around that topic to try to reach a consensus on management in the area. This was then repeated for each individual area of immunosuppression. A professional medical writer was in attendance to record the presentations, as well as the associated discussions to subsequently develop a draft manuscript, after which the group used this draft document to refine the recommendations, which were then finalized in consultation with experts in the field.

INTRODUCTION

Hepatitis B virus (HBV), an enveloped DNA virus, causes the most common chronic liver infection in the world. After entering the body, HBV spreads through the bloodstream to the liver, where it enters hepatocytes and replicates.[2] Infection can then lead to liver necrosis and inflammation through activation of the body's immune system and, rarely, via direct cytopathic effects. This can subsequently result in cirrhosis, liver transplant, hepatocellular carcinoma, and death.[3,4] Chronic HBV infection (CHB) is defined as the presence of hepatitis B surface antigen (HBsAg) for 6 months or more. Screening for HBV predominantly involves testing for HBsAg as it can be detected in high levels in serum during acute or chronic HBV infection and indicates that the person is infectious. Other serologic markers of HBV include antibodies to hepatitis B core (anti-HBc) and surface (anti-HBs) antigens. Patients who are HBsAg negative are either anti-HBc positive/anti-HBs negative or anti-HBc positive/anti-HBs positive may have measurable HBV DNA but this is usually low-level (1–3 log IU), which indicates occult HBV infection (OBI). A recent major literature review of studies, with more than 1 million patients who are HBsAg negative tested for HBV DNA, reported an OBI rate of 0.15% overall, but the rate was 10% with the exclusion of blood bank participants (because they are usually a self-selected healthy population), with detectable HBV DNA among patients who are anti-HBc positive of from 8% to 12%.[5] A recent study in which liver tissue from 100 anti-HBc-positive transplant donors was tested for total HBV DNA by nested-polymerase chain reaction (PCR) found that 52% had a positive nested PCR for 2 or more different HBV genomic regions (specifically, 35 were 4/4 targets positive; 9 were 3/4; and 8 were 2/4).[6]

According to international guidelines, treatment of CHB is generally recommended in patients who have a high viral load (>2000 IU/mL) and evidence of inflammation usually determined by increased alanine aminotransferase (ALT) or liver fibrosis on imaging.[4] This suggests that many patients with CHB who do not fulfill these criteria are not being treated.

Because of the persistence of covalently closed circular DNA (cccDNA) in hepatocytes, HBV is never eradicated, even in patients who lose HBsAg and in some cases seroconvert to anti-HBs. In essence, the infection is kept under long-term immune control and the presence of anti-HBc positive is the best current marker of the cccDNA persistence.[7] Immunosuppression or treatment with HCV DAAs may result in loss of immune control of HBV with recurrence of high-level viral replication, a phenomenon known as reactivation, which can be associated with very high ALT levels with hepatic decompensation and death in some patients.[8] Such patients may also occasionally become HBsAg positive again (seroreversion). The definition of HBV reactivation differs between studies, but in general involves a combination of increased HBV replication and increased necroinflammatory activity, as demonstrated by an elevated ALT level. In HBsAg carriers, this is often defined as either the de novo detection of HBV DNA or a 10-fold (1 log10) increase in HBV DNA level compared with the baseline before immunosuppression. A hepatitis flare is usually defined as at least a 2- to 3-fold elevation in ALT level above the patient's baseline level or a predefined multiple of the upper limit of normal. In patients with resolved infection (HBsAg negative but anti-HBc positive), reactivation is usually defined by reverse seroconversion to HBsAg-positive status.[9]

The risk of reactivation following treatment with many different drug classes can be divided into low-risk, moderate-risk, and high-risk based on the expected likelihood of reactivation. Risk may be further subdivided into those individuals who are either (1) HBsAg positive or (2) anti-HBc positive and HBsAg negative with or without anti-HBs, the latter implying better immune control of the HBV infection. HBsAg-positive individuals usually have a higher risk of reactivation compared with HBsAg-negative individuals. A strategy based on risk stratification can be used to prevent hepatitis due to HBV reactivation. Reactivation rates greater than 1% are considered moderate and greater than 10% are considered high. The lowest-risk patients are anti-HBc positive/anti-HBs positive, with high titers indicating the highest level of immune control. In addition, it is important to be aware that, although extremely rare, there have been reports of reactivation in patients who are HBsAg negative/anti-HBc negative/anti-HBs positive with no history of HBV vaccination.[10–14] Neither prophylaxis nor monitoring is currently recommended for such patients with isolated anti-HBs undergoing immunosuppression, but clinicians should be aware of this reactivation possibility and test for HBV DNA by nucleic acid testing when there is unexplained change in liver enzymes in such patients.[14]

IMMUNOLOGY OF REACTIVATION OF HEPATITIS B: ROLES OF INNATE AND ADAPTIVE IMMUNITY

Innate immunity, the body's nonspecific immune system, normally provides an immediate defense in the presence of infection. However, some pathogenic microbes such as the HBV virus have learned to bypass aspects of the innate immune system. Adaptive immunity is more specific than innate immunity and is activated by exposure to an antigen, with the stimulation of lymphocytes, T cells, and B cells (**Fig. 1**). In adaptive immunity, CD4$^+$ T (helper) cells activate macrophages, cytotoxic T cells, and B cells through the release of cytokines. In HBV, the release of interleukin-12 (IL-12) and interferon-γ by T cells stimulates macrophages to clear debris from the liver. Innate lymphoid cells produce many of the same cytokines as CD4$^+$ T cells, including IL-12 and interferon-γ, which recruit the cells that lead to clearance of the infection.

Activation of B cells by CD4$^+$ T cells and other stimuli leads to effector functions, including antibody secretion and memory B-cell differentiation. Antibodies further stimulate phagocytes, natural killer (NK) cells, and complement activation to produce

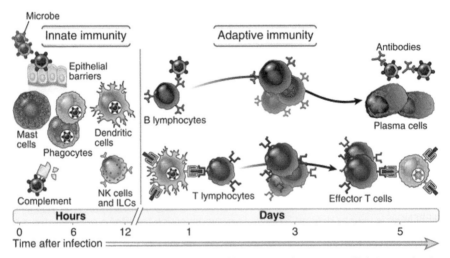

Fig. 1. Innate and adaptive immunity. (*From* Abbas, AK., Lichtman AH, Pillai, S. Introduction to the Immune System: Nomenclature, General Properties, and Components. In: Abbas, AK, Lichtman, AH, Pillai, S, ed. Basic Immunology: Functions and Disorders of the Immune System. 5th ed. St. Louis, MI: Elsevier, Inc; 2016: 1-22, with permission.)

antibody-dependent cellular cytotoxicity and inflammation, as well as neutralizing lysis and phagocytosis of virus particles.

Following acute HBV infection, the virus seems to escape the innate immune response, and adaptive immunity is delayed. Hepatitis B core antibodies (anti-HBc) appear initially 1 to 4 weeks after acute infection, and may be present within the "window" period when hepatitis B surface antigen (HBsAg) is cleared and surface antibody (anti-HBs) is not yet detectable. Anti-HBc usually persists for life and its presence indicates previous or ongoing infection with HBV. The presence of anti-HBs indicates recovery and immunity from HBV infection, or successful vaccination against HBV.

Immune Mechanisms of Viral Clearance

HBV-specific T cells are the principal effector mechanism of viral clearance in acute HBV infection. During acute infection, programmed death-1, IL-10, arginase, myeloid suppressor cells, and T regulatory cells regulate the response of the HBV-specific T cells, providing potential targets for therapeutic intervention. The incidence of HBV-specific T cells declines over time and after serum HBV clearance; however, memory T-cell response remains weakly detectable for 20 to 30 years after infection.

Although nucleic acid sensors, such as Toll-like receptors, are capable of recognizing HBV components, HBV is an active repressor of innate proinflammatory pathways and cytokines in hepatocytes. NK cells have defective noncytolytic antiviral functions in HBV but can amplify liver damage by killing hepatocytes and impairing antiviral immunity by eliminating HBV-specific T cells. NK cells may also play a role in promoting liver fibrosis regression by killing stellate cells.

RECOMMENDATIONS FOR SCREENING AND PROPHYLAXIS TO PREVENT HEPATITIS B REACTIVATION

In the following articles in this issue, we provide specific recommendations for preventing hepatitis B reactivation in various populations based on the most recent data or, where data are limited or missing, on expert opinion: Joe Sasadeusz and colleagues' article, "Screening and Prophylaxis to Prevent Hepatitis B Reactivation: Patients with Hematological and Solid Tumor Malignancies", Joe Sasadeusz and colleagues' article, "Screening and Prophylaxis to Prevent Hepatitis B Reactivation: Transplant Recipients", and Joe Sasadeusz and colleagues' article, "Screening and Prophylaxis to Prevent Hepatitis B Reactivation: Other Populations and Newer Agents," in this issue.

ACKNOWLEDGMENTS

Meetings to discuss and develop recommendations presented in this manuscript and medical writing services provided in the preparation of this manuscript were funded by Gilead Sciences. Neither the medical writer or Gilead in any way influenced the content or the conclusions of the position paper. None of the authors had any direct financial support from Gilead Sciences or any other companies.

REFERENCES

1. Terrault NA, Lok ASF, McMahon BJ, et al. Update on prevention, diagnosis, and treatment of chronic hepatitis B: AASLD 2018 hepatitis B guidance. Hepatology 2018;67(4):1560–99.
2. Hepatitis Australia. About Hep B. Available at: http://www.hepatitisaustralia.com/hepatitis-b-facts/about-hep-b. Accessed: November 16, 2016.

3. World Health Organization. Guidelines for the prevention, care and treatment of persons with chronic hepatitis B infection. Geneva (Switzerland): World Health Organization; 2015.

4. Terrault NA, Bzowej NH, Chang KM, et al. AASLD guidelines for treatment of chronic hepatitis B. Hepatology 2016;63(1):261–83.

5. Mortensen E, Kamali A, Schirmer PL, et al. Are current screening protocols for chronic hepatitis B virus infection adequate? Diagn Microbiol Infect Dis 2016; 85(2):159–67.

6. Caviglia GP, Abate ML, Tandoi F, et al. Quantitation of HBV cccDNA in anti-HBc-positive liver donors by droplet digital PCR: a new tool to detect occult infection. J Hepatol 2018;69(2):301–7.

7. Rehermann B, Ferrari C, Pasquinelli C, et al. The hepatitis B virus persists for decades after patients' recovery from acute viral hepatitis despite active maintenance of a cytotoxic T-lymphocyte response. Nat Med 1996;2(10):1104–8.

8. Lok AS, Liang RH, Chiu EK, et al. Reactivation of hepatitis B virus replication in patients receiving cytotoxic therapy. Report of a prospective study. Gastroenterology 1991;100(1):182–8.

9. Perrillo RP, Gish R, Falck-Ytter YT. American Gastroenterological Association Institute technical review on prevention and treatment of hepatitis B virus reactivation during immunosuppressive drug therapy. Gastroenterology 2015;148(1):221–44.

10. Awerkiew S, Daumer M, Reiser M, et al. Reactivation of an occult hepatitis B virus escape mutant in an anti-HBs positive, anti-HBc negative lymphoma patient. J Clin Virol 2007;38(1):83–6.

11. Ceccarelli L, Salpini R, Sarmati L, et al. Late hepatitis B virus reactivation after lamivudine prophylaxis interruption in an anti-HBs-positive and anti-HBc-negative patient treated with rituximab-containing therapy. J Infect 2012;65(2):180–3.

12. Hui CK, Cheung WW, Zhang HY, et al. Kinetics and risk of de novo hepatitis B infection in HBsAg-negative patients undergoing cytotoxic chemotherapy. Gastroenterology 2006;131(1):59–68.

13. Ferreira R, Carvalheiro J, Torres J, et al. Fatal hepatitis B reactivation treated with entecavir in an isolated anti-HBs positive lymphoma patient: a case report and literature review. Saudi J Gastroenterol 2012;18(4):277–81.

14. Law MF, Ho R, Cheung CK, et al. Prevention and management of hepatitis B virus reactivation in patients with hematological malignancies treated with anticancer therapy. World J Gastroenterol 2016;22(28):6484–500.

Screening and Prophylaxis to Prevent Hepatitis B Reactivation

Transplant Recipients

Joe Sasadeusz, MBBS, PhD, FRACP[a,b,*], Andrew Grigg, MBBS, FRACP, FRCPA, MD[c],
Peter D. Hughes, MBBS, PhD, FRACP[b,d], Seng Lee Lim, MBBS, FRACP, FRCP, MD[e],
Michaela Lucas, MD, Dr Med, FRACP, FRCPA[f],
Geoff McColl, MBBS, BMedSc, MEd, PhD, FRACP[g],
Sue Anne McLachlan, MBBS, MSc, FRACP[h], Marion G. Peters, MD, MBBS[i],
Nicholas Shackel, MB, FRACP, PhD[j], Monica Slavin, MBBS, FRACP, MD[d,k],
Vijaya Sundararajan, MD, MPH[b,h,l], Alexander Thompson, PhD, FRACP[b,h],
Joseph Doyle, MBBS, MPH, PhD, FRACP, FAFPHM[m,n], James Rickard, PhD[c],
Peter De Cruz, MBBS, PhD, FRACP[b], Robert G. Gish, MD[o,1],
Kumar Visvanathan, MBBS, PhD, FRACP[b,h,1]

KEYWORDS

- Hepatitis B • Transplantation • Reactivation • Transmission • Prophylaxis

[a] Peter Doherty Institute for Infection and Immunity, Elizabeth Street, Melbourne, Victoria 3000, Australia; [b] University of Melbourne, Grattan Street, Parkville, Victoria 3010, Australia; [c] Olivia Newton John Cancer Research Institute, Austin Hospital, 145 Studley Road, Heidelberg, Victoria 3084, Australia; [d] Royal Melbourne Hospital, 300 Grattan Street, Parkville, Victoria 3050, Australia; [e] National University of Singapore, 21 Lower Kent Ridge Road, Singapore 119077, Singapore; [f] University of Western Australia, 35 Stirling Highway, Crawley, Western Australia 6009, Australia; [g] University of Queensland Oral Health Centre, 288 Herston Road, Queensland 4006, Australia; [h] St Vincent's Hospital, 41 Victoria Street, Fitzroy, Victoria 3065, Australia; [i] University of California, San Francisco, S357 Parnassus Avenue, San Francisco, CA 94143, USA; [j] Ingham Institute, 1 Campbell Street, Liverpool, Sydney, New South Wales 2170, Australia; [k] Victorian Comprehensive Cancer Centre, 305 Grattan Street, Melbourne, Victoria 3000, Australia; [l] Department of Public Health, La Trobe University, Plenty Road, Bundoora, Victoria 3086, Australia; [m] The Alfred and Monash University, 85 Commercial Road, Melbourne, Victoria 3004, Australia; [n] Burnet Institute, 85 Commercial Road, Melbourne, Victoria 3004, Australia; [o] Division of Gastroenterology and Hepatology, Department of Medicine, Stanford University, Stanford University Medical Center, 300 Pasteur Drive, Stanford, CA 94305, USA
[1] Co-Senior Authors.
* Corresponding author. Peter Doherty Institute for Infection and Immunity, 792 Elizabeth Street, Melbourne, Victoria 3000, Australia.
E-mail address: j.sasadeusz@mh.org.au

Clin Liver Dis 23 (2019) 493–509
https://doi.org/10.1016/j.cld.2019.04.010
1089-3261/19/© 2019 Elsevier Inc. All rights reserved.

liver.theclinics.com

KEY POINTS

- The immunosuppression associated with transplantation may result in reactivation of hepatitis B in individuals with markers of hepatitis B exposure.
- Individuals at risk of reactivation should be given antiviral prophylaxis, ideally using a drug with a high barrier to resistance.
- Because many transplant recipients suffer renal impairment and tenofovir disoproxil fumarate is nephrotoxic, entecavir or tenofovir alafenamide is preferred.
- Individuals who are susceptible and receive a donation from an individual with markers of hepatitis B may suffer hepatitis B transmission.

INTRODUCTION

As is discussed in Joe Sasadeusz and colleagues' article, "Screening and Prophylaxis to Prevent Hepatitis B Reactivation: Introduction and Immunology," in this issue, immunosuppression or treatment with hepatitis C virus (HCV) direct-acting antivirals may result in loss of immune control of hepatitis B virus (HBV) with recurrence of high-level viral replication, a phenomenon known as reactivation, which can be associated with very high alanine aminotransferase (ALT) levels with hepatic decompensation and death in some patients.[1] We focus here on guidelines for patients with HBV infection, both chronic HBV and occult hepatitis B infection as defined in that earlier article, who are transplant recipients. We discuss screening and prophylaxis in patients who would not normally require treatment for chronic HBV and do not directly address management of patients who do need ongoing treatment because well-developed guidelines for treatment of those patients are available elsewhere.[2]

MANAGEMENT OF HEPATITIS B IN LIVER TRANSPLANT RECIPIENTS

During liver transplantation, the HBV status of both the donor and recipient needs to be considered. There is consensus that in liver transplants in which recipients and/or donors are hepatitis B core antibody-positive (anti-HBc positive) there is a requirement for long-term HBV prophylaxis in recipients along with immunosuppression, but no need for hepatitis B immune globulin (HBIG). HBV vaccination of all patients on the transplant waiting list who are negative for all 3 HBV seromarkers should be considered; it could potentially be based on a threshold titer of hepatitis B surface antibody (anti-HBs), the lower effective limit of which is yet to be determined.[3,4] In the absence of prophylaxis, the risk of developing hepatitis B infection is greatest when the recipient is HBV naïve but the donor has anti-HBc (47.8%). When the recipient has anti-HBc, the risk is reduced to 15.2% without prophylaxis; and if the recipient has anti-HBs, the risk is further decreased to 9.7%. The addition of oral nucleos(t)ide prophylaxis in these patients can reduce this risk to 12%, 3.4%, and 0%, respectively (**Table 1**).[5,6]

This variability in risk suggests that there may be a threshold level of anti-HBs required to protect against the development of hepatitis B in liver transplant recipients. However, early studies of passive immunization with HBIG did not clearly define the threshold anti-HBs titer for immune control and cutoffs varied between 20, 100, 200, and 1000 IU/L.[7] Although the risk of recurrence after prophylaxis with HBIG decreases to 20%, the addition of nucleos(t)ide analogues can further decrease the risk to less than 10%.[8,9]

Studies have also shown that oral antiviral therapy alone, using a nucleos(t)ide analogue with a high barrier to resistance, may prevent reactivation and obviate the

Table 1
Risk of de novo hepatitis B in recipients of anti-HBc–positive solid organs

Recipient Status	Naïve	Anti-HBc–positive Anti-HBs⁻	Anti-HBc–positive Anti-HBs⁺	Anti-HBc⁻ Anti-HBs⁺
No prophylaxis	>40%	13%	<2%	10%
With prophylaxis	12%	<4%	<2%	<2%
Risk	High	Intermediate	Low	Intermediate

Data from Jimenez-Perez M, Gonzalez-Grande R, Mostazo Torres J, et al. Management of hepatitis B virus infection after liver transplantation. World J Gastroenterol 2015;21(42):12083-12090.

need for HBIG. A study that assessed the long-term outcome of an HBIG-free regimen consisting only of entecavir in a cohort of 265 chronic HBV liver transplant recipients found it to be highly effective for prevention of HBV reactivation, with a 91.7% HBV surface antigen (HBsAg)-negative rate and a 100% HBV DNA undetectable rate at 8 years after transplantation.[10] Long-term survival was 85% at 9 years, with no retransplantation or deaths related to HBV reactivation.

The patients most likely to benefit from HBIG in combination with antiviral therapy are liver transplant recipients who are HBV DNA positive before liver transplant (hazard ratio [HR], 0.42; 95% confidence interval [CI], 0.32–0.52) compared with patients with undetectable HBV DNA (HR, 0.06; 95% CI, -0.03 to 0.14).[11] An HBIG only solution is cost prohibitive in the long term and a historical protocol would use initial HBIG combined with long-term antiviral prophylaxis or antiviral prophylaxis alone.[12] The net benefit of HBIG in addition to antiviral prophylaxis in anti-HBc–positive donors is marginal, with 1 study showing a de novo recurrence rate of 2.7% with lamivudine alone with no significant difference seen in the combination HBIG/lamivudine group, where the recurrence rate was 3.6%.[13] Although the routine use of lamivudine has been demonstrated to be effective, this agent has been replaced in clinical practice by the use of entecavir or tenofovir (either tenofovir disoproxil fumarate [TDF] or tenofovir alafenamide [TAF]) with their superior high genetic barriers to resistance without HBIG.[14,15] Stratification of risk based on DNA levels and HBsAg has been proposed in clinical care. For example, if the recipient has fulminant liver failure and the donor has a normally functioning liver with low HBV DNA expression, short-term prophylaxis with HBIG may be a clinically appropriate option to enable a life-saving procedure. HBIG combination therapy has also been shown to be beneficial in patients with prior exposure to lamivudine. Interestingly, studies of 3-year survival found that the addition of HBIG to antiviral therapy improved survival (HR, 0.17; 95% CI, 0.05–0.28), but the same benefit was not seen after 1 year or 5 years in other studies.[11]

A study of a new treatment regimen compared with the European dosing schedule of entecavir with HBIG did not demonstrate any difference when HBIG was added during transplantation, with a lower HBIG dose 1 week after surgery and slightly higher doses from 6 weeks to 12 months.[14] Patients with hepatocellular carcinoma (HCC) are at greatest risk of HBV recurrence and should receive HBIG routinely, especially if they have experienced immune reactivation through treatment for HCC. In these patients, there may be a role for HBIG regardless of the HBV DNA status. A study of 30 patients followed for at least 6 years after liver transplantation found that 6 patients had HBV recurrence, 1 patient after HBIG interruption and 5 patients after stopping both HBIG and antiviral therapy. Only 3 patients restarted HBV "prophylaxis" because of persistent HBV replication, and all 6 patients achieved optimal control of HBV infection without any clinical events.[16] In a larger study in which 296 patients were followed for a mean of 46 months, HBV recurrence was associated with the presence of HCC before transplantation (HR, 12.3, 95% CI, 1.5–101.1; P = .02). In addition, survival was significantly better in patients receiving entecavir or tenofovir than in those receiving lamivudine or adefovir, in combination with HBIG.[17] Furthermore, entecavir and tenofovir are now preferred because outcomes, including liver histology and patient and graft survival, are superior when compared with lamivudine.[15]

Recommendations for the Screening and Management of Liver Transplant Recipients

- In recipients of an anti-HBc–positive graft or anti-HBc–positive recipients of an anti-HBc–negative graft:
  - Start prophylaxis with a drug with a high barrier to resistance; because many transplant recipients suffer renal impairment and TDF is nephrotoxic, entecavir or TAF is preferred.
  - There is no role for HBIG.

MANAGEMENT OF HEPATITIS B IN RENAL TRANSPLANT RECIPIENTS

Screening Before Transplantation

- All patients with chronic kidney disease should have testing for HBsAg, anti-HBc, and anti-HBs. Patients testing positive for anti-HBc but negative for HBsAg should also have HBV DNA testing by nucleic acid testing to detect occult HBV infection. Screening for HBV should be conducted regularly while the patient is on the transplant waiting list because they can become infected while on dialysis or lose vaccine-related immunity. There are no data to support vaccination of anti-HBc–positive patients

---

Kidneys from deceased donors should be tested for HBsAg, anti-HBs, and anti-HBc IgG. Nucleic acid testing (NAT) for HBV, hepatitis C virus, and human immunodeficiency virus (HIV) before transplantation should also be conducted for donors with high-risk behaviors.

Living donors account for around 30% of kidney transplants. These donors should undergo serum testing of HBsAg, anti-HBs, and anti-HBc. Donors with high-risk behaviors should also undergo regular NAT testing for HBV, hepatitis C virus, and HIV with repeat testing in the last one to 2 weeks before living donation. NAT testing for HIV one to 2 weeks before transplantation was recommended by the US Centers for Disease Control and Prevention in 2011 and is becoming more common in patients with high-risk behaviors.[18] However, a review by participants at the Optimal Testing of the Live Organ Donor Consensus Conference in 2013 concluded that NAT testing for hepatitis C virus, HBV, and HIV should not be required for live donor evaluation.[19] Several scenarios are possible from the combinations of serology between donor and recipient.

Hepatitis B Surface Antigen–Positive Recipients

In patients in the immune control phase immunosuppression confers a risk of reactivation with increased HBV DNA, hepatic flares and hepatic decompensation or death in some patients.[20] A metaanalysis of 6 studies with 6050 patients compared death and graft loss rates between HBsAg-positive and HBsAg-negative recipients.[21] The analysis found that the relative risk of all-cause mortality was 2.49 (95% CI, 1.64–3.78) and the relative risk of allograft loss was 1.44 (95% CI, 1.02–2.04) in HBsAg-positive recipients. The rate of liver-related mortality is further increased if the recipient has detectable HBV DNA or is hepatitis B e antigen (HBeAg) positive.[22] Significantly worse outcomes are seen compared with matched patients on hemodialysis.[23] In addition, 85% of HBsAg-positive recipients had histologic progression and 28% developed cirrhosis, of whom 23% had developed HCC at 5 years after transplantation.[24] Finally, such patients can occasionally develop fibrosing cholestatic hepatitis, a rapidly progressive form of HBV.[25]

As a result of all these factors, historically transplantation into HBsAg-positive patients was considered an absolute contraindication. In the era of antiviral therapy, this scenario has changed. In a metaanalysis of 14 cohort studies evaluating lamivudine prophylaxis in 184 renal transplant recipients, 87% had detectable HBV DNA, 64% had elevated ALT, and 60% were HBeAg positive.[26] All patients started treatment with lamivudine between 8 and 156 months after transplantation and continued for between 6 and 35 months. The mean rate of HBV DNA negativity was 91% (95% CI, 86%–96%), HBeAg clearance was 27% (95% CI, 16%–39%), and ALT returned to normal levels in 81% of patients (95% CI, 70%–92%). Lamivudine resistance was seen in 18% of patients (95% CI, 10%–37%).

The timing of antivirals after transplant has been studied in a group of HBsAg-positive Korean patients.[27] Six patients were treated with lamivudine after an increase in ALT of 2 times the upper limit of normal. Before undergoing transplantation, they all had normal ALT, were HBV DNA negative, and had mild hepatitis; 5 of the patients were HBeAg negative. After transplantation, ALT increased to a mean level of 186 U/L after a mean 9.8 months. Two of the 5 patients who were HBeAg negative before transplantation and seroreverted to HBeAg positivity. All patients became HBV DNA positive; 4 had moderate to severe hepatitis, 1 had fibrosing cholestatic hepatitis, and 1 developed cirrhosis. In the same study, 10 patients received prophylaxis before or at the time of transplant and before an increase in ALT. Four of these patients were HBeAg positive; 7 were HBV DNA positive. After 10 months, 1 patient had a mild rebound of ALT. All 7 of the patients who were HBV DNA positive became negative.

Entecavir, a more potent drug with a high barrier to resistance, has also been used as prophylaxis in renal transplant recipients.[28] In 27 HBsAg-positive renal transplant recipients, 9 had previously received lamivudine without documented evidence of resistance and 18 were nucleoside analogue naïve. All patients received 0.5 mg entecavir daily and were followed to week 104. There was a rapid viral response to entecavir with all patients becoming HBV DNA negative at the end of follow-up, with no change in the glomerular filtration rate or lactic acidosis or myopathy. This cohort was compared with a historical control group of 19 patients treated with lamivudine, of which only 63% were negative at 104 weeks, suggesting the superiority of entecavir.

Recent data in the era of effective antiviral therapy have shown that patient and graft survival in patients with compensated cirrhosis is similar to that in noncirrhotic patients.[29]

Recommendations for Hepatitis B Surface Antigen–Positive Renal Transplant Recipients

- All HBsAg-positive individuals should undergo review by a specialist in viral hepatitis and should undergo fibrosis assessment, usually with noninvasive means such as transient elastography.

- Treat with oral prophylactic antiviral therapy at the time of transplantation to prevent reactivation.

- Ideally, patients should receive a drug with a high barrier to resistance; TAF and entecavir are preferred given that TDF is nephrotoxic.

- Interferon should not be used after transplantation owing to the high risk of rejection.[30]

- There is no consensus on the duration of antiviral prophylaxis, but it is probably required lifelong owing to a high relapse rate when prophylaxis is ceased.

- Cirrhotic patients should be considered for renal transplant on a case by case basis, and decompensated cirrhotics should be considered for combined renal and liver transplantation.

- There are no data to support vaccination of anti-HBc–positive patients.

- Vaccinate all susceptible patients for HBV if the HBV panel is negative for all 3 markers.

Anti-Hepatitis B Core Antibody–Positive Renal Transplant Recipients

Recipients who are HBsAg negative and anti-HBc positive have an up to 5% risk of reactivation after renal transplantation unrelated to HBV DNA viral load before transplantation.[31–33] A retrospective study of 322 HBsAg-negative, anti-HBc–positive, HBV DNA-negative patients reviewed all kidney transplant recipients at the First Affiliated Hospital of Sun Yat-sen University in China between January 1998 and June 2008. From 2002 onward, patients were given lamivudine prophylaxis at 100 mg/d for 3 months as standard of care. The study found that 15 patients (4.7%) experienced reactivation, with serum HBsAg becoming positive in 13 of the 15 patients (86.7%) and serum HBV DNA becoming positive in 10 patients (66.7%); 12 patients (80%) developed liver function impairment.[34] In 60% of patients, the reactivation occurred in the first 6 months after transplantation and reactivation resulted in decreased patient but not graft survival. The risk of reactivation was higher in older recipients and those who received T-cell–depleting therapy and the risk was significantly lower in patients who received lamivudine. Patient survival was decreased (72.2% vs 91.5% at 5 years and 65% vs 84.5% at 10 years), although there was no difference in graft survival.

Recommendations for Anti-Hepatitis B Core Antibody–Positive Renal Transplant Recipients

- At present, there are insufficient data to recommend routine prophylaxis in this group, although it can be considered in higher risk groups such as those receiving T-cell–depleting therapy and those with negative anti-HBs levels.

- If anti-HBs positive, monitor anti-HBs titers every 3 months for the first year after transplantation, then every 6 to 12 months thereafter.

- Commence antiviral therapy if anti-HBs falls below 10 IU/mL or if HBsAg or DNA becomes detectable.

- If anti-HBs negative, give antiviral prophylaxis, preferably with a drug with a high barrier to resistance such as TAF or entecavir; lamivudine can be considered in resource-constrained countries.

- Continue prophylaxis for at least 12 months and until rejection and immunosuppression are minimized.

- There are no data to support HBV vaccination of anti-HBc–positive patients.

Hepatitis B Surface Antigen–Positive Renal Transplant Donors

There is a high rate of transmission from an HBsAg-positive donor to a susceptible recipient.[35,36] Sixty percent of patients who acquire HBV infection after transplantation will die from liver disease.[37] Transplantation of kidneys from HBsAg-positive patients is not performed in the United States or Australia, but is conducted in some other countries under certain circumstances. Outcomes are variable, but may be favorable in carefully selected recipients. In a prospective Thai study of 43 recipients with an anti-HBs titer of greater than 100 U/L (an immunity level that was possibly vaccine induced after 4 double immunologic doses of vaccine) who received kidneys from HBsAg-positive donors,[38] only one of the HBsAg-positive donors was HBV DNA-positive by polymerase chain reaction, and 100% were NAT positive and HBeAg negative. Lamivudine prophylaxis (100 mg/d for 12 months) was provided to 23 of the 43 recipients of organs from HBsAg-positive donors (lamivudine alone to 21 and lamivudine combined with 1 dose of HBIG to 2 patients); the remaining 20 patients did not receive prophylactic treatment. No recipients developed markers of HBV infection, including HBsAg, anti-HBc, HBeAg or HBV DNA or evidence of hepatitis. There was no difference in patient or graft survival compared with a control group of 86 recipients who received kidneys from an HBsAg-negative donor.[38]

Jiang and colleagues[39] compared 65 patients who received kidney transplants from HBsAg-positive donors to 308 patients who received organs from HBsAg-negative donors. All recipients were anti-HBs positive and 33 patients were also anti-HBc positive. The 58 patients who received kidneys from donors who were HBsAg-positive and HBV DNA-negative were treated with HBIG at surgery and 1 month later. The 7 patients who received kidneys from HBsAg-positive, HBV DNA-positive donors received HBIG (400 U weekly for 3 months) and lamivudine (100 mg/d for 6 months). All 7 recipients who were anti-HBc-negative pre-transplant and received organs from HBsAg-positive donors became anti-HBc positive, indicating an immunologic response to the HBV exposure and HBV infection. One patient each in the groups receiving kidneys from HBsAg-positive and HBsAg-negative donors and each became HBsAg-positive, but no patient became HBV DNA positive or HBeAg positive. The HBsAg-positive donor for the patient who became HBsAg positive was HBV DNA negative and the recipient's anti-HBs titer was 64 U/mL at the time of transplant. There were no cases of severe hepatitis and no difference in survival between recipients of HBsAg-negative and HBsAg-positive donors.

Fatal fulminant HBV infection has been reported 16 months after kidney transplant from a donor who was HBsAg positive transplanted to an immunized anti-HBs–positive recipient.[40] The recipient also received prophylaxis with HBIG and received a supplemental HBV vaccination. An extensively mutated virus was found post mortem.

Recommendations for Hepatitis B Surface Antigen–Positive Donors

- In general, HBsAg-positive donors are not recommended without fully informed consent for HBsAg-negative recipients.

  ○ Donation from HBsAg-positive donors to HBsAg-positive recipients can take place under institutional protocols.

- HBsAg-positive donors can occasionally be considered under exceptional circumstances if they are HBV DNA negative and the recipient has protective levels of anti-HBs (ideally >100 IU/mL).

- If HBsAg-positive donors are used, then recipients should be given antiviral prophylaxis for 12 months from the time of transplantation. Ideally, this should be with an agent with a high barrier to resistance. Given the renal issues with TDF, TAF or entecavir is preferred; lamivudine can be considered in resource-constrained countries.

- There is no role for HBIG in this clinical setting.

Anti-Hepatitis B Core Antibody–Positive Renal Transplant Donors

In anti-HBc–positive donors, the risk of transmission depends on the organ transplanted, recipient immunity, and prophylaxis. The greatest risk is in liver transplantation (46% risk of virus transmission without prophylaxis) with 77% transmission in nonimmune recipients.[41] Compared with this, the risk with kidney transplantation is lower, and even less risk is associated with transplantation of thoracic organs. It follows, therefore, that guidelines for HBV prophylaxis should be organ specific. Different definitions of transmission have been studied. A review of 1385 patients in 9 studies examined seroconversion of HBV markers (HBsAg, anti-HBs, or anti-HBc) in previously seronegative patients with end-stage renal disease after transplantation.[42] Donors who were HBsAg negative/anti-HBc positive, irrespective of anti-HBs status, were included. Four patients converted to HBsAg positive, one of whom was anti-HBc positive before transplantation, resulting in an HBsAg seroconversion rate of 0.28% (95% CI, 0.006–0.570). Anti-HBc seroconversion occurred in 32 patients, a rate of 2.3%; 2 of these patients were also anti-HBs positive and 9 were reported to have anti-HBs seroconversion, although this factor was not reported in most papers. None of the patients had symptomatic hepatitis and there was no increase in mortality or decrease in graft survival. Data also show that the risk of HBV reactivation is lower in recipients with higher levels of immune control, as signified by higher anti-HBs levels or titers.[43]

The role of prophylaxis strategies has received very limited study. In a study of 46 recipients of anti-HBc–positive kidneys, anti-HBs–negative recipients received lamivudine prophylaxis (150 mg/d) for 1 year without HBIG.[44] No prophylaxis was provided to anti-HBs–positive recipients. After a median follow-up of 36 months (range, 6–66 months), no patients developed HBV DNA positivity or seroconverted to HBsAg-positive or anti-HBs positive. However, HBV serology and DNA were only tested in those who developed abnormal liver enzymes. There were no data provided regarding anti-HBc conversion, the best marker of HBV infection. The study concluded that kidneys from anti-HBc–positive donors can be transplanted into anti-HBs–negative recipients with lamivudine prophylaxis without HBIG. Another study found that, of 54 patients who received anti-HBc–positive kidneys, the 18 patients who received prophylaxis with single-dose 2000 IU HBIG did not undergo seroconversion. Of the 36 patients who did not receive prophylaxis, 1 patient became HBsAg positive and 5 patients became anti-HBc positive.[45]

Recommendations for Recipients of Kidneys from Anti-Hepatitis B Core Antibody–Positive Donors

- Vaccinate all patients on renal transplant waiting list or those undergoing renal dialysis, aiming for an anti-HBs titer of greater than 100 IU/mL in patients who are seronegative for all 3 HBV tests.
- Test for HBV DNA by NAT in anti-HBc–positive donors.
- Although transmission rates are low, data suggest a low risk in susceptible individuals of transmission of this virus, which has oncogenic potential and is present lifelong if there is HBsAg positivity or anti-HBc positivity; accordingly, preventive strategies should be considered.
- It is unclear which, if any, strategy is preferred to prevent transmission.
- Consider the use of antiviral prophylaxis in anti-HBs–negative recipients with daily TAF or entecavir, adjusted for renal function until 12 months after transplantation if there are no financial constraints; lamivudine can be considered in resource-constrained countries.

HEPATITIS B REACTIVATION IN HEMATOPOIETIC STEM CELL TRANSPLANTATION

Hematopoietic stem cell transplantation (HSCT) has become the standard curative treatment for various hematologic and oncologic malignancies and some nonmalignant diseases. In principle, very high-dose chemotherapy is used to treat the underlying disease, resulting in ablation of the bone marrow, which then requires rescue by stem cells. Patients undergoing HSCT are among the most immunosuppressed populations. HSCT can be either allogeneic (allografts), where individuals receive stem cells from another individual, or autologous (autografts), where they are rescued with their own stored stem cells. It is estimated that more than 50,000 HSCT procedures are performed annually worldwide, one-half of which are allogeneic and one-half autologous. Recipients of allografts may develop graft-versus-host disease (GvHD), which requires ongoing immunosuppression, but also results in further immunosuppression itself.

Given the necessity of HSCT to improve the overall survival of patients owing to their underlying disease, HBsAg positivity should not be considered a contraindication to HSCT. Donor HBV status also has a bearing on outcome, so donor and recipient serostatus need to be considered as a pair, resulting in several scenarios for their combined HBV status and subsequent management. It should also be remembered that elevated liver enzymes can also be caused by GvHD, other viruses including herpes viruses, and drug toxicity in addition to HBV. Data for HBV reactivation associated with HSCT are very limited. **Fig. 1** shows a suggested pathway for assessing HBV status in patients donating or undergoing HSCT.

Allogeneic Hematopoietic Stem Cell Transplantation in a Chronically Infected Recipient (Hepatitis B Surface Antigen)

In allograft recipients, HBV reactivation has been reported in more than 50% of individuals who are HBsAg positive.[46–48] The risk of fulminant hepatic failure and death among patients who are persistently HBsAg positive after transplantation is approximately 12%.[49] Long-term sequelae in a study of 82 HBsAg-positive patients described a 9.8% cumulative probability of cirrhosis within 7 years of receiving HSCT.[50] HBV-related hepatitis was reported in 19.5% of HBsAg-positive patients (n = 16) and 0.8% of anti-HBc–positive patients (n = 2). Ten of the patients with HBV-related hepatitis had received HBV prophylaxis for 6 to 12 months after transplantation.

Another study of 40 patients demonstrated that HBV prophylaxis decreases reactivation in recipients of allogenic HSCT.[51] The probability of survival without hepatitis owing to exacerbation of HBV was lower in HBsAg-positive patients receiving lamivudine than in those without prophylaxis (54.3% vs 94.1%; $P = .002$). In this study, HSCT recipients receiving prophylactic lamivudine also had a much higher cumulative incidence of sustained HBsAg clearance compared with HSCT recipients without prophylaxis ($P = .011$).

A retrospective review of 216 patients receiving either lamivudine (n = 119) or entecavir (n = 97) found that entecavir treatment was associated with a lower cumulative rate of severe HBV-related hepatitis than lamivudine.[52] Drug resistance mutations were found in 25 patients receiving lamivudine and 1 patient receiving entecavir.

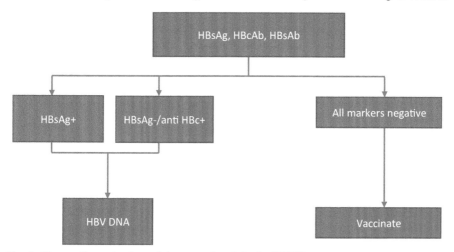

Fig. 1. Diagnostic evaluation of donor and recipient of HSCT.

HBsAg seroclearance was seen in 84.2% of patients (16 of 19) in the lamivudine group and 87.5% of patients (14 of 16) in the entecavir group ($P = .781$). Median times to serologic clearance of HBsAg after transplantation were 2.3 months in the lamivudine group versus 2.5 months in the entecavir group ($P = .745$). All patients who achieved HBsAg seroclearance remained HBsAg negative and HBV DNA undetectable to the end of follow-up, and none developed HBV reactivation.

Another phenomenon reported in allogeneic transplant recipients is adoptive transfer of HBV immune control, whereby stem cells from a patient with resolved HBV can result in HBsAg clearance owing to the transmission of immune control from the donor.[52,53]

Recommendations for Hepatitis B Surface Antigen–Positive Recipients of Hematopoietic Stem Cell Transplants

- Try to identify a donor who is anti-HBc and anti-HBs positive to facilitate donor-derived immune control, although this is not usually feasible. Anti-HBc positivity may indicate enhanced donor-derived immune control, provided the donor is HBV DNA negative.
- Request testing for HBV DNA by NAT in the donor.
- Assess liver fibrosis (either by the aspartate aminotransferase platelet ratio index, the Fibrosis-4 calculator, liver biopsy, transient elastography, or noninvasive serum markers).
- Provide antiviral prophylaxis, ideally with a drug with a high barrier to resistance such as TAF, TDF, or ETV. Because many transplant recipients have renal impairment, entecavir or TAF is preferred. Lamivudine can be considered in resource-constrained countries.
- Start prophylaxis at the time of conditioning and continue for at least 12 months after stopping all immunosuppressive treatment, and indefinitely for patients deemed at the greatest risk of reactivation (those with ongoing GvHD or immunosuppression).

ALLOGENEIC HEMATOPOIETIC STEM CELL TRANSPLANTATION IN A RECIPIENT WITH RESOLVED HEPATITIS B VIRUS INFECTION (HEPATITIS B SURFACE ANTIGEN NEGATIVE AND ANTI–HEPATITIS B CORE ANTIGEN POSITIVE)

Patients with resolved HBV are at risk of reverse seroconversion to HBsAg positivity owing to loss of immune control after transplantation. A retrospective review of HBV serology in 14 anti-HBs–positive individuals receiving HSCT from anti-HBs–negative donors found that a decrease in anti-HBs can predict HBV reactivation.[54] In 12 patients, the anti-HBs titer decreased to less than 10 IU/mL. Seven patients had reverse seroconversion to HBsAg positivity after loss of anti-HBs antibodies and all had chronic GvHD. Of these, 5 patients seroconverted back to HBsAg negativity and 2 had ongoing chronic infection. Rates of between 14.0% and 85.7% have been reported with median follow-up periods of between 16 and 53 months; studies with longer follow-up periods have reported higher reactivation rates.[55,56] There are no data to support vaccination of anti-HBc–positive patients to prevent reactivation. Risk factors for reverse seroconversion include the following[57–59]:

- Low anti-HBs level (<10 IU/mL);
- Decreasing anti-HBs titers;
- Extensive chronic GvHD;
- Matched unrelated donors;
- Corticosteroid exposure;
- Length of cyclosporine therapy;
- Rituximab therapy;
- Donor immunity; and
- GvHD.

One study showed that donor immune control was associated with decreased risk of HBV reactivation in HBsAg-negative and anti-HBc–positive HSCT recipients when compared with nonimmune donors (HR, 0.12; 95% CI, 0.02–0.96; P = .045), although it did not prevent it altogether.[59] Another study attempted to determine whether vaccine-induced anti-HBs response or increased titers in the recipient could prevent reactivation. This study compared 21 individuals who underwent an HBV vaccination course after cessation of immunosuppression with 25 nonvaccinated transplant recipients. Vaccine resulted in a positive anti-HBs titer in 9 of 21 patients. None of the vaccinated patients developed reverse seroconversion, whereas 12 of the 25 nonvaccinated recipients did develop reverse seroconversion, suggesting that immune control can be augmented by vaccine.[60]

Recommendations for Hepatitis B Surface Antigen–Negative/Anti-Hepatitis B Core Antigen–Positive Hematopoietic Stem Cell Transplant Recipients

- Perform HBV DNA NAT test; if positive, treat as is recommended for HBsAg-positive patients.

- Attempt to find donor with vaccine-induced immunity or HBV exposure who is HBV DNA negative and HBsAg negative, although this is frequently not possible.

- Consider vaccination if the donor is HBV naïve and there is time to initiate vaccination.

- Start prophylaxis, ideally with a drug with a high barrier to resistance such as entecavir, TDF, or TAF.

- The ideal duration of prophylaxis is not known. Cessation can be considered if HBsAg seroconversion occurs and all immunosuppression is ceased in the absence of GvHD.

- There are current data to support HBV vaccination of anti-HBc–positive patients, which suggests that vaccination may enhance immune control.

ALLOGENEIC HEMATOPOIETIC STEM CELL TRANSPLANTATION FROM A DONOR WITH PRIOR HEPATITIS B VIRUS INFECTION (HEPATITIS B SURFACE ANTIGEN NEGATIVE AND ANTI–HEPATITIS B CORE ANTIGEN POSITIVE)

There is very little evidence regarding HBV transmission after HSCT from a donor with exposure to HBV infection manifested by anti-HBc. There is known to be a much smaller risk of HBV transmission from a donor whose is HBsAg negative but positive for anti-HBc, especially if they are anti-HBs positive and the donor is unlikely to be viremic or to transmit HBV through hematopoietic stem cell infusion. Stem cells and bone marrow–derived cells are not considered sanctuaries for HBV infection. Negative HBV DNA in the donor serum and hematopoietic cells should virtually eliminate the risk of transmission of HBV; there is a negligible risk of transmission from a donor who is anti-HBs and anti-HBc positive.[49] In an early study, a graft from a donor who was HBsAg negative with prior exposure resulted in transient HBsAg positivity in 1 patient and chronic HBsAg positivity in another. In another small series, none of 5 HBV-naïve recipients of HSCT from an anti-HBc–positive donor who were not given antiviral prophylaxis developed hepatitis, and 1 patient became anti-HBc positive without reactivation.[61] Another study of 17 HBsAg-negative, anti-HBc–positive allogenic HSCTs were performed in 13 HBV-naïve children. Four of the donors were also HBsAg positive. Peritransplant management included various combinations of vaccination, polyvalent immune globulin, HBIG, and lamivudine prophylaxis for between 3 and 8 months in 8 cases. No cases of HBV transmission were observed after a median follow-up period of 22 months.[62] In a further study from Turkey of 7 HBV marker-naïve recipients receiving a bone marrow transplant from HBsAg-negative, anti-HBc–positive donors, 1 patient developed HBsAg with an elevation of ALT.[63]

> **Recommendations for Hepatitis B Surface Antigen–Negative/Anti–Hepatitis B Core Antigen–Positive Donors**
>
> - Perform HBV DNA by NAT to exclude occult HBV; if positive, start prophylaxis as if the patient is HBsAg positive.
> - If possible, test the graft for HBV DNA.
> - Given the very limited data suggesting the potential for transmission in this setting and the severity of immunosuppression, it is suggested to give antiviral prophylaxis regardless of HBV DNA level and continue for at least 12 months after transplantation and until the patient has completed all immunosuppressive treatment with no GvHD.
> - Ideally, use a drug with a high barrier to resistance; because many transplant recipients have renal impairment and TDF is nephrotoxic, entecavir or TAF is preferred; lamivudine could be considered in resource-constrained countries.
> - Consider HBIG at the time of infusion of the graft.

ALLOGENEIC HEMATOPOIETIC STEM CELL TRANSPLANTATION FROM A HEPATITIS B VIRUS–INFECTED DONOR (HEPATITIS B SURFACE ANTIGEN POSITIVE)

A retrospective review found that 24 of 2586 recipients (0.9%) of HSCT were from HBsAg-positive donors.[64] Eighteen of the 24 recipients were HBsAg negative; of those, 4 (22%) became HBsAg positive and 1 (5.5%) became a chronic carrier. Acute hepatitis occurred in 7 patients (29%); 8 patients (33%) developed chronic hepatitis. Fatal severe liver failure occurred in 5 recipients (21%), 4 of whom were due to HBV. Transmission rates were lower in anti-HBs–positive patients (10.0% vs 37.5%).

The development of HBV-related hepatitis is more likely to be associated with HSCT from a donor with precore/core promoter mutations compared with donors with other HBV variants (62.5% vs 0% ($P = .007$).[65] Recipients of HBsAg-positive HSCT were more likely to have anti-HBs than those receiving an HBsAg-negative transplant (50.0% vs 12.5%). HBV-related hepatitis is significantly less likely to develop in recipients of HBsAg-positive HSCT when both the donor and the recipient receive lamivudine prophylaxis compared with those who do not receive antiviral prophylaxis (48.0% vs 6.9%; HR, 7.27; 95% CI, 1.62–32.58; $P = .01$).[66] The rate of fatal hepatic failure has been reported to be higher in patients who did not receive prophylaxis (24% vs 0%; $P = .01$).

> **Recommendations for Hepatitis B Surface Antigen–Positive Donors**
>
> - Donate to an HBsAg-positive recipient if possible.
> - If the recipient is negative for all 3 biomarkers, attempt vaccination before conditioning. The schedule should be short interval (baseline, first, and second month intervals) using a high dose of vaccine (40 μg) to induce earlier immunization or use 2 dose vaccine Heplisav B (Dynavax, Emeryville, CA).
> - If the postvaccine anti-HBs titer is less than 10 IU/mL or the patient is unable to be vaccinated, give HBIG (0.06 mL/kg or 400 IU) immediately before HSCT.
> - If the donor is HBV DNA positive, give antiviral treatment until HBV DNA is negative by polymerase chain reaction if feasible.
> - Ideally, use a potent antiviral with a high barrier to resistance; entecavir or TAF is preferred owing to potential renal toxicity of TDF.
> - Reduce the stem cell harvest volume to the minimum possible and test the aliquot for HBV DNA before infusion.

- Start antiviral therapy in the recipient and continue until at least 12 months after transplantation and after cessation of immunosuppression with no GvHD.
- Monitor HBsAg, anti-HBs, liver enzymes, and HBV DNA every 3 months.
- Monitor carefully after cessation of antiviral for evidence of transmission.

AUTOLOGOUS HEMATOPOIETIC STEM CELL TRANSPLANTATION

Current guidelines do not differentiate between autologous and allogeneic HSCT. The risk of HBV reactivation is lower in autologous transplants, although there is heterogeneity between different patient populations. Consequently, we propose stratification of recommendations for prophylaxis. There are few data in this area. In 1 study of 137 patients undergoing autologous HSCT, 23 were HBsAg positive, 37 were anti-HBs positive (28 of whom were also anti-HBc positive), and 77 patients were negative for any HBV markers. Overall, the cumulative incidence rates of HBV-related hepatitis reactivation were 4.2%, 10.5%, and 11.7% at 3, 6, and 24 months, respectively. Seven patients (54%) developed severe hepatitis. Patients who were HBsAg positive before HSCT had a higher cumulative incidence of hepatitis owing to HBV reactivation (51.9%) than patients who were HBsAg negative (2.5%; $P < .0001$; n = 2). Nine patients (90%) with detectable serum HBV DNA and only 4 (4%) without detectable serum HBV DNA had hepatitis owing to HBV reactivation ($P < .0001$). In a more recent study, in 230 patients with multiple myeloma and resolved HBV who received an autograft, there were cumulative rates of reactivation at 2 and 5 years of 2% and 8%, respectively, with anti-HBs negativity being a predictive factor.[67] Approximately 60% of these patients received bortezomib, an agent known to result in viral reactivation, which may have resulted in higher rates in HBsAg-negative patients.

Recommendations for Autologous Hematopoietic Stem Cell Transplantation

- All HBsAg-positive patients should receive antiviral prophylaxis from conditioning until 12 months after transplantation, ideally using a drug with a high barrier to resistance; because many transplant recipients have renal impairment and TDF is nephrotoxic, entecavir or TAF is preferred.
- HBsAg-negative/anti-HBc–positive patients should have HBV DNA assessed by NAT.
- If positive, treat as if HBsAg positive.
- If negative, monitor carefully with 3 monthly tests of HBsAg, liver enzymes, and HBV DNA.
- Consider prophylaxis if bortezomib therapy is used.
- There are no data to support vaccination of anti-HBc–positive patients.

ACKNOWLEDGMENTS

Meetings to discuss and develop recommendations presented in this manuscript and medical writing services provided in the preparation of this manuscript were funded by Gilead Sciences. Neither the medical writer or Gilead in any way influenced the content or the conclusions of the position paper. None of the authors had any direct financial support from Gilead Sciences or any other companies.

REFERENCES

1. Lok AS, Liang RH, Chiu EK, et al. Reactivation of hepatitis B virus replication in patients receiving cytotoxic therapy. Report of a prospective study. Gastroenterology 1991;100(1):182–8.

2. Terrault NA, Lok ASF, McMahon BJ, et al. Update on prevention, diagnosis, and treatment of chronic hepatitis B: AASLD 2018 hepatitis B guidance. Hepatology 2018;67(4):1560–99.

3. Jankowska I, Pawlowska J, Teisseyre M, et al. Prevention of de novo hepatitis B virus infection by vaccination and high hepatitis B surface antibodies level in children receiving hepatitis B virus core antibody-positive living related donor liver: case reports. Transplant Proc 2007;39(5):1511–2.

4. Onoe T, Tahara H, Tanaka Y, et al. Prophylactic managements of hepatitis B viral infection in liver transplantation. World J Gastroenterol 2016;22(1):165–75.

5. Cholongitas E, Papatheodoridis GV, Burroughs AK. Liver grafts from anti-hepatitis B core positive donors: a systematic review. J Hepatol 2010;52(2):272–9.

6. Jimenez-Perez M, Gonzalez-Grande R, Mostazo Torres J, et al. Management of hepatitis B virus infection after liver transplantation. World J Gastroenterol 2015;21(42):12083–90.

7. Lin CC, Yong CC, Chen CL. Active vaccination to prevent de novo hepatitis B virus infection in liver transplantation. World J Gastroenterol 2015;21(39):11112–7.

8. Manne V, Allen RM, Saab S. Strategies for the prevention of recurrent hepatitis B virus infection after liver transplantation. Gastroenterol Hepatol (N Y) 2014;10(3):175–9.

9. Angus PW, McCaughan GW, Gane EJ, et al. Combination low-dose hepatitis B immune globulin and lamivudine therapy provides effective prophylaxis against posttransplantation hepatitis B. Liver Transpl 2000;6(4):429–33.

10. Fung J, Wong T, Chok K, et al. Long-term outcomes of entecavir monotherapy for chronic hepatitis B after liver transplantation: results up to 8 years. Hepatology 2017;66(4):1036–44.

11. Wang P, Tam N, Wang H, et al. Is hepatitis B immunoglobulin necessary in prophylaxis of hepatitis B recurrence after liver transplantation? A meta-analysis. PLoS One 2014;9(8):e104480.

12. Akcam AT, Ulku A, Rencuzogullari A, et al. Antiviral combination therapy with low-dose hepatitis B immunoglobulin for the prevention of hepatitis B virus recurrence in liver transplant recipients: a single-center experience. Transplant Proc 2015;47(5):1445–9.

13. Saab S, Dong MH, Joseph TA, et al. Hepatitis B prophylaxis in patients undergoing chemotherapy for lymphoma: a decision analysis model. Hepatology 2007;46(4):1049–56.

14. Chen G, Liu H, Hu ZQ, et al. A new scheme with infusion of hepatitis B immunoglobulin combined with entecavir for prophylaxis of hepatitis B virus recurrence among liver transplant recipients. Eur J Gastroenterol Hepatol 2015;27(8):901–6.

15. Fung J, Lo R, Chan SC, et al. Outcomes including liver histology after liver transplantation for chronic hepatitis B using oral antiviral therapy alone. Liver Transpl 2015;21(12):1504–10.

16. Lenci I, Baiocchi L, Tariciotti L, et al. Complete hepatitis B virus prophylaxis withdrawal in hepatitis B surface antigen-positive liver transplant recipients after long-term minimal immunosuppression. Liver Transpl 2016;22(9):1205–13.

17. Idilman R, Akyildiz M, Keskin O, et al. The long-term efficacy of combining nucleos(t)ide analog and low-dose hepatitis B immunoglobulin on post-transplant hepatitis B virus recurrence. Clin Transplant 2016;30(10):1216–21.

18. Centers for Disease Control and Prevention. HIV transmitted from a living organ donor — New York City, 2009. MMWR Morb Mortal Wkly Rep 2011;60(10):297–301.

19. Blumberg EA, Ison MG, Pruett TL, et al. Optimal testing of the live organ donor for blood-borne viral pathogens: the report of a consensus conference. Am J Transplant 2013;13(6):1405–15.

20. Degos F, Lugassy C, Degott C, et al. Hepatitis B virus and hepatitis B-related viral infection in renal transplant recipients. A prospective study of 90 patients. Gastroenterology 1988;94(1):151–6.

21. Fabrizi F, Martin P, Dixit V, et al. HBsAg seropositive status and survival after renal transplantation: meta-analysis of observational studies. Am J Transplant 2005; 5(12):2913–21.

22. Fairley CK, Mijch A, Gust ID, et al. The increased risk of fatal liver disease in renal transplant patients who are hepatitis Be antigen and/or HBV DNA positive. Transplantation 1991;52(3):497–500.

23. Parfrey PS, Forbes RD, Hutchinson TA, et al. The impact of renal transplantation on the course of hepatitis B liver disease. Transplantation 1985;39(6):610–5.

24. Fabrizi F, Lunghi G, Poordad FF, et al. Management of hepatitis B after renal transplantation: an update. J Nephrol 2002;15(2):113–22.

25. Chen CH, Chen PJ, Chu JS, et al. Fibrosing cholestatic hepatitis in a hepatitis B surface antigen carrier after renal transplantation. Gastroenterology 1994;107(5): 1514–8.

26. Fabrizi F, Dulai G, Dixit V, et al. Lamivudine for the treatment of hepatitis B virus-related liver disease after renal transplantation: meta-analysis of clinical trials. Transplantation 2004;77(6):859–64.

27. Han DJ, Kim TH, Park SK, et al. Results on preemptive or prophylactic treatment of lamivudine in HBsAg (+) renal allograft recipients: comparison with salvage treatment after hepatic dysfunction with HBV recurrence. Transplantation 2001; 71(3):387–94.

28. Hu TH, Tsai MC, Chien YS, et al. A novel experience of antiviral therapy for chronic hepatitis B in renal transplant recipients. Antivir Ther 2012;17(4):745–53.

29. Nho KW, Kim YH, Han DJ, et al. Kidney transplantation alone in end-stage renal disease patients with hepatitis B liver cirrhosis: a single-center experience. Transplantation 2015;99(1):133–8.

30. Rostaing L, Modesto A, Baron E, et al. Acute renal failure in kidney transplant patients treated with interferon alpha 2b for chronic hepatitis C. Nephron 1996; 74(3):512–6.

31. Knoll A, Pietrzyk M, Loss M, et al. Solid-organ transplantation in HBsAg-negative patients with antibodies to HBV core antigen: low risk of HBV reactivation. Transplantation 2005;79(11):1631–3.

32. Roberts RC, Lane C, Hatfield P, et al. All anti-HBc-positive, HBsAg-negative dialysis patients on the transplant waiting list should be regarded as at risk of hepatitis B reactivation post-renal transplantation–report of three cases from a single centre. Nephrol Dial Transplant 2006;21(11):3316–9.

33. Berger A, Preiser W, Kachel HG, et al. HBV reactivation after kidney transplantation. J Clin Virol 2005;32(2):162–5.

34. Chen GD, Gu JL, Qiu J, et al. Outcomes and risk factors for hepatitis B virus (HBV) reactivation after kidney transplantation in occult HBV carriers. Transpl Infect Dis 2013;15(3):300–5.

35. Wolf JL, Perkins HA, Schreeder MT, et al. The transplanted kidney as a source of hepatitis B infection. Ann Intern Med 1979;91(3):412–3.

36. Lutwick LI, Sywassink JM, Corry RJ, et al. The transmission of hepatitis B by renal transplantation. Clin Nephrol 1983;19(6):317–9.

37. Scott D, Mijch A, Lucas CR, et al. Hepatitis B and renal transplantation. Transplant Proc 1987;19(1 Pt 3):2159–60.
38. Chancharoenthana W, Townamchai N, Pongpirul K, et al. The outcomes of kidney transplantation in hepatitis B surface antigen (HBsAg)-negative recipients receiving graft from HBsAg-positive donors: a retrospective, propensity score-matched study. Am J Transplant 2014;14(12):2814–20.
39. Jiang H, Wu J, Zhang X, et al. Kidney transplantation from hepatitis B surface antigen positive donors into hepatitis B surface antibody positive recipients: a prospective nonrandomized controlled study from a single center. Am J Transplant 2009;9(8):1853–8.
40. Magiorkinis E, Paraskevis D, Pavlopoulou ID, et al. Renal transplantation from hepatitis B surface antigen (HBsAg)-positive donors to HBsAg-negative recipients: a case of post-transplant fulminant hepatitis associated with an extensively mutated hepatitis B virus strain and review of the current literature. Transpl Infect Dis 2013;15(4):393–9.
41. Yen RD, Bonatti H, Mendez J, et al. Case report of lamivudine-resistant hepatitis B virus infection post liver transplantation from a hepatitis B core antibody donor. Am J Transplant 2006;6(5 Pt 1):1077–83.
42. Mahboobi N, Tabatabaei SV, Blum HE, et al. Renal grafts from anti-hepatitis B core-positive donors: a quantitative review of the literature. Transpl Infect Dis 2012;14(5):445–51.
43. Fytili P, Ciesek S, Manns MP, et al. Anti-HBc seroconversion after transplantation of anti-HBc positive nonliver organs to anti-HBc negative recipients. Transplantation 2006;81(5):808–9.
44. Akalin E, Ames S, Sehgal V, et al. Safety of using hepatitis B virus core antibody or surface antigen-positive donors in kidney or pancreas transplantation. Clin Transplant 2005;19(3):364–6.
45. Veroux M, Corona D, Ekser B, et al. Kidney transplantation from hepatitis B virus core antibody-positive donors: prophylaxis with hepatitis B immunoglobulin. Transplant Proc 2011;43(4):967–70.
46. Lau GK, Lee CK, Liang R. Hepatitis B virus infection and bone marrow transplantation. Crit Rev Oncol Hematol 1999;31(1):71–6.
47. Liang R. How I treat and monitor viral hepatitis B infection in patients receiving intensive immunosuppressive therapies or undergoing hematopoietic stem cell transplantation. Blood 2009;113(14):3147–53.
48. Yeo W, Johnson PJ. Diagnosis, prevention and management of hepatitis B virus reactivation during anticancer therapy. Hepatology 2006;43(2):209–20.
49. Strasser SI, McDonald GB. Hepatitis viruses and hematopoietic cell transplantation: a guide to patient and donor management. Blood 1999;93(4):1127–36.
50. Hui CK, Lie A, Au WY, et al. A long-term follow-up study on hepatitis B surface antigen-positive patients undergoing allogeneic hematopoietic stem cell transplantation. Blood 2005;106(2):464–9.
51. Lau GK, He ML, Fong DY, et al. Preemptive use of lamivudine reduces hepatitis B exacerbation after allogeneic hematopoietic cell transplantation. Hepatology 2002;36(3):702–9.
52. Shang J, Wang H, Sun J, et al. A comparison of lamivudine vs entecavir for prophylaxis of hepatitis B virus reactivation in allogeneic hematopoietic stem cell transplantation recipients: a single-institutional experience. Bone Marrow Transplant 2016;51(4):581–6.
53. Lau GK, Liang R, Lee CK, et al. Clearance of persistent hepatitis B virus infection in Chinese bone marrow transplant recipients whose donors were anti-hepatitis B

core- and anti-hepatitis B surface antibody-positive. J Infect Dis 1998;178(6): 1585–91.

54. Onozawa M, Hashino S, Izumiyama K, et al. Progressive disappearance of anti-hepatitis B surface antigen antibody and reverse seroconversion after allogeneic hematopoietic stem cell transplantation in patients with previous hepatitis B virus infection. Transplantation 2005;79(5):616–9.

55. Knoll A, Boehm S, Hahn J, et al. Long-term surveillance of haematopoietic stem cell recipients with resolved hepatitis B: high risk of viral reactivation even in a recipient with a vaccinated donor. J Viral Hepat 2007;14(7):478–83.

56. Seth P, Alrajhi AA, Kagevi I, et al. Hepatitis B virus reactivation with clinical flare in allogeneic stem cell transplants with chronic graft-versus-host disease. Bone Marrow Transplant 2002;30(3):189–94.

57. Hammond SP, Borchelt AM, Ukomadu C, et al. Hepatitis B virus reactivation following allogeneic hematopoietic stem cell transplantation. Biol Blood Marrow Transplant 2009;15(9):1049–59.

58. Vigano M, Vener C, Lampertico P, et al. Risk of hepatitis B surface antigen seroreversion after allogeneic hematopoietic SCT. Bone Marrow Transplant 2011; 46(1):125–31.

59. Mikulska M, Nicolini L, Signori A, et al. Hepatitis B reactivation in HBsAg-negative/HBcAb-positive allogeneic haematopoietic stem cell transplant recipients: risk factors and outcome. Clin Microbiol Infect 2014;20(10):O694–701.

60. Takahata M, Hashino S, Onozawa M, et al. Hepatitis B virus (HBV) reverse seroconversion (RS) can be prevented even in non-responders to hepatitis B vaccine after allogeneic stem cell transplantation: long-term analysis of intervention in RS with vaccine for patients with previous HBV infection. Transpl Infect Dis 2014; 16(5):797–801.

61. Giaccone L, Festuccia M, Marengo A, et al. Hepatitis B virus reactivation and efficacy of prophylaxis with lamivudine in patients undergoing allogeneic stem cell transplantation. Biol Blood Marrow Transplant 2010;16(6):809–17.

62. Frange P, Leruez-Ville M, Neven B, et al. Safety of hematopoietic stem cell transplantation from hepatitis B core antibodies-positive donors with low/undetectable viremia in HBV-naive children. Eur J Clin Microbiol Infect Dis 2014;33(4):545–50.

63. Ustun C, Koc H, Karayalcin S, et al. Hepatitis B virus infection in allogeneic bone marrow transplantation. Bone Marrow Transplant 1997;20(4):289–96.

64. Locasciulli A, Alberti A, Bandini G, et al. Allogeneic bone marrow transplantation from HBsAg+ donors: a multicenter study from the Gruppo Italiano Trapianto di Midollo Osseo (GITMO). Blood 1995;86(8):3236–40.

65. Lau GK, Lie AK, Kwong YL, et al. A case-controlled study on the use of HBsAg-positive donors for allogeneic hematopoietic cell transplantation. Blood 2000; 96(2):452–8.

66. Hui CK, Lie A, Au WY, et al. Effectiveness of prophylactic Anti-HBV therapy in allogeneic hematopoietic stem cell transplantation with HBsAg positive donors. Am J Transplant 2005;5(6):1437–45.

67. Lee JY, Lim SH, Lee MY, et al. Hepatitis B reactivation in multiple myeloma patients with resolved hepatitis B undergoing chemotherapy. Liver Int 2015; 35(11):2363–9.

Screening and Prophylaxis to Prevent Hepatitis B Reactivation

Patients with Hematological and Solid Tumor Malignancies

Joe Sasadeusz, MBBS, PhD, FRACP[a,b,*], Andrew Grigg, MBBS, FRACP, FRCPA, MD[c],
Peter D. Hughes, MBBS, PhD, FRACP[b,d], Seng Lee Lim, MBBS, FRACP, FRCP, MD[e],
Michaela Lucas, MD, Dr Med, FRACP, FRCPA[f],
Geoff McColl, MBBS, BMedSc, MEd, PhD, FRACP[g],
Sue Anne McLachlan, MBBS, MSc, FRACP[h], Marion G. Peters, MD, MBBS[i],
Nicholas Shackel, FRACP, PhD[j], Monica Slavin, MBBS, FRACP, MD[d,k],
Vijaya Sundararajan, MD, MPH[b,h,l], Alexander Thompson, PhD, FRACP[b,h],
Joseph Doyle, MBBS, MPH, PhD, FRACP, FAFPHM[m,n], James Rickard, PhD[c],
Peter De Cruz, MBBS, PhD, FRACP[b], Robert G. Gish, MD[o,1],
Kumar Visvanathan, MBBS, PhD, FRACP[b,h,1]

KEYWORDS

- Hematological malignancy • Solid tumors • Cancer • Hepatitis B • Reactivation
- Prophylaxis • Rituximab

[a] Peter Doherty Institute for Infection and Immunity, Elizabeth Street, Melbourne, Victoria 3000, Australia; [b] University of Melbourne, Grattan Street, Parkville, Victoria 3010, Australia; [c] Olivia Newton John Cancer Research Institute, Austin Hospital, 145 Studley Road, Heidelberg, Victoria 3084, Australia; [d] Royal Melbourne Hospital, 300 Grattan Street, Parkville, Victoria 3050, Australia; [e] National University of Singapore, 21 Lower Kent Ridge Road, Singapore 119077, Singapore; [f] University of Western Australia, 35 Stirling Highway, Crawley, Western Australia 6009, Australia; [g] University of Queensland Oral Health Centre, 288 Herston Road, Queensland 4006, Australia; [h] St Vincent's Hospital, 41 Victoria Street, Fitzroy, Victoria 3065, Australia; [i] University of California, San Francisco, S357 Parnassus Avenue, San Francisco, CA 94143, USA; [j] Ingham Institute, 1 Campbell Street, Liverpool, Sydney, North South Wales 2170, Australia; [k] Victorian Comprehensive Cancer Centre, 305 Grattan Street, Melbourne, Victoria 3000, Australia; [l] Department of Public Health, La Trobe University, Plenty Road, Bundoora, Victoria 3086, Australia; [m] The Alfred and Monash University, 85 Commercial Road, Melbourne, Victoria 3004, Australia; [n] Burnet Institute, 85 Commercial Road, Melbourne, Victoria 3004, Australia; [o] Division of Gastroenterology and Hepatology, Department of Medicine, Stanford University, Stanford University Medical Center, 300 Pasteur Drive, Stanford, CA 94305, USA
[1] Co-senior authors.
* Corresponding author. Peter Doherty Institute for Infection and Immunity, 792 Elizabeth Street, Melbourne, Victoria 3000, Australia.
E-mail address: j.sasadeusz@mh.org.au

Clin Liver Dis 23 (2019) 511–519
https://doi.org/10.1016/j.cld.2019.04.011
1089-3261/19/© 2019 Elsevier Inc. All rights reserved.

liver.theclinics.com

KEY POINTS

- The immunosuppression associated with chemotherapy for hematological and solid tumor malignancies may result in hepatitis B reactivation, which can be fatal.
- Reactivation is most likely to occur with the use of B cell–active agents such as rituximab and it can occur even in hepatitis B surface antigen–negative patients.
- Flares may result in delay of chemotherapy, which can negatively affect the outcome of the underlying malignancy.
- It is critical to assess patients for markers of hepatitis B before starting chemotherapy.
- Antiviral prophylaxis is highly effective in preventing flares and should be used, ideally using an agent with a high barrier to resistance, such as entecavir, tenofovir disoproxil fumarate (TDF), or tenofovir alafenamide (TAF); in patients with renal impairment, entecavir or TAF is preferred because TDF is nephrotoxic.

INTRODUCTION

As is discussed in Joe Sasadeusz and colleagues' article, "Screening and Prophylaxis to Prevent Hepatitis B Reactivation: Introduction and Immunology," in this issue, immunosuppression or treatment with hepatitis C virus direct-acting antivirals may result in loss of immune control of hepatitis B virus (HBV) with recurrence of high-level viral replication, a phenomenon known as reactivation, which can be associated with very high alanine aminotransferase (ALT) levels with hepatic decompensation and death in some patients.[1] This article focuses on guidelines for patients who are undergoing treatment of cancer, either hematological malignancies or solid tumors, who have ever been exposed to hepatitis B, including not only those diagnosed with chronic hepatitis B (CHB) but also those who are hepatitis B core antibody (HBcAb) positive (anti-HBc+); this includes patients who are anti-HBc+ only or both anti-HBc+ and hepatitis B surface antibody positive (anti-HBs+). Screening and prophylaxis in patients who would not normally require treatment of CHB are discussed, and management of patients who do need ongoing treatment is not directly addressed because well-developed guidelines for treatment of those patients are available elsewhere.[2]

MANAGEMENT OF INDIVIDUALS RECEIVING CHEMOTHERAPY FOR HEMATOLOGICAL MALIGNANCIES

Non-Hodgkin lymphoma (NHL) is the best-characterized form of hematological malignancy associated with HBV reactivation. Two randomized controlled trials describe experience with antiviral treatment during cancer chemotherapy, comparing prophylactic antiviral therapy started before or at the time of initiation of chemotherapy with deferred or on-demand treatment.[3,4] In a study of 30 hepatitis B surface antigen (HBsAg)–positive patients with NHL given chemotherapy, reactivation occurred in 8 of 15 patients (53%) for whom treatment was deferred until there was serologic evidence of reactivation and in none of the 15 patients given prophylactic lamivudine.[4] In a later study of 52 patients with NHL treated with chemotherapy, 30.8% of patients given prophylactic lamivudine experienced reactivation compared with 60.0% of patients in the group only given lamivudine if serum ALT levels increased to more than 1.5-fold of the upper limit of normal.[3]

For HBsAg-positive patients with NHL, the use of corticosteroids with other agents doubles the risk of HBV reactivation. The effect of high-dose prednisolone was evaluated in a small randomized controlled study of 2 chemotherapy regimens for NHL.[5] The only difference between regimens was the use of high-dose prednisolone in 1 of the arms. The cumulative incidence of HBV reactivation at 9 months was 73% in the high-dose prednisolone cohort and 38% in the steroid-free cohort ($P = .03$). There was a suggestion that the prednisolone-free regimen may have resulted in decreased remission of tumors and a trend to decreased survival suggesting an adverse effect on the malignancy outcome.

In a study of 401 HBsAg-negative, anti-HBc–positive patients with NHL, none were given prophylactic antiviral therapy, and most were treated with rituximab.[6] The mean rate of HBV reactivation was 12.2% (range, 3.2%–23.8%). In a controlled comparison between rituximab, cyclophosphamide, doxorubicin, vincristine, and prednisone (R-CHOP) and cyclophosphamide, doxorubicin, vincristine, and prednisone (CHOP) in 46 patients with NHL, a significantly greater number of patients given R-CHOP developed HBV reactivation: 5 of 21 versus 0 of 25, respectively ($P = .015$).[7] Death caused by reactivation was uncommon but occurred in 1 patient (2.1%). Most of these patients were treated with rituximab in addition to CHOP or other combination regimens. In another study, 85 newly diagnosed patients with NHL aged more than 65 years received rituximab-containing regimens between 2007 and 2014.[8] All patients were HBsAg negative and anti-HBc positive and received lamivudine prophylaxis starting 1 week before rituximab. Nine (10%) patients experienced HBV reactivation or hepatitis that resolved following treatment with entecavir. Just more than half (55%) of patients with reactivation had anti-HBs at baseline compared with 80% of patients who did not experience reactivation. HBV reactivation was seen in patients at a median of 5 cycles of R-CHOP or fludarabine.

Late reactivation of HBV has been reported in patients treated with anti-CD20 antibodies. A patient with Waldenström macroglobulinemia was treated with chlorambucil (4 mg oral daily for 7 months) and rituximab (375 mg/m^2 intravenous monthly for 4 months and then once every 3 months for 2 more years, for a total of 12 doses).[9] He was HBsAg positive, anti-HBc positive, and HBV DNA negative with normal liver function tests (LFTs). Despite prophylaxis with lamivudine from commencement of treatment until 12 months after the last dose of rituximab, 6 months after discontinuing lamivudine (18 months after the final dose of rituximab) he experienced a hepatitis flare with jaundice, increased ALT level (2260 U/L), and increased HBV DNA viral load (28,812 IU/mL). An additional case was described of reactivation in a woman treated with rituximab and fludarabine who was HBsAg negative, anti-HBs positive, and HBV DNA positive.[10] Despite prophylaxis with lamivudine that was continued for 12 months after the discontinuation of chemotherapy, she experienced reactivation 18 months after the completion of chemotherapy. Taken together, these reports suggest a need for long-term vigilance in monitoring for HBV reactivation and longer duration of prophylaxis in the case of rituximab therapy.

The pooled overall risk of reactivation in resolved HBV is 16.9%.[6] More than two-thirds of anti-HBc–positive/HBsAg-negative patients in various studies had detectable anti-HBs.[6] In one study, HBV reactivation was observed in 2.7% of patients who had detectable anti-HBs (1 out of 37), a frequency that was significantly lower than the total group of anti-HBc–positive patients (21.1%, 4/19).[11] The small number of cases did not allow comparison as to whether the patients who had anti-HBs had clinically less severe hepatitis. The effect of anti-HBs titer on HBV reactivation has not been well reported. However, at present there is insufficient evidence to support the use of anti-HBs titers in making a recommendation regarding prophylaxis.

In a review of 5 studies, the overall risk ratio for the use of prophylaxis for HBV reactivation was 0.13 (95% confidence interval [CI], 0.06, 0.30) in favor of the use of antiviral therapy in patients with NHL receiving chemotherapy, which equates to 44 fewer cases per 1000 moderate-risk patients and 435 fewer per 1000 low-risk patients.[3,4,12–14] The risk ratio for prophylaxis to prevent an HBV hepatitis flare was 0.16 (95% CI, 0.06, 0.42), equating to 42 fewer per 1000 moderate-risk patients and 420 fewer per 1000 low-risk patients. A randomized study comparing the frequency of HBV reactivation and hepatitis in patients treated with entecavir or lamivudine suggests that the rates are lower with entecavir; however, further studies are needed to confirm this.[15]

RITUXIMAB AND OTHER B CELL–DEPLETING AGENTS

As shown earlier in the description of several studies, rituximab is often used for the treatment of hematological malignancies. The effect of rituximab and other medications on B cells warrants a separate discussion. Rituximab is an anti-CD20 monoclonal chimeric antibody that depletes B cells, leading to antibody-mediated cytotoxicity, complement-mediated cell lysis, B-cell apoptosis, and B-cell growth arrest. B-cell depletion tends to start within days of starting treatment and levels decrease to 20% of baseline within 8 to 12 weeks.[16,17] B-cell recovery follows original ontogeny and is similar to recovery following hematopoietic stem cell transplant.

During reconstitution, most peripheral B cells have immature transitional phenotype and recovery of CD27+ memory cells is delayed.[18] Factors influencing this delay include baseline immune deficit, concomitant immunosuppressive drugs, longer duration of rituximab therapy, and age.[17] Transitional B cells are predominant for at least 15 months after the start of immune recovery and in response to stimulation they mature from B cells into T2 and then T1 cells, during which time they are more susceptible to apoptosis. For 12 months after stopping rituximab, B cells are immature and less effective than normal. Because of the potential late reactivation that may occur after rituximab and other B cell–depleting agent use,[19] it is recommended that antiviral prophylaxis be administered at least 12 months after completion of rituximab.

Therapy with other antibodies and small molecules involved in B-cell depletion or B-cell receptor signaling include the following: other anti-CD20 antibodies such as ocrelizumab, ofatumumab, and obinutuzumab; the anti-CD52 agent alemtuzumab when used for more than 12 months[20]; the Bruton tyrosine kinase (BTK) inhibitor ibrutinib; and the Pi3Kδ (phosphatidylinositol-4,5-bisphosphate 3-kinase catalytic subunit delta) inhibitor idealisib.[21] Obinutuzumab has a greater capacity for B-cell depletion than rituximab, ocrelizumab, and ofatumumab, with enhanced Fc-Fcγ receptor interaction, antibody-dependent cytotoxicity, and phagocytosis.[22,23] Ibrutinib blocks pathways that regulate survival, proliferation, adhesion, and homing of cancerous cells.[24]

Recommendations for Screening and Prophylaxis of Patients with Hematological Malignancies Receiving Chemotherapy

Screen all patients for HBsAg, anti-HBc, and anti-HBs. Test for HBV DNA by nucleic acid test (NAT) if anti-HBc positive and HBsAg negative.

Vaccinate patients with no evidence of HBV exposure.

Assess HBsAg-positive patients for liver fibrosis, ideally by noninvasive methods such as transient elastography or serum markers. Refer patients with cirrhosis for specialist care.

Provide antiviral prophylaxis in HBsAg-positive patients from 1 week before starting immunosuppressive agent and until 12 months after discontinuation. In the case of rituximab, this should be extended to 18 months. This advice may apply to the other drugs that affect B cells but there are currently no data on this.

Ideally, use a drug with a high barrier to resistance, such as tenofovir disoproxil fumarate (TDF), tenofovir alafenamide (TAF), or entecavir; lamivudine could be considered in resource-constrained countries.

Monitor patients every 3 months for HBsAg, anti-HBs, HBV DNA, and liver panel (liver enzymes and LFTs, including bilirubin, albumin, and International Normalized Ratio [INR]) for 6 months after cessation of the antiviral therapy.

Patients should be reviewed by a clinician with experience in treating patients with CHB before discontinuing therapy.

There are no data to support vaccination of anti-HBc+ patients; although it may increase anti-HBs titers, there are no data showing clinical benefit or improved clinical outcomes.

Management of Hepatitis B Reactivation in Solid Tumor Populations

A systematic review and meta-analysis by Paul and colleagues[25] determined the risk for HBV reactivation with and without antiviral prophylaxis and the effectiveness of prophylaxis in adults with chronic or resolved HBV receiving chemotherapy for solid tumors. The absolute risk of HBV reactivation without prophylaxis was between 4% and 68% with a median rate of HBV reactivation of 25%. There is variable but appreciable risk in patients with cancers of the gastrointestinal tract, breast, lung, and head and neck, ranging from 5% to 68%. However, of greater relevance are the different rates of HBV reactivation in patients receiving different chemotherapy regimens in the absence of prophylaxis. Reactivation risk varied from 3.0% with taxane treatment to 88% in an anthracycline-based study. Most studies (15 out of 16) had a reactivation risk greater than 10%. All but 1 anthracycline-based study involved patients with breast cancer. The median reactivation rates were 25% with platinum-based chemotherapy, 19% to 25% with FOLFOX (folinic acid, fluorouracil [5FU], and oxaliplatin) or FOLFIRI (folinic acid, 5FU, and irinotecan), 17% to 23% with antimetabolites, and 3% with taxanes.

In 4 studies reporting their use, of 94 patients receiving concomitant glucocorticoids 20% had reactivation compared with 14% reactivation in those not receiving glucocorticoids. Paul and colleagues[25] also reported on clinically important complications of reactivation as secondary outcomes, including HBV-related hepatitis, interrupted or delayed chemotherapy, acute liver failure (with coagulopathy and hepatic encephalopathy), and death. The presence of anti-HBs was protective, with higher titers more protective and declining anti-HBs titers indicating a higher risk of reactivation.[6]

The odds ratio for HBV reactivation across the 14 studies was 0.12 (95% CI, 0.06–0.11; $P = .49$) in favor of using antiviral prophylaxis.[25] HBV reactivation risk was lower with both entecavir and lamivudine. For entecavir, relative risk was 0.14 (95% CI, 0.02–1.05; $P = .06$) and for lamivudine it was 0.13 (95% CI, 0.06–0.32; $P = .00001$). The use of prophylaxis also significantly reduced the rate of hepatitis (odds ratio [OR], 0.18; 95% CI, 0.10–1.32; $P = .62$) and interruption of chemotherapy (OR, 0.10; 95% CI, 0.04–0.27; $P = .079$). In addition, the OR favored prophylaxis for reducing the risk of acute liver failure (OR, 0.31; CI, 0.09–1.02) and death (OR, 0.43; CI, 0.15–1.20).

The clinical spectrum of oncological treatments that potentially induce HBV reactivation has recently expanded with the development of biologic agents. One of the main classes in use for solid tumors are the tyrosine kinase inhibitors such as sorafenib for hepatocellular carcinoma, gefitinib for epidermal growth factor receptor–mutated adenocarcinoma of the lung, imatinib for gastrointestinal stromal tumors, and sunitinib for renal cell carcinoma. The risks and recommendations for these newer agents are covered in "Screening and Prophylaxis to Prevent Hepatitis B Reactivation: Other Populations and Newer Agents" in this issue.

Recommendations for Screening and Prophylaxis of Patients with Solid Tumors Receiving Chemotherapy

> Screen all patients with solid tumors receiving chemotherapy for HBsAg as a minimum. Additional serologic testing for anti-HBc and anti-HBs can be decided at an institutional level, although cost-effectiveness for this is lacking. HBV DNA testing by NAT should be done in patients who are HBsAg positive or anti-HBc positive in the absence of anti-HBs.
>
> Vaccinate patients with no evidence of HBV infection or exposure (triple panel negative).
>
> Provide antiviral prophylaxis in HBsAg-positive patients from 1 week before starting an immunosuppressive agent until 12 months after discontinuation of the agent.
>
> Ideally, use a drug with a high barrier to resistance, such as TDF, TAF, or entecavir; lamivudine could be considered in resource-constrained countries.
>
> Monitor patients every 3 months with testing for HBsAg, anti-HBs, HBV DNA by NAT and liver panel (liver enzymes and LFTs, including bilirubin, albumin, and INR) for 6 months after cessation of the antiviral therapy.
>
> Patients should be reviewed by a clinician with experience in treating patients with CHB before discontinuing therapy.
>
> At present there are insufficient data to recommend prophylaxis in HBsAg-negative but anti-HBc–positive individuals. In addition, there is no evidence that vaccinating such individuals improves immune control and modulates reactivation risk.

Cost-effectiveness of Hepatitis B Viral Suppressive Therapy

Cost-effectiveness analyses have been conducted for the use of prophylaxis to prevent HBV reactivation in lymphoma, breast cancer, and solid tumors.[26–29] Zurawska and colleagues[27] in 2012 focused on patients with diffuse large B-cell lymphoma undergoing first-line treatment with 6 cycles of R-CHOP every 3 weeks with curative intent. All-cause mortality at 12 months was estimated at 15%, increasing by an OR of 5.32 in patients experiencing a severe hepatitis flare and a chemotherapy course reduction. The perspective of the model was that of a third-party payer.

The model considered 3 scenarios:

Screen none: no screening
Screen high risk (HR): screen HR patients with HBsAg. HR was defined as patients born in countries with intermediate (2%–8%) or high (>8%) prevalence (equivalent to approximately 20% of Canadian population)
Screen all: screen all patients with HBsAg before chemotherapy

Base probabilities for hepatitis as a result of HBV reactivation without prophylaxis were 51% and, for severe HBV-related hepatitis, 26%. Meta-analysis of 6 controlled studies conducted for the analysis showed that antiviral prophylaxis reduced the rate of hepatitis by 95% (OR, 0.05; 95% CI, 0.02–0.15). In all scenarios modeled, HBsAg-positive patients received prophylaxis with lamivudine 100 mg daily or entecavir 0.5 mg daily until 6 months after completion of chemotherapy if baseline HBV DNA level was greater than 2000 IU/mL. Costs included in the model were those related to outpatient clinic follow-up, laboratory tests, and hospitalizations. Using the screen-all strategy compared with the screen-none strategy, the rate of HBV hepatitis was estimated to be 10 times lower (0.6 vs 5.9 per 1000 patients); the rate of HBV hepatitis-related hospitalizations was projected to be 30 times lower (0.1 vs 3.0 per 1000 patients); the rate of hepatitis-related deaths was reduced to zero (0 vs 0.8 per 1000 patients); and the costs were somewhat lower ($32,589 vs $32,667 in 2010 Canadian dollars). As such, the screen-all strategy was dominant, having both the highest effectiveness and the lowest cost.

The other analysis in patients with lymphoma, from Saab and colleagues[26] in 2007, did not show that an HBV prophylaxis strategy was dominantly cost-effective, but did show an incremental cost-effectiveness ratio for lamivudine prophylaxis of US$33,514 per life year saved.

For patients with early-stage breast cancer receiving adjuvant chemotherapy, the Canadian team of Wong and colleagues[29] modeled the use of antiviral prophylaxis for 3 scenarios, using a third-party payer perspective:

- Screen none: no screening
- Screen HR: screen and treat foreign-born individuals
- Screen all: screen and treat to prevent reactivation with either lamivudine or tenofovir or entecavir if baseline HBV DNA level exceeds 2000 IU/mL

The analysis estimated the incremental cost-effectiveness ratio of the screen-all scenario with lamivudine or tenofovir versus the screen-none scenario to be $47,808 (2014 Canadian dollars) per quality-adjusted life year (QALY) gained; for entecavir it was $76,527 per QALY.

A comparable Australian analysis by Day and colleagues[28] estimated the cost-effectiveness of universal screening with both HBsAg and HBcAb versus no screening in patients receiving adjuvant chemotherapy for early breast cancer to be AU$88,244 per life year saved; if screening were limited to HBsAg only, the ratio decreased to AU$30,126 per life year saved.

Overall, HBV screening using HBsAg and prophylaxis with lamivudine seems cost-effective in lymphoma and early-stage breast cancer with adjuvant chemotherapy at cost-effective thresholds of $50,000 per life year saved. At current prices, prophylaxis with entecavir may be cost-effective at a threshold of $100,000. The addition of anti-HBcAb testing to screening increases the cost; its use with entecavir at current prices may not be cost-effective. The clinical relevance and costs of differing tests for HBV infection require additional investigation. Further analyses are also needed to clarify the impact of decreasing medication and screening costs, and HBV reactivation risk with rituximab and a broader range of immunosuppressive medications and diseases.

ACKNOWLEDGEMENTS

Meetings to discuss and develop recommendations presented in this manuscript and medical writing services provided in the preparation of this manuscript were funded by Gilead Sciences. Neither the medical writer or Gilead in any way influenced the content or the conclusions of the position paper. None of the authors had any direct financial support from Gilead Sciences or any other companies.

REFERENCES

1. Lok AS, Liang RH, Chiu EK, et al. Reactivation of hepatitis B virus replication in patients receiving cytotoxic therapy. Report of a prospective study. Gastroenterology 1991;100(1):182–8.

2. Terrault NA, Lok ASF, McMahon BJ, et al. Update on prevention, diagnosis, and treatment of chronic hepatitis B: AASLD 2018 hepatitis B guidance. Hepatology 2018;67(4):1560–99.

3. Hsu C, Hsiung CA, Su IJ, et al. A revisit of prophylactic lamivudine for chemotherapy-associated hepatitis B reactivation in non-Hodgkin's lymphoma: a randomized trial. Hepatology 2008;47(3):844–53.

4. Lau GK, Yiu HH, Fong DY, et al. Early is superior to deferred preemptive lamivudine therapy for hepatitis B patients undergoing chemotherapy. Gastroenterology 2003;125(6):1742–9.

5. Cheng AL, Hsiung CA, Su IJ, et al. Steroid-free chemotherapy decreases risk of hepatitis B virus (HBV) reactivation in HBV-carriers with lymphoma. Hepatology 2003;37(6):1320–8.

6. Perrillo RP, Gish R, Falck-Ytter YT. American Gastroenterological Association Institute technical review on prevention and treatment of hepatitis B virus reactivation during immunosuppressive drug therapy. Gastroenterology 2015;148(1): 221–44.e3.

7. Yeo W, Chan TC, Leung NW, et al. Hepatitis B virus reactivation in lymphoma patients with prior resolved hepatitis B undergoing anticancer therapy with or without rituximab. J Clin Oncol 2009;27(4):605–11.

8. Castelli R, Ferraris L, Pantaleo G, et al. High rate of hepatitis B viral breakthrough in elderly non-Hodgkin lymphomas patients treated with Rituximab based chemotherapy. Dig Liver Dis 2016;48(11):1394–7.

9. Chew E, Thursky K, Seymour JF. Very late onset hepatitis-B virus reactivation following rituximab despite lamivudine prophylaxis: the need for continued vigilance. Leuk Lymphoma 2014;55(4):938–9.

10. Ceccarelli L, Salpini R, Sarmati L, et al. Late hepatitis B virus reactivation after lamivudine prophylaxis interruption in an anti-HBs-positive and anti-HBc-negative patient treated with rituximab-containing therapy. J Infect 2012;65(2): 180–3.

11. Matsue K, Kimura S, Takanashi Y, et al. Reactivation of hepatitis B virus after rituximab-containing treatment in patients with CD20-positive B-cell lymphoma. Cancer 2010;116(20):4769–76.

12. Huang YH, Hsiao LT, Hong YC, et al. Randomized controlled trial of entecavir prophylaxis for rituximab-associated hepatitis B virus reactivation in patients with lymphoma and resolved hepatitis B. J Clin Oncol 2013;31(22):2765–72.

13. Jang JW. Hepatitis B virus reactivation in patients with hepatocellular carcinoma undergoing anti-cancer therapy. World J Gastroenterol 2014;20(24):7675–85.

14. Long M, Jia W, Li S, et al. A single-center, prospective and randomized controlled study: can the prophylactic use of lamivudine prevent hepatitis B virus reactivation in hepatitis B s-antigen seropositive breast cancer patients during chemotherapy? Breast Cancer Res Treat 2011;127(3):705–12.

15. Huang H, Li X, Zhu J, et al. Entecavir vs lamivudine for prevention of hepatitis B virus reactivation among patients with untreated diffuse large B-cell lymphoma receiving R-CHOP chemotherapy: a randomized clinical trial. JAMA 2014; 312(23):2521–30.

16. Kado R, Sanders G, McCune WJ. Suppression of normal immune responses after treatment with rituximab. Curr Opin Rheumatol 2016;28(3):251–8.
17. Ghielmini M, Rufibach K, Salles G, et al. Single agent rituximab in patients with follicular or mantle cell lymphoma: clinical and biological factors that are predictive of response and event-free survival as well as the effect of rituximab on the immune system: a study of the Swiss Group for Clinical Cancer Research (SAKK). Ann Oncol 2005;16(10):1675–82.
18. Anolik JH, Friedberg JW, Zheng B, et al. B cell reconstitution after rituximab treatment of lymphoma recapitulates B cell ontogeny. Clin Immunol 2007;122(2): 139–45.
19. Seto WK, Chan TS, Hwang YY, et al. Hepatitis B reactivation in patients with previous hepatitis B virus exposure undergoing rituximab-containing chemotherapy for lymphoma: a prospective study. J Clin Oncol 2014;32(33):3736–43.
20. Thursky KA, Worth LJ, Seymour JF, et al. Spectrum of infection, risk and recommendations for prophylaxis and screening among patients with lymphoproliferative disorders treated with alemtuzumab. Br J Haematol 2006;132(1):3–12.
21. Bai B, Huang HQ. Individualized management of follicular lymphoma. Chin Clin Oncol 2015;4(1):7.
22. Gabellier L, Cartron G. Obinutuzumab for relapsed or refractory indolent non-Hodgkin's lymphomas. Ther Adv Hematol 2016;7(2):85–93.
23. Reddy V, Dahal LN, Cragg MS, et al. Optimising B-cell depletion in autoimmune disease: is obinutuzumab the answer? Drug Discov Today 2016;21(8):1330–8.
24. de Jesus Ngoma P, Kabamba B, Dahlqvist G, et al. Occult HBV reactivation induced by ibrutinib treatment: a case report. Acta Gastroenterol Belg 2015; 78(4):424–6.
25. Paul S, Saxena A, Terrin N, et al. Hepatitis B virus reactivation and prophylaxis during solid tumor chemotherapy: a systematic review and meta-analysis. Ann Intern Med 2016;164(1):30–40.
26. Saab S, Dong MH, Joseph TA, et al. Hepatitis B prophylaxis in patients undergoing chemotherapy for lymphoma: a decision analysis model. Hepatology 2007; 46(4):1049–56.
27. Zurawska U, Hicks LK, Woo G, et al. Hepatitis B virus screening before chemotherapy for lymphoma: a cost-effectiveness analysis. J Clin Oncol 2012;30(26): 3167–73.
28. Day FL, Karnon J, Rischin D. Cost-effectiveness of universal hepatitis B virus screening in patients beginning chemotherapy for solid tumors. J Clin Oncol 2011;29(24):3270–7.
29. Wong WW, Hicks LK, Tu HA, et al. Hepatitis B virus screening before adjuvant chemotherapy in patients with early-stage breast cancer: a cost-effectiveness analysis. Breast Cancer Res Treat 2015;151(3):639–52.

Screening and Prophylaxis to Prevent Hepatitis B Reactivation

Other Populations and Newer Agents

Joe Sasadeusz, MBBS, PhD, FRACP[a,b,]*, Andrew Grigg, MBBS, FRACP, FRCPA, MD[c],
Peter D. Hughes, MBBS, PhD, FRACP[b,d], Seng Lee Lim, MBBS, FRACP, FRCP, MD[e],
Michaela Lucas, MD, Dr Med, FRACP, FRCPA[f],
Geoff McColl, MBBS, BMedSc, MEd, PhD, FRACP[g],
Sue Anne McLachlan, MBBS, MSc, FRACP[h], Marion G. Peters, MD, MBBS[i],
Nicholas Shackel, FRACP, PhD[j], Monica Slavin, MBBS, FRACP, MD[d,k],
Vijaya Sundararajan, MD, MPH[b,h,l], Alexander Thompson, PhD, FRACP[b,h],
Joseph Doyle, MBBS, MPH, PhD, FRACP, FAFPHM[m,n], James Rickard, PhD[c],
Peter De Cruz, MBBS, PhD, FRACP[b], Robert G. Gish, MD[o,1],
Kumar Visvanathan, MBBS, PhD, FRACP[b,h,1]

KEYWORDS

- Hepatitis B • Rheumatoid arthritis • Inflammatory bowel diseases • Reactivation
- Anti-CD20 • Direct-acting antivirals

[a] Peter Doherty Institute for Infection and Immunity, Elizabeth Street, Melbourne, Victoria 3000, Australia; [b] University of Melbourne, Grattan Street, Parkville, Victoria 3010, Australia; [c] Olivia Newton John Cancer Research Institute, Austin Hospital, 145 Studley Road, Heidelberg, Victoria 3084, Australia; [d] Royal Melbourne Hospital, 300 Grattan Street, Parkville, Victoria 3050, Australia; [e] National University of Singapore, 21 Lower Kent Ridge Road, Singapore 119077, Singapore; [f] University of Western Australia, 35 Stirling Highway, Crawley, Western Australia 6009, Australia; [g] University of Queensland Oral Health Centre, 288 Herston Road, Queensland 4006, Australia; [h] St Vincent's Hospital, 41 Victoria Street, Fitzroy, Victoria 3065, Australia; [i] University of California, San Francisco, S357 Parnassus Avenue, San Francisco, CA 94143, USA; [j] Ingham Institute, 1 Campbell Street, Liverpool, Sydney, North South Wales 2170, Australia; [k] Victorian Comprehensive Cancer Centre, 305 Grattan Street, Melbourne, Victoria 3000, Australia; [l] Department of Public Health, La Trobe University, Plenty Road, Bundoora, Victoria 3086, Australia; [m] The Alfred and Monash University, 85 Commercial Road, Melbourne, Victoria 3004, Australia; [n] Burnet Institute, 85 Commercial Road, Melbourne, Victoria 3004, Australia; [o] Division of Gastroenterology and Hepatology, Department of Medicine, Stanford University, Stanford University Medical Center, 300 Pasteur Drive, Stanford, CA 94305, USA
[1] Co-Senior authors.
* Corresponding author. Peter Doherty Institute for Infection and Immunity, 792 Elizabeth Street, Melbourne, Victoria 3000, Australia.
E-mail address: j.sasadeusz@mh.org.au

Clin Liver Dis 23 (2019) 521–534
https://doi.org/10.1016/j.cld.2019.04.012
1089-3261/19/© 2019 Elsevier Inc. All rights reserved.

liver.theclinics.com

KEY POINTS

- Treatment of inflammatory arthritis with azothiaprine and methotrexate without steroids had a low risk of reactivation, whereas this risk increases with anti–tumor necrosis factor (anti-TNF) inhibitors, rituximab, and abatacept.
- Moderate-risk and high-risk patients require prophylaxis with anti-HBV agents.
- The TNF inhibitors, adalimumab, infliximab, and certolizumab, which are central to inflammatory bowel disease management confer a moderate risk of HBV reactivation, especially when associated with steroid therapy.
- Newer drugs with immunosuppressive activity are likely to be important risk factors for HBV reactivation, including, in particular, BTK, PI3K, and T-cell inhibitors.
- Treatment of hepatitis C with direct-acting antivirals can result in HBV reactivation, with the highest risk in patients who are HBsAg positive.

INTRODUCTION

As is discussed in "Screening and Prophylaxis to Prevent Hepatitis B Reactivation: Introduction and Immunology" (in this issue), immunosuppression or treatment with hepatitis C virus (HCV) direct-acting antivirals (DAAs) may result in loss of immune control of hepatitis B virus (HBV) with recurrence of high-level viral replication, a phenomenon known as reactivation, which can be associated with very high alanine aminotransferase (ALT) levels with hepatic decompensation, liver transplant, or death in some patients.[1] We focus here on guidelines for patients with HBV infection, chronic hepatitis B (CHB) and occult hepatitis B infection, as defined in the above-mentioned article, who are receiving immunosuppressive therapy for treatment of autoimmune inflammatory arthritis or inflammatory bowel disease (IBD). We also discuss recommendations for patients being treated with DAAs or any of the newer immunosuppressive agents, whether approved or still in development, including monoclonal antibodies, fusion antibodies, treatments for hepatocellular carcinoma (HCC), Bruton kinase inhibitors (BKIs), phosphatidylinositol 3-kinase (PI3K) inhibitors, JAK inhibitors, hypomethylating agents, and others. We discuss screening and prophylaxis in patients who would not normally require treatment of CHB and do not directly address management of patients who do need ongoing treatment, because well-developed guidelines for treatment of those patients are available elsewhere.[2]

MANAGEMENT OF HEPATITIS B IN RHEUMATOLOGY

The relatively high prevalence of both hepatitis B infection/exposure and various forms of autoimmune inflammatory arthritis (rheumatoid arthritis, psoriatic arthritis, ankylosing spondylitis, and others) in some parts of the world will result in the coexistent diagnoses of both diseases in a substantial number of patients. The exact frequency of this association will vary according to the prevalence and incidence of each disease in each country.

Disease-Modifying Antirheumatic Drugs

In a prospective study of 476 patients with rheumatoid arthritis, there were 4 reactivation events, 2/27 (7.4%) HBsAg positive and 2/188 (1.1%) HBsAg negative/anti-HBc positive. No HBV reactivation events were observed in patients receiving disease-modifying antirheumatic drugs (DMARDs) alone, including methotrexate. However, the addition of corticosteroids and negative anti-HBs status at baseline increased the risk of reactivation. Notably, all 4 cases of reactivation occurred in patients receiving concomitant corticosteroids.[3] Isolated cases of HBV reactivation have been reported during treatment with methotrexate, leflunomide, azathioprine, chloroquine, and sulphasalazine.[4] Overall, the risk of reactivation seems low and may be greatest in those who receive corticosteroids, lack anti-HBs, or have high levels of HBV DNA.

Corticosteroids

Glucocorticoids, also called glucocorticosteroids or corticosteroids, and including prednisolone and prednisone, are used frequently in patients with inflammatory arthritis, generally for symptom control, whereas DMARDs are initiated for long-term treatment. Glucocorticoids have been reported to reactivate HBV both at high and low doses, alone and in combination with DMARDs.[5] Corticosteroids are known to have dual effects of increasing HBV replication while suppressing T-cell function. Long-term doses of prednisolone (in excess of 10 mg) have previously been shown to negatively affect the natural history of HBV.[6] In a study of patients with obstructive respiratory disease 11% of patients receiving systemic corticosteroids developed reactivation. Those receiving continuous chronic systemic use for more than 3 months suffered more reactivations than those on intermittent therapy, while those on continuous dosing greater than 20 mg/day had higher rates compared with those on lower doses.[7] Intra-articular steroids do not seem to carry an increased risk. Accordingly, a risk-stratification approach should be used to determine whether monitoring or prophylaxis is appropriate.

Anti–Tumor Necrosis Factor Inhibitors

The most commonly used biological DMARDs (bDMARDs) in patients with inflammatory arthritis are those that inhibit tumor necrosis factor alpha (TNF-α) (etanercept, adalimumab, infliximab, certolizumab, and golimumab). Patients treated with anti-TNF-α agents for rheumatoid arthritis have a reactivation rate of 15.4% with overt HBV infection (HBsAg-positive) and 3% with HBsAg-negative/anti-HBc-positive HBV infection, suggesting the need for prophylaxis in HBsAg-positive patients receiving anti-TNF-α agents.[8] In an analysis of 89 previously reported cases who were HBsAg-positive and received TNF-α inhibitors for their inflammatory arthritis, 35 patients (39%) reactivated their HBV; 5 developed acute liver failure, 4 of whom died.[9] Reactivation was significantly less common in individuals who received antiviral prophylaxis, and infliximab was associated with a higher rate of reactivation than etanercept. In the same analysis, 168 patients with anti-HBc serology who were HBsAg-negative were treated with TNF-α inhibitors and 9 (5%) had reactivated HBV, with 1 patient dying of liver failure. It is notable, however, that some case series with modest numbers showed no reactivation.[10–12]

In a subsequent review of 35 cases of HBV reactivation in patients who were HBsAg positive, most of whom received TNF-α inhibitors for rheumatological conditions, 17 were treated with infliximab, 12 with etanercept, and 6 with adalimumab. Infliximab was associated with a higher number of cases of ALT $> 2\times$ upper limit of normal (6/9) and a 1000-fold increase in HBV DNA (3/4), with only 2 deaths reported.[13] Although it is not a controlled study, this also suggests that infliximab may be more potent in reactivation than other TNF inhibitors. Like other clinical scenarios, antiviral prophylaxis has been shown to be effective in prevention of reactivation.[14]

Rituximab

Rituximab is also an effective treatment for patients with active rheumatoid arthritis. HBV reactivation has been reported in patients with rheumatoid arthritis receiving rituximab.[15–17] A multicenter observational study of 234 patients with moderate or severe rheumatoid arthritis and inadequate response or intolerance to anti-TNF treatment evaluated the long-term safety of rituximab.[16] Three cases of HBV reactivation were reported (2 in patients with chronic HBV, 1 despite lamivudine prophylaxis, and 1 in a patient who was HBsAg negative, anti-HBc positive, and anti-HBs positive). All patients responded to tenofovir. In a retrospective study of 33 HBsAg-negative, anti-HBs-positive patients with rheumatoid arthritis and undetectable HBV DNA, none became HBsAg positive during rituximab treatment.[18] Six of the 28 patients with anti-HBs at baseline (21%) had a greater than 50% decrease in anti-HBs and 2 patients became negative. One patient (3%) became HBV DNA positive after 6 months of rituximab and was successfully treated with lamivudine. Of the 14 patients monitored for 18 months (range 0–70 months) after stopping rituximab, none had HBV reactivation.

Other Agents

Abatacept is a fusion protein composed of the Fc region of the immunoglobulin IgG1 fused to the extracellular domain of CTLA-4. In order for a T cell to be activated and produce an immune response, an antigen-presenting cell must present 2 signals to the T cell. One of those signals is the major histocompatibility complex, combined with the antigen, and the other signal is the CD80 or CD86 molecule (also known as B7-1 and B7-2). Abatacept binds to the CD80 and CD86 molecule, and prevents the second signal. Without the second signal, the T cell cannot be activated. In a study of 8 patients who were HBsAg positive treated with abatacept for rheumatoid arthritis, 4 patients did not receive prophylactic antiviral therapy and all had HBV reactivation, whereas none of the 4 patients who received prophylactic antiviral therapy reactivated.[19] In addition, a further case report identified reactivation in an HBsAg-negative, anti-HBc-positive individual.[20]

Tocilizumab is a monoclonal antibody that binds IL-6 and is effective in the treatment of patients with active rheumatoid arthritis. At this time there is limited evidence about the safety of using tocilizumab in patients with HBV and therefore it would be prudent to follow the guidelines for the other bDMARDS until further evidence is accrued.

Recommendations for Screening and Prophylaxis of Patients in Rheumatological Settings

Perform HBV serology for HBsAg, anti-HBs, and anti-HBc in patients with inflammatory arthritis commencing therapy in whom there is a high risk of reactivation of HBV, which includes the following:

o All bDMARDs

o cDMARDS used in combination with corticosteroids

o Patients starting corticosteroid therapy at, or in excess of, 10 mg daily

In patients who are HBsAg positive:

o Carry out HBV DNA testing by nucleic acid testing, test liver enzymes, and perform fibrosis assessment:

o Start prophylactic antiviral therapy before rheumatology therapy, preferably using an agent with a high barrier to resistance.

If HBsAg negative but anti-HBc positive:

o Start antiviral prophylaxis if using bDMARD

o Monitor monthly for 3 months with HBsAg, liver enzymes, and HBV DNA when using other agents.

Recommendation for Rheumatological Diseases and Rituximab

If HBsAg positive, start antiviral prophylaxis.

Recommendations are less clear with suggestion of lower risk for HBV reactivation than with hematological malignancy. In the absence of large datasets, recommend antiviral prophylaxis with entecavir or tenofovir for patients who are anti-HBc positive (whether HBsAg positive or HBsAg negative), 1 week before rituximab treatment and for 12 to 18 months after the last dose.

Monitor HBsAg and anti-HBs titers, HBV DNA quantification, and liver enzymes and liver function for 18 months after cessation of rituximab.

• There are no data to support vaccination of patients who are anti-HBc positive

Chronic hepatitis B and immune suppression in inflammatory bowel disease

IBD, comprised largely of Crohn disease and ulcerative colitis, often requires immuno-suppressive medication to induce and maintain remission. Immunosuppressive treatment can increase susceptibility to infections, including latent CHB reactivation, which may culminate in acute liver failure or death.[21,22] HBV screening rates have, however, been found to be suboptimal.[23–26]

If CHB is identified in an IBD patient requiring immunosuppressive treatment, then the need for antiviral prophylaxis must be considered. Patients who are HBsAg-positive are at higher risk of HBV reactivation than HBsAg-negative/anti-HBc-positive patients, some of whom will have occult CHB.[23] As already mentioned above, moderate-dose to high-dose corticosteroids are estimated to pose the greatest risk for HBV reactivation of all IBD medications, with a predicted greater than 10% risk for patients who are HBsAg positive receiving 10 mg or more of prednisolone for 4 or more weeks.[6] Shorter courses, smaller doses, and being HBsAg negative were estimated to reduce the risk. With 6-mercaptopurine, an active metabolite of azathioprine with similar effects on the immune system, there have been no reports in the literature of HBV reactivation either when used on its own or in combination with other immunomodulatory agents. Methotrexate use is covered in the section on rheumatological agents.

The TNF inhibitors adalimumab, infliximab and certolizumab are central to IBD management, and many of the data around these agents are already covered in the section on rheumatological agents where most of the evidence is found. One study dedicated to IBD evaluated 23 HBV-infected individuals, of whom 65% received infliximab and 59% received concomitant immunosuppressive agents, while 64% received corticosteroids; no patient suffered viral reactivation.[27]

Recommendations for Hepatitis B Virus Infection in Patients with Inflammatory Bowel Disease

• Screen all patients with IBD, ideally at the time of diagnosis, with HBsAg, anti-HBs, and anti-HBc serology, and, in the event of a positive HBsAg test, also test HBeAg, anti-HBe, and HBV DNA viral load quantification, and treat all patients who are HBsAg positive according to local guidelines.

• All patients seronegative for HBsAg and anti-HBc should be vaccinated, preferably during IBD remission and in the absence of immunosuppression, if possible.

• There are no data to support vaccination of patients who are anti-HBc positive.

Recommendations for Antiviral Prophylaxis in HBsAg-Negative, Anti-HBc-Positive Inflammatory Bowel Disease Patients Scheduled for Immunosuppressive Therapy

---

For HBsAg-positive individuals about to receive biologic agents (infliximab, adalimumab, certolizumab, golimumab, vedolizumab, or ustekinumab), or 4 or more weeks of corticosteroid treatment, check baseline HBV DNA levels and then treat with a nucleos(t)ide agent with a high barrier to resistance during immunosuppression and for 1 year after it is ceased.

For patients who are HBsAg negative/anti-HBc positive, also treat with prophylactic antiviral agents, as with patients who are HBsAg positive.

Neither thiopurines nor methotrexate pose a significant HBV reactivation risk, and antiviral prophylaxis is generally not required.

- There are no data to support vaccination of patients who are anti-HBc positive

---

Hepatitis B reactivation and new drugs

Reactivation of hepatitis B has been observed with many emerging immunosuppressive treatments, including monoclonal antibodies, fusion antibodies, treatments of HCC, BKIs, and PI3K inhibitors, JAK inhibitors, and hypomethylating agents. The risk of reactivation depends on the degree and duration of immunosuppression. Reactivation with these agents is currently limited to case reports, which are listed below in **Table 1**. Reactivation has also been reported to occur in patients given DAAs for the treatment of HCV infection, although the rates of reactivation have varied widely across studies.[28–38] In a recent review that assessed a pooled sample of data from 10 studies carried out from 2015 to 2018, the average rate of reactivation in patients given DAA therapy was 8%.[28] For patients who are HBsAg positive, the European Association for the Study of the Liver (EASL) recommends prophylactic HBV treatment with nucleos(t)ide analog antivirals during, and for 12 weeks after, completion of DAA treatment; in patients who are HBsAg negative/anti-HBc positive, EASL recommends monitoring and testing for HBV reactivation in case of ALT elevation, with treatment if reactivation is detected.[39]

There are many agents that have the potential to cause HBV reactivation based on their mechanism of action, their ability to cause myelosuppression, or by direct action on the virus. Obinutuzumab is a newer-generation anti-CD-20 monoclonal antibody that produces more profound B-cell depletion than rituximab. Daratumumab is a human IgG1k monoclonal antibody targeting CD38 in patients with refractory myeloma. Vascular endothelial growth factor inhibitors, epidermal growth factor receptor inhibitors, and hormone therapies are used for the treatment of HCC. The PI3Kδ inhibitor idelalisib inhibits B-cell receptor signaling. The hypomethylating agents decitabine and azacitidine have the potential for developing myelosuppression. A summary of recommendations for newer drugs based on their mechanism of action and class effects are listed in **Table 2**.

In summary, newer drugs with immunosuppressive activity are likely to be important risk factors for HBV reactivation, in particular, BTK, PI3K, and T-cell inhibitors. As yet, there are insufficient data to firmly establish the need for prophylaxis in patients receiving these newer agents. Where case reports have been published and there is a clear mechanism to trigger HBV reactivation, the clinical benefit of prophylaxis should be considered in the context of liver function and comorbidities for the individual.

Table 1
Agents with reported cases of HBV reactivation

Agent	Target	Use	Reports of Reactivation	Timing of Reactivation
Tocilizumab	IL-6	Rheumatoid arthritis Castleman disease	7 cases[a,40–44]	8 wk to 5 y
Mogamulizumab[45]	Anti-CCR4	T-cell leukemia and lymphoma	2 cases[b,45,46]	Following X cycles of CHOP and THP-CHOP
Brentuximab vedotin	CD30	Relapsed or refractory Hodgkin lymphoma and T-cell lymphoma	1 case[47]	
Abatacept	CTLA-4	Rheumatoid arthritis	17 cases[c,19,20,48,49]	
TACE[50,51]	HCC		80+ cases[d,52]	
Ibrutinib	IL2	B-cell non-Hodgkin lymphoma	4 cases[53,54]	5 mo
Ruxolitinib[55]	JAK1 JAK2	Myelofibrosis	1 case[56]	4 wk
Pomalidomide[57]	Angiogenesis	Multiple myeloma	1 case[e,57]	6 cycles
Bortezomib	T cells	Hematopoietic stem cell transplantation	11 cases[58–61]	1–3 y

[a] Two cases were from the same retrospective study of 9 patients treated with tocilizumab for rheumatoid arthritis. In that study, reactivation was defined as anti-HBc positive, HBV DNA negative. Neither patient was treated, and they remained with subclinical levels of infection.
[b] One occurred despite prophylaxis with entecavir.
[c] Patients did not receive antiviral prophylaxis; also 1 occult HBV case.
[d] Risk factors include high-level viremia, intensity of treatment, and combination with doxorubicin; risk higher following hepatic resection than with radiofrequency ablation.
[e] In combination with doxorubicin and dexamethasone.[57]

Table 2
Immunosuppressive drugs and risk of HBV reactivation

Drug Class	Drug	Risk of Reactivation		Recommendations
		HBsAg+	HBsAg −/anti-HBc+	
B-Cell depleting agents	Rituximab[62] Ofatumumab Alemtuzumab Ibrutinib	30%–60%	24.00%	Prophylaxis
Checkpoint inhibitors	Nivolumab Ipilimumab			
Anthracycline derivatives	Doxorubicin[63] Epirubicin	15%–30%	>10%	Prophylaxis
TNF-α inhibitors	Infliximab Etanercept[64] Adalimumab[65] Certolizumab Golimumab	39% 1%–5% 12%–39%	5%	Prophylaxis Prophylaxis
Cytokine and integrin inhibitors	Abatacept[19,20,48,66] Ustekinumab Natalizumab Mogamulizumab[22] Vedolizumab	1%–10%	1% 12.50%	Prophylaxis
Immunophilin inhibitors	Cyclosporine			
Tyrosine kinase inhibitors	Imatinib[67] Nilotinib Dasatinib Ibrutinib Erlotinib	1%–10%	1%	Monitor/ prophylaxis
Steroids duration >4 wk	High dose >20 mg[68] Moderate dose 10–20 mg orally >4 wk[69,70] Low dose <10 mg orally >4 wk or less	10%–15% 5%–10% <1%	<1%	Prophylaxis if HBsAg+ Monitor/ prophylaxis Monitor/ prophylaxis
Duration <2 wk	Intra-articular[71]	<1%	<0.1%	Usual care
Antimetabolites	Azathioprine[72] 6-MP Methotrexate	<1% <1%	<0.1% <0.1%	Usual care Usual care Usual care

Diabetes, liver cirrhosis, and allogenic transplantation and anti-HBs titers <100 U/mL are independent risk factors. Steroids significantly increased the risk for all other regimens by up to 75%.

Recommendations with newer agents now approved or in development

---

Clearly it is difficult to assess newer drugs that have insufficient data on use, but there are some classes of drugs that, based on their mechanism of action, are thought likely to reactivate HBV, suggesting the need for a low threshold for prophylaxis. Newer drugs that will probably need prophylaxis include the following.

- B-cell inhibitors, including ofatumamab, ustekinamab, natalizumab, ibrotumomab, and obinuzumab
- PI3Kδ inhibitors, including idelasib
- Anti-CD38 agents, including daratumumab
- JAK inhibitors, including ruxolitinib
- T-cell inhibitors (CTLA-4), including abatacept
- Cytokine and chemokine inhibitors, including tocilizumab and mogamulizumab
- Proteasome inhibitors, including bortezomib
- DAAs used for treatment of hepatitis C in patients who are HBsAg positive

---

SUMMARY

Further research and data collection are needed to more clearly address the questions of risk-based screening and HBV prophylaxis in immunosuppressed patients. Possibilities include a registry to collect reports of HBV reactivation; a mechanism to follow-up patients with previous HBV infection who receive immunosuppressive therapy; 1 year follow-up of patients after receiving rituximab to assess B-cell and T-cell activity; and collection of cost-effectiveness data in a broader range of diseases and with different therapies. A better understanding of the public health issues related to prophylaxis for patients who are anti-HBc-positive is needed.

ACKNOWLEDGMENTS

Meetings to discuss and develop recommendations presented in this manuscript and medical writing services provided in the preparation of this manuscript were funded by Gilead Sciences. Neither the medical writer or Gilead in any way influenced the content or the conclusions of the position paper. None of the authors had any direct financial support from Gilead Sciences or any other companies.

REFERENCES

1. Lok AS, Liang RH, Chiu EK, et al. Reactivation of hepatitis B virus replication in patients receiving cytotoxic therapy. Report of a prospective study. Gastroenterology 1991;100(1):182–8.
2. Terrault NA, Lok ASF, McMahon BJ, et al. Update on prevention, diagnosis, and treatment of chronic hepatitis B: AASLD 2018 hepatitis B guidance. Hepatology 2018;67(4):1560–99.
3. Tan J, Zhou J, Zhao P, et al. Prospective study of HBV reactivation risk in rheumatoid arthritis patients who received conventional disease-modifying antirheumatic drugs. Clin Rheumatol 2012;31(8):1169–75.
4. Felis-Giemza A, Olesinska M, Swierkocka K, et al. Treatment of rheumatic diseases and hepatitis B virus coinfection. Rheumatol Int 2015;35(3):385–92.

5. Koutsianas C, Thomas K, Vassilopoulos D. Hepatitis B reactivation in rheumatic diseases: screening and prevention. Rheum Dis Clin North Am 2017;43(1): 133–49.

6. Lam KC, Lai CL, Trepo C, et al. Deleterious effect of prednisolone in HBsAg-positive chronic active hepatitis. N Engl J Med 1981;304(7):380–6.

7. Kim TW, Kim MN, Kwon JW, et al. Risk of hepatitis B virus reactivation in patients with asthma or chronic obstructive pulmonary disease treated with corticosteroids. Respirology 2010;15(7):1092–7.

8. Cantini F, Boccia S, Goletti D, et al. HBV reactivation in patients treated with anti-tumor necrosis factor-alpha (TNF-alpha) agents for rheumatic and dermatologic conditions: a systematic review and meta-analysis. Int J Rheumatol 2014;2014: 926836.

9. Perez-Alvarez R, Diaz-Lagares C, Garcia-Hernandez F, et al. Hepatitis B virus (HBV) reactivation in patients receiving tumor necrosis factor (TNF)-targeted therapy: analysis of 257 cases. Medicine (Baltimore) 2011;90(6):359–71.

10. Charpin C, Guis S, Colson P, et al. Safety of TNF-blocking agents in rheumatic patients with serology suggesting past hepatitis B state: results from a cohort of 21 patients. Arthritis Res Ther 2009;11(6):R179.

11. Vassilopoulos D, Apostolopoulou A, Hadziyannis E, et al. Long-term safety of anti-TNF treatment in patients with rheumatic diseases and chronic or resolved hepatitis B virus infection. Ann Rheum Dis 2010;69(7):1352–5.

12. Caporali R, Bobbio-Pallavicini F, Atzeni F, et al. Safety of tumor necrosis factor alpha blockers in hepatitis B virus occult carriers (hepatitis B surface antigen negative/anti-hepatitis B core antigen positive) with rheumatic diseases. Arthritis Care Res (Hoboken) 2010;62(6):749–54.

13. Carroll MB, Forgione MA. Use of tumor necrosis factor alpha inhibitors in hepatitis B surface antigen-positive patients: a literature review and potential mechanisms of action. Clin Rheumatol 2010;29(9):1021–9.

14. Zingarelli S, Frassi M, Bazzani C, et al. Use of tumor necrosis factor-alpha-blocking agents in hepatitis B virus-positive patients: reports of 3 cases and review of the literature. J Rheumatol 2009;36(6):1188–94.

15. Salman-Monte TC, Lisbona MP, Garcia-Retortillo M, et al. Reactivation of hepatitis virus B infection in a patient with rheumatoid arthritis after treatment with rituximab. Reumatol Clin 2014;10(3):196–7.

16. Vassilopoulos D, Delicha EM, Settas L, et al. Safety profile of repeated rituximab cycles in unselected rheumatoid arthritis patients: a long-term, prospective real-life study. Clin Exp Rheumatol 2016;34(5):893–900.

17. Gigi E, Georgiou T, Mougiou D, et al. Hepatitis B reactivation in a patient with rheumatoid arthritis with antibodies to hepatitis B surface antigen treated with rituximab. Hippokratia 2013;17(1):91–3.

18. Varisco V, Vigano M, Batticciotto A, et al. Low risk of hepatitis B virus reactivation in HBsAg-negative/anti-HBc-positive carriers receiving rituximab for rheumatoid arthritis: a retrospective multicenter Italian study. J Rheumatol 2016;43(5): 869–74.

19. Kim PS, Ho GY, Prete PE, et al. Safety and efficacy of abatacept in eight rheumatoid arthritis patients with chronic hepatitis B. Arthritis Care Res (Hoboken) 2012; 64(8):1265–8.

20. Germanidis G, Hytiroglou P, Zakalka M, et al. Reactivation of occult hepatitis B virus infection, following treatment of refractory rheumatoid arthritis with abatacept. J Hepatol 2012;56(6):1420–1.

21. Karvellas CJ, Cardoso FS, Gottfried M, et al. HBV-associated acute liver failure after immunosuppression and risk of death. Clin Gastroenterol Hepatol 2017; 15(1):113–22.

22. Loomba R, Liang TJ. Hepatitis B reactivation associated with immune suppressive and biological modifier therapies: current concepts, management strategies, and future directions. Gastroenterology 2017;152(6):1297–309.

23. Rahier JF, Magro F, Abreu C, et al. Second European evidence-based consensus on the prevention, diagnosis and management of opportunistic infections in inflammatory bowel disease. J Crohns Colitis 2014;8(6):443–68.

24. Jiang HY, Wang SY, Deng M, et al. Immune response to hepatitis B vaccination among people with inflammatory bowel diseases: a systematic review and meta-analysis. Vaccine 2017;35(20):2633–41.

25. Walsh AJ, Weltman M, Burger D, et al. Implementing guidelines on the prevention of opportunistic infections in inflammatory bowel disease. J Crohns Colitis 2013; 7(10):e449–56.

26. Vaughn BP, Doherty GA, Gautam S, et al. Screening for tuberculosis and hepatitis B prior to the initiation of anti-tumor necrosis therapy. Inflamm Bowel Dis 2012; 18(6):1057–63.

27. Papa A, Felice C, Marzo M, et al. Prevalence and natural history of hepatitis B and C infections in a large population of IBD patients treated with anti-tumor necrosis factor-alpha agents. J Crohns Colitis 2013;7(2):113–9.

28. Mavilia MG, Wu GY. HBV-HCV coinfection: viral interactions, management, and viral reactivation. J Clin Transl Hepatol 2018;6(3):296–305.

29. Calvaruso V, Ferraro D, Licata A, et al. HBV reactivation in patients with HCV/HBV cirrhosis on treatment with direct-acting antivirals. J Viral Hepat 2018;25(1):72–9.

30. Collins JM, Raphael KL, Terry C, et al. Hepatitis B virus reactivation during successful treatment of hepatitis C virus with sofosbuvir and simeprevir. Clin Infect Dis 2015;61(8):1304–6.

31. Sato K, Kobayashi T, Yamazaki Y, et al. Spontaneous remission of hepatitis B virus reactivation during direct-acting antiviral agent-based therapy for chronic hepatitis C. Hepatol Res 2017;47(12):1346–53.

32. Belperio PS, Shahoumian TA, Mole LA, et al. Evaluation of hepatitis B reactivation among 62,920 veterans treated with oral hepatitis C antivirals. Hepatology 2017; 66(1):27–36.

33. Gane EJ, Hyland RH, An D, et al. Ledipasvir and sofosbuvir for HCV infection in patients coinfected with HBV. Antivir Ther 2016;21(7):605–9.

34. Wang C, Ji D, Chen J, et al. Hepatitis due to reactivation of hepatitis B virus in endemic areas among patients with hepatitis C treated with direct-acting antiviral agents. Clin Gastroenterol Hepatol 2017;15(1):132–6.

35. Kawagishi N, Suda G, Onozawa M, et al. Comparing the risk of hepatitis B virus reactivation between direct-acting antiviral therapies and interferon-based therapies for hepatitis C. J Viral Hepat 2017;24(12):1098–106.

36. Ogawa E, Furusyo N, Murata M, et al. Potential risk of HBV reactivation in patients with resolved HBV infection undergoing direct-acting antiviral treatment for HCV. Liver Int 2018;38(1):76–83.

37. Doi A, Sakamori R, Tahata Y, et al. Frequency of, and factors associated with, hepatitis B virus reactivation in hepatitis C patients treated with all-oral direct-acting antivirals: analysis of a Japanese prospective cohort. Hepatol Res 2017; 47(13):1438–44.

38. Yeh ML, Huang CF, Hsieh MH, et al. Reactivation of hepatitis B in patients of chronic hepatitis C with hepatitis B virus infection treated with direct acting antivirals. J Gastroenterol Hepatol 2017;32(10):1754–62.
39. European Association for the Study of the Liver. EASL 2017 clinical practice guidelines on the management of hepatitis B virus infection. J Hepatol 2017; 67(2):370–98.
40. Chen LF, Mo YQ, Jing J, et al. Short-course tocilizumab increases risk of hepatitis B virus reactivation in patients with rheumatoid arthritis: a prospective clinical observation. Int J Rheum Dis 2017;20(7):859–69.
41. Barone M, Notarnicola A, Lopalco G, et al. Safety of long-term biologic therapy in rheumatologic patients with a previously resolved hepatitis B viral infection. Hepatology 2015;62(1):40–6.
42. Nagashima T, Minota S. Long-term tocilizumab therapy in a patient with rheumatoid arthritis and chronic hepatitis B. Rheumatology (Oxford) 2008;47(12): 1838–40.
43. Mitroulis I, Hatzara C, Kandili A, et al. Long-term safety of rituximab in patients with rheumatic diseases and chronic or resolved hepatitis B virus infection. Ann Rheum Dis 2013;72(2):308–10.
44. Nakamura J, Nagashima T, Nagatani K, et al. Reactivation of hepatitis B virus in rheumatoid arthritis patients treated with biological disease-modifying antirheumatic drugs. Int J Rheum Dis 2016;19(5):470–5.
45. Ifuku H, Kusumoto S, Tanaka Y, et al. Fatal reactivation of hepatitis B virus infection in a patient with adult T-cell leukemia-lymphoma receiving the anti-CC chemokine receptor 4 antibody mogamulizumab. Hepatol Res 2015;45(13):1363–7.
46. Nakano N, Kusumoto S, Tanaka Y, et al. Reactivation of hepatitis B virus in a patient with adult T-cell leukemia-lymphoma receiving the anti-CC chemokine receptor 4 antibody mogamulizumab. Hepatol Res 2014;44(3):354–7.
47. Drgona L, Gudiol C, Lanini S, et al. ESCMID Study Group for Infections in Compromised Hosts (ESGICH) consensus document on the safety of targeted and biological therapies: an infectious diseases perspective (Agents targeting lymphoid or myeloid cells surface antigens [II]: CD22, CD30, CD33, CD38, CD40, SLAMF-7 and CCR4). Clin Microbiol Infect 2018;24(Suppl 2):S83–94.
48. Talotta R, Atzeni F, Sarzi Puttini P. Reactivation of occult hepatitis B virus infection under treatment with abatacept: a case report. BMC Pharmacol Toxicol 2016;17:17.
49. De Nard F, Todoerti M, Grosso V, et al. Safety of the newer biological Dmards, tocilizumab and abatacept, in rheumatoid arthritis (RA) patients with a history of HBV infection: a real life experience. Ann Rheum Dis 2014;73(Suppl 2):499.
50. Perrillo RP, Gish R, Falck-Ytter YT. American Gastroenterological Association Institute technical review on prevention and treatment of hepatitis B virus reactivation during immunosuppressive drug therapy. Gastroenterology 2015;148(1):221–44.e3.
51. Liu F, Dan J, Zhang Y, et al. Hepatitis B reactivation after treatment for HBV-related hepatocellular carcinoma: comparative analysis of radiofrequency ablation versus hepatic resection. Zhonghua Gan Zang Bing Za Zhi 2014;22(1): 38–42 [in Chinese].
52. Wang K, Jiang G, Jia Z, et al. Effects of transarterial chemoembolization combined with antiviral therapy on HBV reactivation and liver function in HBV-related hepatocellular carcinoma patients with HBV-DNA negative. Medicine (Baltimore) 2018;97(22):e10940.
53. Molica S, Levato L, Mirabelli R, et al. Feasibility and safety of therapy with ibrutinib after antiviral control of hepatitis B virus (HBV) reactivation in chronic lymphocytic leukemia patients. Leuk Lymphoma 2018;59(11):2734–6.

54. de Jesus Ngoma P, Kabamba B, Dahlqvist G, et al. Occult HBV reactivation induced by ibrutinib treatment: a case report. Acta Gastroenterol Belg 2015; 78(4):424–6.
55. Caocci G, Murgia F, Podda L, et al. Reactivation of hepatitis B virus infection following ruxolitinib treatment in a patient with myelofibrosis. Leukemia 2014; 28(1):225–7.
56. Kirito K, Sakamoto M, Enomoto N. Elevation of the hepatitis B virus DNA during the treatment of polycythemia vera with the JAK kinase inhibitor ruxolitinib. Intern Med 2016;55(10):1341–4.
57. Danhof S, Schreder M, Strifler S, et al. Long-term disease control by pomalidomide-/dexamethasone-based therapy in a patient with advanced multiple myeloma: a case report and review of the literature. Case Rep Oncol 2015; 8(1):189–95.
58. Almaghrabi MM, Fortinsky KJ, Wong D. Severe acute hepatitis B in HBV-vaccinated partner of a patient with multiple myeloma treated with cyclophosphamide, bortezomib, and dexamethasone and autologous stem cell transplant. Case Reports Hepatol 2017;2017:2463953.
59. Hussain S, Jhaj R, Ahsan S, et al. Bortezomib induced hepatitis B reactivation. Case Rep Med 2014;2014:964082.
60. Tanaka H, Sakuma I, Hashimoto S, et al. Hepatitis B reactivation in a multiple myeloma patient with resolved hepatitis B infection during bortezomib therapy: case report. J Clin Exp Hematop 2012;52(1):67–9.
61. Li J, Huang B, Li Y, et al. Hepatitis B virus reactivation in patients with multiple myeloma receiving bortezomib-containing regimens followed by autologous stem cell transplant. Leuk Lymphoma 2015;56(6):1710–7.
62. Hsu C, Tsou HH, Lin SJ, et al. Chemotherapy-induced hepatitis B reactivation in lymphoma patients with resolved HBV infection: a prospective study. Hepatology 2014;59(6):2092–100.
63. Kim MK, Ahn JH, Kim SB, et al. Hepatitis B reactivation during adjuvant anthracycline-based chemotherapy in patients with breast cancer: a single institution's experience. Korean J Intern Med 2007;22(4):237–43.
64. Nobile S, Gionchetti P, Rizzello F, et al. Mucosal healing in pediatric Crohn's disease after anti-TNF therapy: a long-term experience at a single center. Eur J Gastroenterol Hepatol 2014;26(4):458–65.
65. Abramson A, Menter A, Perrillo R. Psoriasis, hepatitis B, and the tumor necrosis factor-alpha inhibitory agents: a review and recommendations for management. J Am Acad Dermatol 2012;67(6):1349–61.
66. Nard FD, Todoerti M, Grosso V, et al. Risk of hepatitis B virus reactivation in rheumatoid arthritis patients undergoing biologic treatment: extending perspective from old to newer drugs. World J Hepatol 2015;7(3):344–61.
67. Yeo W, Lam KC, Zee B, et al. Hepatitis B reactivation in patients with hepatocellular carcinoma undergoing systemic chemotherapy. Ann Oncol 2004;15(11):1661–6.
68. Cheng AL, Hsiung CA, Su IJ, et al. Steroid-free chemotherapy decreases risk of hepatitis B virus (HBV) reactivation in HBV-carriers with lymphoma. Hepatology 2003;37(6):1320–8.
69. Hoofnagle JH, Davis GL, Pappas SC, et al. A short course of prednisolone in chronic type B hepatitis. Report of a randomized, double-blind, placebo-controlled trial. Ann Intern Med 1986;104(1):12–7.
70. Perrillo RP, Schiff ER, Davis GL, et al. A randomized, controlled trial of interferon alfa-2b alone and after prednisone withdrawal for the treatment of chronic

hepatitis B. The Hepatitis Interventional Therapy Group. N Engl J Med 1990; 323(5):295–301.

71. Habib GS. Systemic effects of intra-articular corticosteroids. Clin Rheumatol 2009;28(7):749–56.

72. Sagnelli E, Manzillo G, Maio G, et al. Serum levels of hepatitis B surface and core antigens during immunosuppressive treatment of HBsAg-positive chronic active hepatitis. Lancet 1980;2(8191):395–7.

Drugs in the Pipeline for HBV

Uri Lopatin, MD

KEYWORDS

- HBV cure • cccDNA • Core protein inhibitor • siRNA • Entry inhibitor • TLR agonist
- Immunotherapy

KEY POINTS

- The primary goal of current therapeutic research for chronic hepatitis B is to achieve a functional cure after a finite course of therapy.
- Both direct-acting antivirals, targeting different aspects of the hepatitis B virus (HBV) replication cycle, and immunotherapeutic approaches are being explored as monotherapies and/or in combination with other agents. The key molecular objective is elimination of HBV covalently closed circular DNA, which is the source of viral transcripts associated with chronic infection, but minimally affected by current therapies.
- Direct-acting antivirals under clinical investigation include entry inhibitors, core protein inhibitors, and RNA silencers.
- Immunotherapeutic approaches include TLR-7 and TLR-8 agonists, therapeutic vaccines, checkpoint inhibitors, RIG-I agonist, and anti-HBV antibodies.
- Results of preclinical and early clinical studies are promising; in the next few years, anticipated phase 2 and phase 3 data will establish which drugs or drug combinations may contribute to a functional cure.

INTRODUCTION
Global Burden

Despite the introduction of an effective vaccine almost 40 years ago, hepatitis B virus (HBV) remains a major cause of chronic liver disease. Globally, an estimated 257 million people have chronic hepatitis B (CHB), and 600,000 to 1 million deaths occur annually because of the end-stage complications of cirrhosis and hepatocellular carcinoma.[1] The global burden of disease attributable to chronic viral hepatitis (B and C combined) has increased over the last 2 decades. Viral hepatitis was the seventh leading cause of death worldwide in 2013, compared with tenth in 1990.[2]

Hepatitis B Virus Life Cycle

The complex HBV life cycle has recently been extensively reviewed and presents multiple potential antiviral targets.[3,4] Replication begins when circulating HBV binds to a

Disclosure Statement: U. Lopatin is an employee of Assembly Biosciences.
Assembly Biosciences, 331 Oyster Point Boulevard, South San Francisco, CA 94080, USA
E-mail address: uri@assemblybio.com

https://doi.org/10.1016/j.cld.2019.04.006
liver.theclinics.com
1089-3261/19/© 2019 The Author. Published by Elsevier Inc. This is an open access article under the
CC BY-NC-ND license (http://creativecommons.org/licenses/by-nc-nd/4.0/).

hepatocyte through interactions between hepatitis B surface antigen (HBsAg) and sodium taurocholate cotransporting polypeptide (NTCP) as a receptor.[5,6] Subsequently, the viral capsid is released into the cell and traffics to the nuclear pore, where the HBV relaxed circular DNA (rcDNA) can be delivered to the nucleus. In the nucleus, the rcDNA is converted by host polymerases to covalently closed circular DNA (cccDNA), which is a nuclear mini-chromosome-like moiety that exists in low copy numbers in infected hepatocyte nuclei.[7] cccDNA is thought to be relatively stable in quiescent hepatocytes but may be lost during cell division.[8,9]

cccDNA molecules function as templates for transcription of full-length pregenomic RNA (pgRNA) and subgenomic messenger RNAs (mRNAs) that encode viral proteins. These proteins include HBV polymerase/reverse transcriptase (pol/RT), hepatitis B x-protein, core protein, hepatitis B e-antigen (HBeAg), and HBsAg. HBV pol/RT binds to pgRNA and is encapsidated within 120 core protein dimers to form a nascent viral capsid, where the pgRNA is reverse transcribed to produce viral rcDNA. The capsid can then either acquire an HBsAg-containing envelope and be secreted as infectious virus or traffic back to the nucleus and replenish the cccDNA pool.[10] The lifespan of individual cccDNA molecules is not well understood and in the setting of an antiviral immune response may be shorter than the life of a hepatocyte.[11] In cell culture systems, cccDNA has been estimated to have a half-life of approximately 40 days,[10,12] whereas human studies evaluating cccDNA turnover have suggested that populations of cccDNA can convert from mutant to wild type (or via versa) in as little as 12 weeks.[13] However, cccDNA may persist longer in a residual pool of quiescent nondividing hepatocytes.[9] cccDNA is not known to tether to the nuclear spindle, and most cccDNA is thought to be lost during hepatocyte expansion, as occurs, for example, following an immune response and clearance of infected cells. Importantly, HBV is not a cytopathic virus; thus, in the absence of an adequate antiviral immune response, there is not thought to be a virus-derived trigger to drive hepatocyte loss or proliferation.

Possible targets for therapeutic intervention include HBV binding and absorption, capsid dissociation, cccDNA formation, gene expression, protein synthesis, capsid assembly, viral DNA synthesis, capsid envelopment, and virion release (**Fig. 1**). Most of these targets are being addressed by ongoing therapeutic research programs. In addition, because attenuation of the HBV-specific immune response is a key feature of chronic HBV infection, multiple approaches are being explored to restore immune responsiveness to allow immune-mediated clearance of HBV-infected hepatocytes.

Goal of New Therapies

The ultimate goal of ongoing research for novel HBV therapeutics is eradication of the cccDNA viral reservoir. Because measurement of cccDNA itself is challenging, requiring a biopsy and sophisticated assays that have not yet been standardized, surrogates for cccDNA loss or inactivation are required. These surrogates must include a sustained viral response (SVR), lack of viral rebound with persistent normal liver function and lack of inflammation, after a finite course of therapy. In addition to loss of detectable serum HBV DNA, additional biomarker changes expected to coincide with such improved off-treatment responses include a loss of serum HBeAg and either loss or a decline to a stable low level of detectable serum HBsAg.[14] Loss of HBsAg in particular, although uncommon with current therapies, has been associated with sustained posttreatment virologic responses and is generally considered a clinical marker of a functional cure, indicating that treatment is no longer required.[14] Although HBsAg clearance is accepted as a desirable

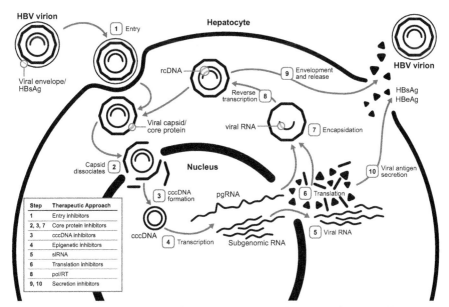

Fig. 1. HBV replication cycle and therapeutic targets. The steps of HBV replication are shown, beginning with viral entry into a hepatocyte. The inset table indicates active therapeutic research targets associated with each step.

endpoint, its achievement has been somewhat confounded by the discovery that, at least in chimpanzees, circulating HBsAg may arise from HBV integrants, which, although unable to produce complete virus, may produce a significant fraction of the total circulating HBsAg.[15] Unfortunately, even in the rare instances in which HBsAg loss has been achieved, reactivation in the setting of immunosuppression is possible. The exact mechanisms by which immune control and escape occur are only partially understood, suggesting that the understanding of even such "functional cures" is still evolving.[16]

Given the challenges of defining what constitutes a "cure" for CHB (functional or otherwise) with today's technology, the author proposes that a more appropriate definition of the clinical goals for current studies may be similar to those used as hepatitis C therapeutics were being developed. An initial objective should be "sustained viral response" as measured by lack of viral DNA or antigen rebound for a fixed period off treatment. Subsequently, "cure" could be declared in individuals in whom SVR is maintained over a more extended time frame.

Current Options

Current options for CHB therapy include nucleos(t)ide analogues and interferons. In brief, nearly all patients respond during treatment with nucleos(t)ide analogues, but beneficial responses are rarely sustained after treatment. Interferons, in contrast, may provide sustained responses more frequently, but only in a limited subset of patients defined primarily by HBV genotype and disease characteristics.[17–19] Although neither of these therapies, alone or in combination, has dramatically increased cure rates in patients with CHB, it is highly likely that a successful curative regimen will entail combinations with either or both of these modalities.

Interferons

In 1991, interferon alfa-2b became the first treatment approved for CHB therapy; pegylated interferon alfa-2a was approved in 2005.[20] Interferons are typically administered by subcutaneous injection for up to 12 months and can elicit durable posttreatment suppression of HBV replication and antigenemia.[21] Tolerability can be poor, however, and clinically significant response rates are generally achievable by only a small subset of patients.

Nucleos(t)ide Analogues

The most commonly used therapies for CHB at present, nucleos(t)ide HBV pol/RT inhibitors, profoundly inhibit HBV DNA synthesis, frequently reducing serum HBV DNA to levels at the limit of quantification. This response is associated with improvement of hepatic fibrosis and reduced risk of hepatocellular carcinoma. All agents in this class have similar modes of action. Lamivudine, approved in the United States in 1998, was the first antiviral nucleos(t)ide analogue available for treatment of CHB.[20] Subsequently, adefovir (2002), entecavir (2005), telbivudine (2006), tenofovir disoproxil fumarate (2008), and tenofovir alafenamide (2016) were approved. Clevudine and besifovir dipivoxil maleate are approved in South Korea but not in the United States. Agents in this class exhibit some differences with respect to potency, safety, and resistance profiles. The most important difference is the superior barrier to resistance exhibited by tenofovir and entecavir, as demonstrated by negligible rates of virologic failure even after years of therapy.[22,23] Tenofovir alafenamide elicits virologic responses similar to those associated with tenofovir disoproxil fumarate, but with reduced risk of bone and renal toxicities.[24–26]

Despite their success in persistently inhibiting HBV pol/RT, because cccDNA formation from rcDNA is catalyzed primarily by cellular polymerases, nucleos(t)ide analogues have minimal effects on cccDNA establishment and affect HBV gene expression only indirectly.[27] Over the last several years, several lines of evidence have also suggested that nucleos(t)ide analogues alone are unable to fully inhibit all HBV replication. For example, analysis of liver biopsies has shown that HBV replication often persists at low levels even after years of nucleos(t)ide analogue therapy.[28] As long as low-level replication persists, new hepatocytes can be reinfected continuously, and it is unlikely that nucleos(t)ide analogues alone will cure most individuals; clinically, this is apparent from the slow HBsAg declines and low cure rates seen on current standards of care.[29] As a result, for most patients, lengthy if not lifelong treatment is likely to be needed. In those few patients in whom both serum antigens and HBV DNA do become undetectable, a sustained posttreatment virologic response is often achieved if therapy is stopped, supporting HBsAg clearance as a possible biomarker of functional cure.[14,30,31]

Combination therapy with a nucleos(t)ide analogue and pegylated interferon has been explored with generally disappointing results.[32,33] Although a few studies have reported higher rates of sustained posttreatment responses with peginterferon combined with entecavir or tenofovir versus interferon alone,[34–36] response rates are typically low and the population likely to benefit appears similar to that with interferon alone.[37] Several Asian studies have reported no incremental benefit from combination therapies.[38–41]

Novel Therapies

Novel therapies in clinical development include both direct-acting antivirals (DAAs), which target viral proteins or viral RNAs, and host-directed antivirals, such as entry inhibitors and immunomodulators (**Table 1**). Additional approaches, such as direct cccDNA targeting, epigenetic modifiers, and RNAse H inhibition, remain preclinical but are anticipated to initiate clinical evaluation over the next few years.

THERAPIES IN CLINICAL DEVELOPMENT

As discussed, inhibition of the HBV pol/RT by nucleos(t)ide analogues is of limited efficacy owing to their primary mode of action, which has little impact on either cccDNA establishment or viral gene expression. They have repeatedly been shown to incompletely suppress intrahepatic viral replication,[28,42,43] resulting in rapid recurrence of viral replication if treatment is stopped. Over the past 5 to 10 years, other aspects of the HBV replication cycle have been explored with the aim of identifying agents that could address these limitations and achieve antiviral effects that persist after treatment.

Direct-Acting Antivirals

Novel DAAs are being developed with the rationale that hepatocytes have a finite lifespan; thus, if new (uninfected) hepatocytes can be protected from infection by a potent antiviral regimen, then the duration of the infection cannot exceed the lifespan of the hepatocytes and may be shorter if cccDNA loss is more rapid than hepatocyte loss.[10,44,45] If current standard-of-care nucleos(t)ide therapies are, in fact, achieving low cure rates as a result of ongoing intrahepatic HBV replication (ie, primary antiviral failure), then combining a nucleos(t)ide analogue with a DAA for a sufficient length of time may be all that is required to achieve a cure for CHB. DAAs in development include entry inhibitors, RNA inhibitors, and core protein inhibitors.

Entry Inhibitors

Blockade of HBV entry into hepatocytes, thus preventing the earliest step of infection, has been explored concurrent with identification of NTCP as the HBV receptor.[6] Bulevirtide (myrcludex B; Hepatera Ltd), a specific NTCP inhibitor, blocks attachment of viral pre-S1 via high-affinity binding to NTCP.[46] Current clinical studies of bulevirtide are focused on patients with hepatitis delta virus (HDV) coinfection. Because infectivity of both HBV and HDV depends on the presence of HBsAg in the viral envelope, these studies will assess virologic responses of both HDV and HBV. Phase 2 data showed a marked reduction of HDV RNA after 24 weeks of bulevirtide combined with tenofovir,[47] and after 48 weeks of bulevirtide with or without peginterferon-alfa.[48] In the latter study, the HBsAg decline was greater with bulevirtide in combination with peginterferon-alfa. Planned phase 3 studies will explore extended therapy with bulevirtide as monotherapy or in combination with peginterferon-alfa in patients with HBV/HDV coinfection, focusing on HDV clearance as the primary objective. Although entry blockers would not be expected to directly interfere with HBV cccDNA formation, entry inhibition with bulevirtide would be anticipated to protect still uninfected cells and thus may contribute to HBV therapy either alone or in combination with other modalities.

RNA Interference

RNA interference (RNAi) is a natural process by which a small interfering RNA (siRNA) duplex directs sequence-specific posttranscriptional silencing by binding to complementary mRNA, triggering its elimination.[49,50] Because the HBV genome is compact with multiple overlapping reading frames, targeting viral transcripts with siRNA has emerged as an attractive approach anticipated to reduce expression of multiple viral

Table 1
Therapeutics in clinical development for chronic hepatitis B

Drug Class	Drug	Company	Phase 1	Phase 2	Phase 3
DAAs					
Core protein inhibitors	AB-506	Arbutus Biopharma	↑		
	ABI-H0731	Assembly Biosciences	→→	↑	
	ABI-H2158	Assembly Biosciences	↑		
	EDP-514	Enanta Pharmaceuticals	↑		
	JNJ-6379	Johnson & Johnson	→→	↑	
	JNJ-0440	Johnson & Johnson	↑		
	RO7049389	Roche	↑		
siRNA, antisense RNA	AB-729	Arbutus Biopharma	↑		
	DCR-HBVS	Dicerna Pharmaceuticals	↑		
	GSK/IONIS-HBV-L$_{Rx}$	Ionis/GlaxoSmithKline	→→	↑	
	IONIS-HBV$_{Rx}$	Ionis/GlaxoSmithKline	→→	↑	
	JNJ-3989 (ARO-HBV)	Johnson & Johnson	→→	↑	
	RO7062931	Roche	↑		
	Vir-2218 (ALN-HBV02)	Vir Biotechnology/Alnylam	↑		
pol/RT inhibitor	Tenofovir exalidex	ContraVir Pharmaceuticals	→→	↑	
HBsAg secretion inhibitors	REP-2139	Replicor	→→	↑	
	REP-2165	Replicor	→→	↑	

Indirect-acting antivirals and immunotherapeutics

HBV entry inhibitor	Bulevirtide	Hepatera Ltd
TLR-7 agonists	AL-034	Johnson & Johnson/Alios
	RG-7854	Roche
	RO7020531	Roche
TLR-8 agonist	GS-9688	Gilead Sciences
Therapeutic vaccines	AIC-649	AiCuris
	INO-1800	Inovio Pharmaceuticals
	TG1050	Transgene
RIG-I and NOD2 agonist	Inarigivir	Spring Bank
Apoptosis inducer	APG-1387	Ascentage Pharma
FXR agonist	EYP-001	Enyo Pharma

Abbreviations: NOD2, nucleotide-binding oligomerization domain-containing protein 2; RIG-I, retinoic acid-inducible gene-I.

antigens. Of particular interest has been the implication of reducing HBsAg, which has been proposed to contribute to specific impairment of an effective anti-HBV immune response.

Various approaches have been taken to safely enhance delivery of the siRNA moiety and to target the HBV genome within hepatocytes. Although most of these programs remain preclinical, several have entered human studies with mixed results. An early siRNA against HBV, ARC-520 (Arrowhead Pharmaceuticals), was composed of 2 siRNAs conjugated to cholesterol and administered with a polymer-based system containing N-acetyl galactosamine; together these conjugates enhance delivery to the hepatocyte cytoplasm.[51,52] Monthly injections of ARC-520 in combination with standard oral entecavir achieved multilog reductions of serum HBsAg concentrations in HBeAg-positive patients that persisted for months after discontinuing ARC-520; lesser (<1 log) reductions of HBsAg were reported in HBeAg-negative patients.[53] These results helped demonstrate the significant percentage of circulating HBsAg that could be derived from integrated HBV sequences in HBeAg-negative patients. Subsequently, 3 monthly subcutaneous injections of a follow-on product, JNJ-3989 (formerly ARO-HBV; Johnson & Johnson/Arrowhead), which targets a different region of the HBV genome, also elicited dose-related reductions of serum HBsAg of 1.3 to 3.8 $\log_{10}$ IU/mL, as well as reductions of HBV DNA, HBV RNA, HBeAg, and hepatitis B core-related antigen.[54,55] Viral antigen responses were similar with or without concomitant nucleos(t)ide analogue therapy and in both HBeAg-positive and HBeAg-negative patients, in contrast to previous results with ARC-520.[53,56]

AB-729 (Arbutus) is a subcutaneously delivered N-acetylgalactosamine-conjugated siRNA moiety that demonstrated significant suppression of HBsAg in mouse models of HBV infection.[57] Initial clinical evaluation is planned for 2019. Clinical development of ARB-1467, Arbutus' initial product in this category, has been discontinued.

Core Protein Inhibitors

The HBV core protein plays several essential roles in the HBV life cycle, including capsid formation.[58–67] The kinetics of core protein assembly are critical for functional capsid formation, encapsidation of pgRNA, and formation of infectious virions. The HBV capsid is also essential for nuclear importation of HBV rcDNA through a regulated interaction with nuclear pore proteins, allowing replenishment of nuclear cccDNA pools from either newly formed capsids or incoming virus.[68] Nuclear forms of the HBV core protein have been implicated in modulating the expression of viral and host genes and contributing to regulated splicing and nuclear export of HBV RNAs, and to cccDNA function.[69,70]

These findings suggest that allosteric modulation of the core protein would allow targeting of multiple aspects of the viral life cycle and predict that HBV core protein inhibitors (also known as core inhibitors, or core protein allosteric modulators) may be potent antivirals. Several classes of core inhibitors have been described across multiple chemotypes[71]; all are thought to bind to the same pocket in the dimer-dimer interface, nucleating inappropriate oligomerization and rendering nascent capsids unable to encapsidate viral RNA. Subtle differences in core oligomer morphologies following addition of core inhibitors in vitro have been described, ranging from empty capsids to "cracked" capsids with potential changes in cellular localization following core protein aggregation.[72] How these may relate to clinical outcomes remains to be demonstrated. Importantly, all core inhibitors in clinical development exhibit a common property: in addition to potent inhibition of new rcDNA formation, all inhibit viral RNA packaging, and at higher doses, may inhibit the establishment of cccDNA. In contrast, nucleos(t)ide analogues inhibit neither of these processes to a significant degree.

Preclinically, several core inhibitors have shown attractive profiles as once-daily oral therapeutics, with potential for additive to synergistic activity in combination with nucleos(t)ide analogues.[73–75] Several core inhibitors are currently in clinical evaluation.[76–83] Early data from phase 1b monotherapy studies suggest that this novel class has the potential to be at least as potent as nucleos(t)ide analogue monotherapy, with single-agent HBV DNA declines of up to 4 $\log_{10}$ IU/mL, as well as 2 to 3 $\log_{10}$ declines in viral RNA over ≤ 28 days.[79,80,83–85] Early data from phase 2 evaluations of core inhibitors are anticipated in 2019, including combinations with other therapeutic modalities. If preclinical data with these combinations, suggesting additive to synergistic interactions,[64,65,86,87] are reflected by anticipated enhanced declines in viral load, it will be extremely interesting to assess whether these effects are followed by viral antigen reductions or loss, which would be predicted if an enhanced antiviral effect reduces cccDNA persistence.

Novel Viral Polymerase Inhibitors

Besifovir dipivoxil maleate has recently been approved in Korea, based on phase 3 data indicating noninferior HBV DNA suppression versus tenofovir disoproxil fumarate, with significantly reduced bone and renal toxicities at 48 weeks.[88] However, further clinical evaluation appears to be limited to studies in Korea, suggesting that broader registration efforts may not be forthcoming. A lipid-conjugated, liver-targeted prodrug of tenofovir (tenofovir exalidex; ContraVir) is in early clinical development, with the primary objective of improving safety over current tenofovir disoproxil fumarate formulations.[89]

Immunotherapeutic Strategies

From an immunologic perspective, it has been shown that a persistent, HBV-specific immunologic dysfunction exists in CHB, with both a paucity and a functional impairment of HBV-specific T cells.[90,91] Although the nature of this dysfunction is only partially understood, multiple potential immunotherapeutic approaches have been suggested as a means to achieve a cure by restoring immune competence against HBV and HBV-infected hepatocytes.[92–96] A thesis underlying immunotherapeutic approaches is that HBV is a disease that can be fully suppressed and functionally cured in the context of most (adult) acute infections. If the deficit that allows CHB persistence could be resolved, then immune restoration may allow a similar clinical cure for CHB. Immunotherapeutics in clinical development include toll-like receptor (TLR)7 AND TLR8 agonists, checkpoint inhibitors (eg, anti-PD-1), an RIG-I agonist, and therapeutic vaccines.

Toll-like Receptor Agonists

TLRs are intracellular pathogen-sensing receptors that, when triggered, can arm the immune response to produce antiviral cytokines, such as interferons alfa and gamma, and induce activation of both natural killer and T cells.[97,98] In animal models, both TLR7 and TLR8 have shown an impressive ability to cure woodchucks of woodchuck hepatitis virus infection, although tolerability has arisen as a potential concern.[99,100] The ability to deliver TLR agonists such as Gilead TLR7 agonist vesatolimod (GS-9620)[101] and TLR8 agonist (GS-9688)[102] orally has led to the hope that a "presystemic" antiviral immune response that was limited to the portal circulation might be generated, potentially providing the benefits seen with injected interferons without systemic side effects. Although early clinical results with vesatolimod in patients with CHB were disappointing,[101] GS-9688 as well as TLR7 agonists from Roche (RO7020531) and Johnson & Johnson (JNJ-4964) are still advancing in clinical trials and have been shown to successfully stimulate immune responses in both healthy volunteers and patients with CHB.[102–105]

Checkpoint Blockers

The presence of an "exhausted" CD8$^+$ T-cell phenotype in patients with CHB has spurred exploration of PD1-PDL1 interactions as a possible strategy for restoration of an anti-HBV immune response.[106] Several checkpoint modulators are approved for use in oncology and are thus already available for exploratory studies in CHB patients. One immunologic study concluded that maturation of HBV-specific B cells is adversely affected by the presence of serum HBsAg regardless of disease stage, and that B-cell maturation could be partially restored by addition of anti-PD1 antibodies.[93] However, in a small study of patients with HBeAg-negative CHB, the addition of nivolumab (Bristol-Myers Squibb), an anti-PD1 monoclonal antibody, to GS-4774 (Gilead Sciences), an experimental therapeutic T-cell vaccine, did not significantly impact HBsAg levels except in a single patient, although changes in T-cell and natural killer cell composition were reported.[107,108] The combination of an anti-PD-L1 antibody with siRNA in a woodchuck model led to sustained reductions of HBsAg in some animals.[106] Whether combinations of checkpoint inhibitors with alternative regimens will significantly improve efficacy in the clinic remains to be seen.

Therapeutic Vaccines

There is an extensive and largely unsuccessful history of therapeutic vaccine development for patients with CHB.[109] Previous failures have prompted more sophisticated approaches designed to broaden HBV-specific immune responses[110] and explore combinations with both immunomodulators (anti-PD-1/anti-PDL1) and DAAs (such as siRNA).[111] Although preclinical work has demonstrated exciting results in nonclinical models, these have yet to be validated in human studies.[111,112]

OTHER CLINICAL STAGE THERAPEUTICS OF INTEREST
Nucleic Acid Polymers

In addition to the development programs mentioned above, several other therapeutic classes are currently being evaluated in the clinic. These therapeutic classes include the nucleic acid polymers being developed by Replicor (REP 2139).[113] In patients coinfected with HDV and HBV, REP 2139 in combination with peginterferon alfa-2a provided marked suppression of plasma HDV RNA and HBsAg concentrations; HDV RNA remained undetectable at 1 year after treatment in 7 of the 12 patients, and, after 1.5 to 2 years, HBsAg remained undetectable in 4 patients.[114,115] In a subsequent study, patients with HBeAg-negative CHB were treated for 48 weeks with combinations of REP 2139 or REP 2165 and both tenofovir and peginterferon alfa-2a.[116,117] At 24 to 48 weeks of posttreatment follow-up, 14 of 34 patients had undetectable HBsAg and HBV DNA; significant alanine aminotransferase flares were common and were correlated with antiviral responses. Positive results have also been reported in an uncontrolled study conducted in Bangladesh.[118]

A different approach is being taken by Spring Bank, which is developing inarigivir (SB9200), an orally administered linear dinucleotide, as an RIG-I agonist with the objective of activating cellular innate immune responses in HBV-infected cells.[119] Inarigivir is also a relatively weak inhibitor of the HBV polymerase.[120] After 12 weeks of dosing in patients with CHB, inarigivir elicited modest declines in both HBV DNA and HBV RNA, with somewhat greater efficacy reported in HBeAg-negative versus HBeAg-positive patients at doses up to 100 mg.[121–123] Data at higher doses are anticipated in 2019. A collaborative study with Gilead Sciences is evaluating inarigivir in combination with tenofovir alafenamide in adults with CHB; other phase 2 and phase 3 combination studies are planned.

Farnesoid X Receptor Agonists

The gene encoding the NTCP receptor, which mediates HBV entry into hepatocytes, contains 2 farnesoid X receptor (FXR) α response elements.[124] FXR agonists reportedly inhibit HBV replication, and at least 1 FXR agonist (EYP001, Enyo Pharma) is entering phase 2 evaluation in patients with CHB, based on preclinical data, suggesting potential to suppress both HBsAg and HBeAg production.[125]

FUTURE THERAPIES (NOT YET IN CLINICAL DEVELOPMENT)

In addition to the studies in clinical development, a growing number of targets are being explored preclinically.

PAPD5/7 Inhibition

Dihydroquinolizinones have been identified as small molecules that can reduce production of both viral DNA and viral antigens.[126] Elucidation of the target for these agents determined that they inhibit the catalytic domain of 2 enzymes, PAPD5 and PAPD7, leading to destabilization of HBV mRNA without impacting production of transcripts. Although this target has accrued significant interest, no compounds of this type have yet progressed to studies in patients with CHB.

RNAse H

RNAse H activity is required for production of new infectious virus and replenishment of nuclear cccDNA through conversion of rcDNA into cccDNA. Ablating HBV RNAse H activity causes accumulation of long RNA:DNA heteroduplexes, truncates minus-polarity DNA strands, and blocks production of the plus-polarity DNA strand.[127] Several chemical leads have been identified, but they also have not yet entered clinical evaluation.[128–130]

Epigenetic Modifiers

Epigenetic regulation of HBV has recently been extensively reviewed.[131] "Epigenetics" refers to (heritable) alterations in gene expression that occur to a chromosome without changes in DNA sequence. Because HBV cccDNA exists as a nucleosome-decorated minichromosome, replete with histones and other host proteins, it can presumably be regulated by small-molecule epigenetic-modifying agents, such as those that target histone deacetylases (HDAC), histone acetyltransferases, methyltransferases, and demethylases (KDMs). Indeed, HDAC inhibitors have been shown to suppress cccDNA transcription in tissue culture under noncytotoxic conditions.[132] Interestingly, transcription from HBV DNA integrated into the host genome was enhanced, suggesting that cccDNA is regulated differently than transcription from an integrated genome.[133] As HDAC inhibitors have been approved for other indications, it may be anticipated that these could be used in patients with CHB as well, perhaps in combination with an immunotherapeutic, should they be useable at a dose that is free of toxicity. Other epigenetic approaches have also been contemplated, and at least 1 company (Gilead Sciences) has explored targeting KDM5, demonstrating potent reductions of viral antigens as well as RNA associated with histone demethylation (H3K4me3:H3)[134]; however, future development for this target indication is uncertain.

Direct cccDNA Targeting

The ability to directly eliminate or silence HBV cccDNA has been considered the "holy grail" of HBV therapies. However, until recently, such direct targeting of the viral reservoir has not been feasible. The emergence of CRISPR-Cas9 and other technologies that can directly edit DNA (zinc finger nucleases and such) has the potential to target cccDNA directly. Several companies have emerged around this exciting platform, and in nonclinical studies, several academic groups have shown that this approach can successfully reduce functional cccDNA.[135–138] Although the data are exciting, several important caveats remain: (1) elimination of off-target effects need to be addressed; (2) the vector for delivery would need to access all infected hepatocytes to remove the potential for reactivation; and (3) although studies have shown that integrated genomes may be targeted, cleavage of such integrants runs the theoretical risk of inducing genomic instability, with the concomitant risk of carcinogenesis. It remains to be seen whether these questions can be addressed before entry into the clinic.

SUMMARY

The last several years have seen a dramatic resurgence of interest in HBV therapeutic research, with multiple novel targets beyond the HBV pol/RT being explored for the first time in almost 20 years. Although it is early, it is anticipated that the next several years will yield important new insights into the underlying biology of HBV in parallel with new treatments that may have the potential to cure substantially more patients than can be achieved today.

ACKNOWLEDGMENTS

The author gratefully acknowledges Jason Deer, MS, for his help, and apologizes to numerous colleagues whose inputs and original contributions could not be included or cited due to space and topical constraints. The author also gratefully acknowledges the editorial assistance provided by Richard Boehme, PhD, of MediTech Media, and funding by Assembly Biosciences.

REFERENCES

1. World Health Organization. Hepatitis B key facts. 2018. Available at: https://www.who.int/news-room/fact-sheets/detail/hepatitis-b. Accessed March 12, 2019.
2. Stanaway JD, Flaxman AD, Naghavi M, et al. The global burden of viral hepatitis from 1990 to 2013: findings from the Global Burden of Disease Study 2013. Lancet 2016;388:1081–8.
3. Seeger C, Mason WS. Molecular biology of hepatitis B virus infection. Virology 2015;479-480:672–86.
4. Ko C, Michler T, Protzer U. Novel viral and host targets to cure hepatitis B. Curr Opin Virol 2017;24:38–45.
5. Seeger C, Mason WS. Sodium-dependent taurocholic cotransporting polypeptide: a candidate receptor for human hepatitis B virus. Gut 2013;62:1093–5.
6. Yan H, Zhong G, Xu G, et al. Sodium taurocholate cotransporting polypeptide is a functional receptor for human hepatitis B and D virus. Elife 2012;1: e00049.
7. Qi Y, Gao Z, Xu G, et al. DNA polymerase κ is a key cellular factor for the formation of covalently closed circular DNA of hepatitis B virus. PLoS Pathog 2016;12: e1005893.

8. Dandri M, Petersen J. Mechanism of hepatitis B virus persistence in hepatocytes and its carcinogenic potential. Clin Infect Dis 2016;62(Suppl 4):S281–8.

9. Yang HC, Kao JH. Persistence of hepatitis B virus covalently closed circular DNA in hepatocytes: molecular mechanisms and clinical significance. Emerg Microbes Infect 2014;3:e64.

10. Ko C, Chakraborty A, Chou WM, et al. Hepatitis B virus genome recycling and de novo secondary infection events maintain stable cccDNA levels. J Hepatol 2018;69:1231–41.

11. Bockmann JH, Stadler D, Xia Y, et al. Comparative analysis of the antiviral effects mediated by type I and III interferons in hepatitis B virus infected hepatocytes. J Infect Dis 2019. [Epub ahead of print].

12. Zhu Y, Yamamoto T, Cullen J, et al. Kinetics of hepadnavirus loss from the liver during inhibition of viral DNA synthesis. J Virol 2001;75:311–22.

13. Huang Q, Zhou B, Zong Y, et al. Rapid turnover of cccDNA in chronic hepatitis B patients who have failed nucleoside treatment due to emerging resistance. The Liver Meeting. Washington, DC, October 20–24, 2017.

14. Vigano M, Lampertico P. Clinical implications of HBsAg quantification in patients with chronic hepatitis B. Saudi J Gastroenterol 2012;18:81–6.

15. Wooddell CI, Yuen MF, Chan HL, et al. RNAi-based treatment of chronically infected patients and chimpanzees reveals that integrated hepatitis B virus DNA is a source of HBsAg. Sci Transl Med 2017;9 [pii:eaan0241].

16. Loomba R, Liang TJ. Hepatitis B reactivation associated with immune suppressive and biological modifier therapies: current concepts, management strategies, and future directions. Gastroenterology 2017;152:1297–309.

17. Flink HJ, van Zonneveld M, Hansen BE, et al. Treatment with peg-interferon alpha-2b for HBeAg-positive chronic hepatitis B: HBsAg loss is associated with HBV genotype. Am J Gastroenterol 2006;101:297–303.

18. Sonneveld MJ, Rijckborst V, Boucher CA, et al. Prediction of sustained response to peginterferon alfa-2b for hepatitis B e antigen-positive chronic hepatitis B using on-treatment hepatitis B surface antigen decline. Hepatology 2010;52:1251–7.

19. Tseng TC, Yu ML, Liu CJ, et al. Effect of host and viral factors on hepatitis B e antigen-positive chronic hepatitis B patients receiving pegylated interferon-alpha-2a therapy. Antivir Ther 2011;16:629–37.

20. Hepatitis B Foundation. Drug Watch. 2019. Available at: http://www.hepb.org/treatment-and-management/drug-watch/. Accessed February 25, 2019.

21. Arends P, Rijckborst V, Zondervan PE, et al. Loss of intrahepatic HBsAg expression predicts sustained response to peginterferon and is reflected by pronounced serum HBsAg decline. J Viral Hepat 2014;21:897–904.

22. Chang TT, Lai CL, Kew Yoon S, et al. Entecavir treatment for up to 5 years in patients with hepatitis B e antigen-positive chronic hepatitis B. Hepatology 2010;51:422–30.

23. Liu Y, Corsa AC, Buti M, et al. No detectable resistance to tenofovir disoproxil fumarate in HBeAg+ and HBeAg- patients with chronic hepatitis B after 8 years of treatment. J Viral Hepat 2017;24:68–74.

24. Buti M, Gane E, Seto WK, et al. Tenofovir alafenamide versus tenofovir disoproxil fumarate for the treatment of patients with HBeAg-negative chronic hepatitis B virus infection: a randomised, double-blind, phase 3, non-inferiority trial. Lancet Gastroenterol Hepatol 2016;1:196–206.

25. Chan HL, Fung S, Seto WK, et al. Tenofovir alafenamide versus tenofovir disoproxil fumarate for the treatment of HBeAg-positive chronic hepatitis B virus

infection: a randomised, double-blind, phase 3, non-inferiority trial. Lancet Gastroenterol Hepatol 2016;1:185–95.

26. Seto WK, Buti M, Izumi N, et al. Bone and renal safety are improved in chronic HBV patients 1 year after switching to tenofovir alafenamide from tenofovir disoproxil fumarate. The Liver Meet. San Francisco, CA, November 9–13, 2018.

27. Moraleda G, Saputelli J, Aldrich CE, et al. Lack of effect of antiviral therapy in nondividing hepatocyte cultures on the closed circular DNA of woodchuck hepatitis virus. J Virol 1997;71:9392–9.

28. Boyd A, Lacombe K, Lavocat F, et al. Decay of ccc-DNA marks persistence of intrahepatic viral DNA synthesis under tenofovir in HIV-HBV co-infected patients. J Hepatol 2016;65:683–91.

29. Alidjinou EK, Michel C, Canva V, et al. Very slow decline of hepatitis B virus surface antigen and core related antigen in chronic hepatitis B patients successfully treated with nucleos(t)ide analogues. J Med Virol 2018;90:989–93.

30. Chi H, Wong D, Peng J, et al. Durability of response after hepatitis B surface antigen seroclearance during nucleos(t)ide analogue treatment in a multiethnic cohort of chronic hepatitis B patients: results after treatment cessation. Clin Infect Dis 2017;65:680–3.

31. Van Hees S, Chi H, Hansen B, et al. Sustained off-treatment viral control is associated with high hepatitis B surface antigen seroclearance rates in Caucasian patients with nucleos(t)ide analogue induced HBeAg seroconversion. J Viral Hepat 2019. https://doi.org/10.1111/jvh.13084.

32. Arends JE, Lieveld FI, Ahmad S, et al. New viral and immunological targets for hepatitis B treatment and cure: a review. Infect Dis Ther 2017;6:461–76.

33. Su TH, Liu CJ. Combination therapy for chronic hepatitis B: current updates and perspectives. Gut Liver 2017;11:590–603.

34. Brouwer WP, Xie Q, Sonneveld MJ, et al. Adding pegylated interferon to entecavir for hepatitis B e antigen-positive chronic hepatitis B: a multicenter randomized trial (ARES study). Hepatology 2015;61:1512–22.

35. Marcellin P, Ahn SH, Ma X, et al. Combination of tenofovir disoproxil fumarate and peginterferon alpha-2a increases loss of hepatitis B surface antigen in patients with chronic hepatitis B. Gastroenterology 2016;150:134–44.e10.

36. Ahn SH, Marcellin P, Ma X, et al. Hepatitis B surface antigen loss with tenofovir disoproxil fumarate plus peginterferon alfa-2a: week 120 analysis. Dig Dis Sci 2018;63:3487–97.

37. Marcellin P, Ahn SH, Chuang WL, et al. Predictors of response to tenofovir disoproxil fumarate plus peginterferon alfa-2a combination therapy for chronic hepatitis B. Aliment Pharmacol Ther 2016;44:957–66.

38. Chi H, Hansen BE, Guo S, et al. Pegylated interferon alfa-2b add-on treatment in hepatitis B virus envelope antigen-positive chronic hepatitis B patients treated with nucleos(t)ide analogue: a randomized, controlled trial (PEGON). J Infect Dis 2017;215:1085–93.

39. Hsu CW, Su WW, Lee CM, et al. Phase IV randomized clinical study: peginterferon alfa-2a with adefovir or entecavir pre-therapy for HBeAg-positive chronic hepatitis B. J Formos Med Assoc 2018;117:588–97.

40. Jun DW, Ahn SB, Kim TY, et al. Efficacy of pegylated interferon monotherapy versus sequential therapy of entecavir and pegylated interferon in hepatitis B e antigen-positive hepatitis B patients: a randomized, multicenter, phase IIIb open-label study (POTENT study). Chin Med J (Engl) 2018;131:1645–51.

41. Xie Q, Zhou H, Bai X, et al. A randomized, open-label clinical study of combined pegylated interferon alfa-2a (40KD) and entecavir treatment for hepatitis B "e" antigen-positive chronic hepatitis B. Clin Infect Dis 2014;59:1714–23.
42. Marcellin P, Buti M, Krastev Z, et al. Kinetics of hepatitis B surface antigen loss in patients with HBeAg-positive chronic hepatitis B treated with tenofovir disoproxil fumarate. J Hepatol 2014;61:1228–37.
43. Burdette D. Evidence for the presence of infectious virus in the serum from chronic hepatitis B patients suppressed on nucleos(t)ide therapy with detectable but not quantifiable HBV DNA. The Int Liver Congress. Vienna, Austria, April 10–14, 2019.
44. Xia Y, Stadler D, Lucifora J, et al. Interferon-gamma and tumor necrosis factor-alpha produced by T cells reduce the HBV persistence form, cccDNA, without cytolysis. Gastroenterology 2016;150:194–205.
45. Guidotti LG, Ishikawa T, Hobbs MV, et al. Intracellular inactivation of the hepatitis B virus by cytotoxic T lymphocytes. Immunity 1996;4:25–36.
46. Urban S, Bartenschlager R, Kubitz R, et al. Strategies to inhibit entry of HBV and HDV into hepatocytes. Gastroenterology 2014;147:48–64.
47. Wedemeyer H, Bogomolov P, Blank A, et al. Final results of a multicenter, open-label phase 2b clinical trial to assess safety and efficacy of Myrcludex B in combination with tenofovir in patients with HBV/HDV coinfection. The Int Liver Congress. Paris, France, April 11–15, 2018.
48. Wedemeyer H, Schoneweis K, Bogomolov P, et al. Interim results of a multicenter, open-label phase 2 clinical trial (MYR203) to assess safety and efficacy of Myrcludex B in combination with PEG-IFNα in patients with chronic HBV/HDV co-infection. The Liver Meeting. San Francisco, CA, November 9–13, 2018.
49. Chen Y, Cheng G, Mahato RI. RNAi for treating hepatitis B viral infection. Pharm Res 2008;25:72–86.
50. Flisiak R, Jaroszewicz J, Lucejko M. siRNA drug development against hepatitis B virus infection. Expert Opin Biol Ther 2018;18:609–17.
51. Schluep T, Lickliter J, Hamilton J, et al. Safety, tolerability, and pharmacokinetics of ARC-520 injection, an RNA interference-based therapeutic for the treatment of chronic hepatitis B virus infection, in healthy volunteers. Clin Pharmacol Drug Dev 2017;6:350–62.
52. Wooddell CI, Rozema DB, Hossbach M, et al. Hepatocyte-targeted RNAi therapeutics for the treatment of chronic hepatitis B virus infection. Mol Ther 2013;21: 973–85.
53. Yuen M-F, Liu K, Given B, et al. RNA interference therapy with ARC-520 injection results in long term off-therapy antigen reductions in treatment naïve, HBeAg positive and negative patients with chronic HBV. The Int Liver Congress. Paris, France, April 11–15, 2018.
54. Gane EJ, Locarnini S, Lim TH, et al. First results with RNA interference (RNAi) in chronic hepatitis B (CHB) using ARO-HBV. The Liver Meeting. San Francisco, CA, November 9–13, 2018.
55. Gane EJ, Locarnini S, Lim TH, et al. RNA interference (RNAi) in chronic hepatitis B (CHB): data from phase 2 study with JNJ-3989. 28th annual Conference of the Asian Pacific Association for the Study of the Liver. Manila, Philippines, February 20–24, 2019.
56. Yuen M-F, Chan HL-Y, Liu K, et al. Differential reductions in viral antigens expressed from cccDNA vs integrated DNA in treatment naive HBeAg positive and negative patients with chronic HBV after RNA interference therapy with

ARC-520. The International Liver Congress. Barcelona, Spain, April 13–17, 2016.

57. Lee ACH. Durable inhibition of hepatitis B virus replication and antigenemia using subcutaneously administered siRNA agent AB-729 in preclinical models. The International Liver Congress. Paris, France, April 11–15, 2018.

58. Mak LY, Wong DK, Seto WK, et al. Hepatitis B core protein as a therapeutic target. Expert Opin Ther Targets 2017;21:1153–9.

59. Selzer L, Zlotnick A. Assembly and release of hepatitis B virus. Cold Spring Harb Perspect Med 2015;5 [pii:a021394].

60. Zlotnick A, Venkatakrishnan B, Tan Z, et al. Core protein: a pleiotropic keystone in the HBV lifecycle. Antiviral Res 2015;121:82–93.

61. Tan Z, Pionek K, Unchwaniwala N, et al. The interface between hepatitis B virus capsid proteins affects self-assembly, pregenomic RNA packaging, and reverse transcription. J Virol 2015;89:3275–84.

62. Huang Q, Mercier A, Zhou Y, et al. Preclinical characterization of potent core protein assembly modifiers for the treatment of chronic hepatitis B. The International Liver Congress. Barcelona, Spain, April 13–17, 2016.

63. Huang Q, Turner WW, Haydar S, et al. Preclinical profile of potent second generation CpAMs capable of inhibiting the generation of HBsAg, HBeAg, pgRNA and cccDNA in HBV-infected cells. The Liver Meeting. Washington, DC, October 20–24, 2017.

64. Rijnbrand R. Preclinical antiviral drug combination studies utilizing novel orally bioavailable agents for chronic hepatitis B infection: AB-506, a next generation HBV capsid inhibitor, and AB-452, an HBV RNA destabilizer. The International Liver Congress. Paris, France, April 11–15, 2018.

65. Zhang Z, Liang B, Jin Q, et al. A novel HBV capsid formation inhibitor that additively inhibits virus replication in combination with tenofovir or IFN-α. The Liver Meeting. San Francisco, CA, November 9–13, 2018.

66. Zhou X, Zhou Y, Tian X, et al. In vitro and in vivo antiviral characterization of RO7049389, a novel small molecule capsid assembly modulator, for the treatment of chronic hepatitis B. The International Liver Congress. Paris, France, April 11–15, 2018.

67. Yang L, Liu F, Tong X, et al. Treatment of chronic hepatitis B virus infection using small molecule modulators of nucleocapsid assembly: recent advances and perspectives. ACS Infect Dis 2019. https://doi.org/10.1021/acsinfecdis.8b00337.

68. Guo F, Zhao Q, Sheraz M, et al. HBV core protein allosteric modulators differentially alter cccDNA biosynthesis from de novo infection and intracellular amplification pathways. PLoS Pathog 2017;13:e1006658.

69. Belloni L, Allweiss L, Guerrieri F, et al. IFN-alpha inhibits HBV transcription and replication in cell culture and in humanized mice by targeting the epigenetic regulation of the nuclear cccDNA minichromosome. J Clin Invest 2012;122:529–37.

70. Diab A, Foca A, Zoulim F, et al. The diverse functions of the hepatitis B core/capsid protein (HBc) in the viral life cycle: implications for the development of HBc-targeting antivirals. Antiviral Res 2018;149:211–20.

71. Zhang X, Cheng J, Ma J, et al. Discovery of novel hepatitis B virus nucleocapsid assembly inhibitors. ACS Infect Dis 2018. https://doi.org/10.1021/acsinfecdis.8b00269.

72. Schlicksup CJ, Wang JC, Francis S, et al. Hepatitis B virus core protein allosteric modulators can distort and disrupt intact capsids. Elife 2018;7 [pii:e31473].

73. Bassit L, Cox B, Ono SK, et al. Novel and potent HBV capsid modulator reduces HBeAg and cccDNA in core-site directed T109I mutant in HepNTCP cells. The International Liver Congress. Paris, France, April 11–15, 2018.

74. Berke JM, Dehertogh P, Vergauwen K, et al. In vitro antiviral activity and mode of action of JNJ-64530440, a novel potent hepatitis B virus capsid assembly modulator in clinical development. The Liver Meeting. San Francisco, CA, November 9–13, 2018.

75. Berke JM, Verbinnen T, Tan Y, et al. The HBV capsid assembly modulator JNJ-379 is a potent inhibitor of viral replication across full length genotype A-H clinical isolates in vitro. The Liver Meeting. Washington, DC, October 20–24, 2017.

76. Eley T, Caamano S, Denning J, et al. Single dose safety, tolerability and pharmacokinetics of AB-423 in healthy volunteers from the ongoing single and multiple ascending dose study AB-423-001. The Liver Meeting. Washington, DC, October 20–24, 2017.

77. Gane E, Liu A, Yuen MF, et al. RO7049389, a core protein allosteric modulator, demonstrates robust anti-HBV activity in chronic hepatitis B patients and is safe and well tolerated. The International Liver Congress. Paris, France, April 11–15, 2018.

78. Kakuda TN, Yogaratnam JZ, Gane EJ, et al. Single-dose pharmacokinetics, safety and tolerability of JNJ-64530440, a novel hepatitis B virus capsid assembly modulator, in healthy volunteers. The Liver Meeting. San Francisco, CA, November 9–13, 2018.

79. Yuen MF, Agarwal K, Gane EJ, et al. Interim safety, tolerability, pharmacokinetics, and antiviral activity of ABI-H0731, a novel core protein allosteric modifier (CpAM), in healthy volunteers and non-cirrhotic viremic subjects with chronic hepatitis B. The International Liver Congress. Paris, France, April 11–15, 2018.

80. Yuen MF, Agarwal K, Gane EJ, et al. Final results of a phase 1B 28-day study of ABI-H0731, a novel core inhibitor, in non-cirrhotic viremic subjects with chronic HBV. The Liver Meeting. San Francisco, CA, November 9–13, 2018.

81. Yuen MF, Gane EJ, Kim DJ, et al. Antiviral activity, safety, and pharmacokinetics of capsid assembly modulator NVR 3-778 in patients with chronic HBV infection. Gastroenterology 2019. https://doi.org/10.1053/j.gastro.2018.12.023.

82. Zoulim F, Yogaratnam JZ, Vandenbossche JJ, et al. Safety, tolerability, pharmacokinetics, and antiviral activity of JNJ-56136379, a novel HBV capsid assembly modulator, in non-cirrhotic, treatment-naïve patients with chronic hepatitis B. The Liver Meeting. Washington, DC, October 20–24, 2017.

83. Zoulim F, Yogaratnam JZ, Vandenbossche JJ, et al. Safety, pharmacokinetics and antiviral activity of novel HBV capsid assembly modulator, JNJ-56136379, in patients with chronic hepatitis B. The Liver Meeting. San Francisco, CA, November 9–13, 2018.

84. Yogaratnam JZ, Zoulim F, Vandenbossche JJ, et al. Safety and antiviral activity of a novel hepatitis B virus capsid assembly modulator, JNJ-56136379, in Asian and non-Asian patients with chronic hepatitis B. 28th Annual Conference of the Asian Pacific Association for the Study of the Liver. Manila, Philippines, February 20–24, 2019.

85. Zoulim F, Yogaratnam JZ, Vandenbossche JJ, et al. Safety, pharmacokinetics, and antiviral activity of a novel hepatitis B virus capsid assembly modulator, JNJ-56136379, in patients with chronic hepatitis B. 28th Annual Conference of the Asian Pacific Association for the Study of the Liver. Manila, Philippines, February 20–24, 2019.

86. Dai L, Yu Y, Zhou X, et al. Combination treatment of a TLR7 agonist RO7020531 and a core protein allosteric modulator RO7049389 achieved sustainable viral load suppression and HBsAg loss in an AAV-HBV mouse model. The International Liver Congress. Paris, France, April 11–15, 2018.

87. Klumpp K, Shimada T, Allweiss L, et al. Efficacy of NVR 3-778, alone and in combination with pegylated interferon, vs entecavir in uPA/SCID mice with humanized livers and HBV infection. Gastroenterology 2018;154:652–62.e8.

88. Ahn SH, Kim W, Jung YK, et al. Efficacy and safety of besifovir dipivoxil maleate compared with tenofovir disoproxil fumarate in treatment of chronic hepatitis B virus infection. Clin Gastroenterol Hepatol 2018. https://doi.org/10.1016/j.cgh.2018.11.001.

89. Tanwandee T, Chatsiricharoenkul S, Tangkijvanich P, et al. Pharmacokinetics, safety and tolerability of tenofovir exalidex, a novel prodrug of tenofovir, administered as ascending multiple doses to healthy volunteers and HBV-infected subjects. The International Liver Congress. Amsterdam, The Netherlands, April 19–23, 2017.

90. Bertoletti A, Maini MK, Ferrari C. The host-pathogen interaction during HBV infection: immunological controversies. Antivir Ther 2010;15(Suppl 3):15–24.

91. Rehermann B, Thimme R. Insights from antiviral therapy into immune responses to hepatitis B and C virus infection. Gastroenterology 2019;156:369–83.

92. Bertoletti A, Le Bert N. Immunotherapy for chronic hepatitis B virus infection. Gut Liver 2018;12:497–507.

93. Salimzadeh L, Le Bert N, Dutertre CA, et al. PD-1 blockade partially recovers dysfunctional virus-specific B cells in chronic hepatitis B infection. J Clin Invest 2018;128:4573–87.

94. Lim SG, Agcaoili J, De Souza NNA, et al. Therapeutic vaccination for chronic hepatitis B: a systematic review and meta-analysis. J Viral Hepat 2019. https://doi.org/10.1111/jvh.13085.

95. Maini MK, Gehring AJ. The role of innate immunity in the immunopathology and treatment of HBV infection. J Hepatol 2016;64:S60–70.

96. Gehring AJ, Protzer U. Targeting innate and adaptive immune responses to cure chronic HBV infection. Gastroenterology 2019;156:325–37.

97. Ma Z, Cao Q, Xiong Y, et al. Interaction between hepatitis B virus and toll-like receptors: current status and potential therapeutic use for chronic hepatitis B. Vaccines (Basel) 2018;6 [pii:E6].

98. Boni C, Vecchi A, Rossi M, et al. TLR7 agonist increases responses of hepatitis B virus-specific T cells and natural killer cells in patients with chronic hepatitis B treated with nucleos(t)ide analogues. Gastroenterology 2018;154:1764–7.e7.

99. Menne S, Tumas DB, Liu KH, et al. Sustained efficacy and seroconversion with the toll-like receptor 7 agonist GS-9620 in the woodchuck model of chronic hepatitis B. J Hepatol 2015;62:1237–45.

100. Lanford RE, Guerra B, Chavez D, et al. GS-9620, An oral agonist of Toll-like receptor-7, induces prolonged suppression of hepatitis B virus in chronically infected chimpanzees. Gastroenterology 2013;144:1508–17, 1517.e1-10.

101. Agarwal K, Ahn SH, Elkhashab M, et al. Safety and efficacy of vesatolimod (GS-9620) in patients with chronic hepatitis B who are not currently on antiviral treatment. J Viral Hepat 2018;25:1331–40.

102. Gane E, Kim HJ, Visvanathan K, et al. Safety, pharmacokinetics, and pharmacodynamics of oral TLR8 agonist GS-9688 in patients with chronic hepatitis B: a randomized, placebo-controlled, double-blind phase 1b study. The Liver Meeting. San Francisco, CA, November 9–13, 2018.

103. Gane E, Agarwal K, Balabanska R, et al. TLR7 agonist RO7020531 triggers immune activation after multiple doses in chronic hepatitis B patients. The Liver Meeting. San Francisco, CA, November 9–13, 2018.

104. Gane E, Kim HJ, Visvanathan K, et al. Safety, pharmacokinetics, and pharmacodynamics of oral TLR8 agonist GS-9688 in patients with chronic hepatitis B: a randomized, placebo-controlled, double-blind phase 1b study. 28th Annual Conference of the Asian Pacific Association for the Study of the Liver. Manila, Philippines, February 20–24, 2019.

105. Luk A, Grippo JF, Folitar I, et al. A single and multiple ascending dose study of toll-like receptor 7 (TLR7) agonist (RO7020531) in Chinese healthy subjects. 28th Annual Conference of the Asian Pacific Association for the Study of the Liver. Manila, Philippines, February 20–24, 2019.

106. Liu J, Zhang E, Ma Z, et al. Enhancing virus-specific immunity in vivo by combining therapeutic vaccination and PD-L1 blockade in chronic hepadnaviral infection. PLoS Pathog 2014;10:e1003856.

107. Verdon D, Brooks AE, Gaggar A, et al. Immunological assessment of HBeAg-negative chronic hepatitis B patient responses following anti-PD-1 treatment. The Liver Meeting. Washington, DC, October 20–24, 2017.

108. Gane EJ, Gaggar A, Nguyen AH, et al. A phase 1 study evaluating anti-PD-1 treatment with or without GS-4774 in HBeAg negative chronic hepatitis B patients. The International Liver Congress. Amsterdam, The Netherlands, April 19–21, 2017.

109. Kosinska AD, Bauer T, Protzer U. Therapeutic vaccination for chronic hepatitis B. Curr Opin Virol 2017;23:75–81.

110. Aguilar JC, Lobaina Y, Penton E, et al. Development of a nasal therapeutic vaccine against chronic hepatitis B. 28th Annual Conference of the Asian Pacific Association for the Study of the Liver. Manila, Philippines, February 20–24, 2019.

111. Michler T, Kosinska A, Bunse T, et al. Preclinical study of a combinatorial RNAi/vaccination therapy as a potential cure for chronic hepatitis B. The International Liver Congress. Amsterdam, The Netherlands, April 19–23, 2017.

112. Dembek C, Protzer U, Roggendorf M. Overcoming immune tolerance in chronic hepatitis B by therapeutic vaccination. Curr Opin Virol 2018;30:58–67.

113. Vaillant A. Nucleic acid polymers: broad spectrum antiviral activity, antiviral mechanisms and optimization for the treatment of hepatitis B and hepatitis D infection. Antiviral Res 2016;133:32–40.

114. Bazinet M, Pântea V, Cebotarescu V, et al. Safety and efficacy of REP 2139 and pegylated interferon alfa-2a for treatment-naive patients with chronic hepatitis B virus and hepatitis D virus co-infection (REP 301 and REP 301-LTF): a non-randomised, open-label, phase 2 trial. Lancet Gastroenterol Hepatol 2017;2: 877–89.

115. Bazinet M, Pantea V, Cebotarescu V, et al. Establishment of persistent functional remission of HBV and HDV infection following REP 2139-Ca and pegylated interferon alpha-2a therapy in patients with chronic HBV/HCV co-infection: 1.5-2 year follow-up results from the REP-301 study. The International Liver Congress. Paris, France, April 11–15, 2018.

116. Bazinet M, Pantea V, Placinta G, et al. Establishment of high rates of functional control and reversal of fibrosis following treatment of HBeAg negative chronic HBV infection with REP 2139-Mg/REP 2165-Mg, tenofovir disoproxil fumarate and pegylated interferon alpha-2a. The Liver Meeting. San Francisco, CA, November 9–13, 2018.

117. Bazinet M, Pantea V, Placinta G, et al. Updated follow-up analysis in the REP 401 protocol: treatment of HBeAg negative chronic HBV infection with REP 2139-Mg or REP 2165-Mg, tenofovir disoproxil fumarate and pegylated interferon alfa-2a. The International Liver Congress. Paris, France, April 11–15, 2018.
118. Al-Mahtab M, Bazinet M, Vaillant A. Safety and efficacy of nucleic acid polymers in monotherapy and combined with immunotherapy in treatment-naive Bangladeshi patients with HBeAg+ chronic hepatitis B infection. PLoS One 2016;11: e0156667.
119. Sato S, Li K, Kameyama T, et al. The RNA sensor RIG-I dually functions as an innate sensor and direct antiviral factor for hepatitis B virus. Immunity 2015; 42:123–32.
120. College D, Jackson K, Sozzi V, et al. Inarigivir is a novel selective inhibitor of the HBV replicase complex in vitro. The Liver Meeting. San Francisco, CA, November 9–13, 2018.
121. Locarnini S, Wong D, Jackson K, et al. Novel antiviral activity of SB 9200 (inarigivir), a RIG-I agonist: results from cohort 1 of the ACHIEVE trial. The Liver Meeting. Washington, DC, October 20–24, 2017.
122. Yuen MF, Elkashab M, Chen CY, et al. Dose response and safety of the daily, oral RIG-I agonist inarigivir (SB 9200) in treatment naïve patients with chronic hepatitis B: results from the 25 mg and 50 mg cohorts in the ACHIEVE trial. The International Liver Congress. Paris, France, April 11–15, 2018.
123. Yuen MF, Elkhashab M, Chen CY, et al. Predictors of inarigivir dose response in HBV treatment-naive patients: role of HBeAg status and baseline HBsAg in antiviral response. 28th Annual Conference of the Asian Pacific Association for the Study of the Liver. Manila, Philippines, February 20–24, 2019.
124. Radreau P, Porcherot M, Ramiere C, et al. Reciprocal regulation of farnesoid X receptor alpha activity and hepatitis B virus replication in differentiated HepaRG cells and primary human hepatocytes. FASEB J 2016;30:3146–54.
125. Joly S, Porcherot M, Radreau P, et al. The selective FXR agonist EYP001 is well tolerated in healthy subjects and has additive anti-HBV effect with nucleoside analogues in HepaRG cells. The International Liver Congress. Amsterdam, The Netherlands, April 19–23, 2017.
126. Mueller H, Lopez A, Tropberger P, et al. PAPD5/7 are host factors that are required for hepatitis B virus RNA stabilization. Hepatology 2018. https://doi.org/10.1002/hep.30329.
127. Tavis JE, Lomonosova E. The hepatitis B virus ribonuclease H as a drug target. Antiviral Res 2015;118:132–8.
128. Cai CW, Lomonosova E, Moran EA, et al. Hepatitis B virus replication is blocked by a 2-hydroxyisoquinoline-1,3(2H,4H)-dione (HID) inhibitor of the viral ribonuclease H activity. Antiviral Res 2014;108:48–55.
129. Edwards TC, Mani N, Dorsey B, et al. Inhibition of HBV replication by N-hydroxyisoquinolinedione and N-hydroxypyridinedione ribonuclease H inhibitors. Antiviral Res 2019;164:70–80.
130. Long KR, Lomonosova E, Li Q, et al. Efficacy of hepatitis B virus ribonuclease H inhibitors, a new class of replication antagonists, in FRG human liver chimeric mice. Antiviral Res 2018;149:41–7.
131. Hong X, Kim ES, Guo H. Epigenetic regulation of hepatitis B virus covalently closed circular DNA: implications for epigenetic therapy against chronic hepatitis B. Hepatology 2017;66:2066–77.
132. Yu HB, Jiang H, Cheng ST, et al. AGK2, a SIRT2 inhibitor, inhibits hepatitis B virus replication in vitro and in vivo. Int J Med Sci 2018;15:1356–64.

133. Liu F, Campagna M, Qi Y, et al. Alpha-interferon suppresses hepadnavirus transcription by altering epigenetic modification of cccDNA minichromosomes. PLoS Pathog 2013;9:e1003613.
134. Gilmore SA, Tam D, Dick R, et al. Antiviral activity of GS-5801, a liver-targeted prodrug of a lysine demethylase-5 inhibitor, in a hepatitis B virus primary human hepatocyte infection model. The International Liver Congress. Amsterdam, The Netherlands, April 19–23, 2017.
135. Kennedy EM, Bassit LC, Mueller H, et al. Suppression of hepatitis B virus DNA accumulation in chronically infected cells using a bacterial CRISPR/Cas RNA-guided DNA endonuclease. Virology 2015;476:196–205.
136. Kennedy EM, Kornepati AV, Cullen BR. Targeting hepatitis B virus cccDNA using CRISPR/Cas9. Antiviral Res 2015;123:188–92.
137. Lin SR, Yang HC, Kuo YT, et al. The CRISPR/Cas9 system facilitates clearance of the intrahepatic HBV templates in vivo. Mol Ther Nucleic Acids 2014;3:e186.
138. Weber ND, Stone D, Sedlak RH, et al. AAV-mediated delivery of zinc finger nucleases targeting hepatitis B virus inhibits active replication. PLoS One 2014;9: e97579.

HBV/HDV Coinfection
A Challenge for Therapeutics

Christopher Koh, MD, MHSc[a],*, Ben L. Da, MD[b],
Jeffrey S. Glenn, MD, PhD[c,d]

KEYWORDS

• Hepatitis D • Hepatitis B • Clinical trials • Therapeutics • Cirrhosis

KEY POINTS

- Hepatitis D virus (HDV) infection represents the most serious form of viral hepatitis in humans.
- Pegylated interferon alfa therapy is currently the recommended therapy but has attenuated efficacy at the cost of substantial side effects.
- With increased understanding of HDV, several promising drugs (pegylated interferon lambda, lonafarnib, bulevirtide, REP2139-Ca) have been developed to target various stages of the HDV lifecycle.
- Clinical trials of combination therapy with investigative drugs and pegylated interferon are currently underway.

INTRODUCTION

The hepatitis D virus (HDV) was first described by Rizzetto and colleagues[1] in 1977 and today is described as the most severe and rapidly progressive form of chronic viral hepatitis despite being an incomplete virus that requires the presence of hepatitis B

Disclosure Statement: Drs C. Koh and B.L. Da have nothing to disclose. Dr J.S. Glenn is a board member and has equity interest in Eiger Biopharmaceutics, Inc.
Financial Support: This research was supported by the Intramural Research Program of the National Institute of Diabetes and Digestive and Kidney Diseases of the National Institutes of Health.
a Liver Diseases Branch, National Institute of Diabetes and Digestive and Kidney Diseases, National Institutes of Health, 10 Center Drive, Building 10, Room 9B-16, MSC 1800, Bethesda, MD 20892, USA; b Digestive Diseases Branch, National Institute of Diabetes and Digestive and Kidney Diseases, National Institutes of Health, 10 Center Drive, CRC, Room 4-5722, Bethesda, MD 20892, USA; c Department of Medicine, Division of Gastroenterology and Hepatology, Stanford University School of Medicine, CCSR Building, Room 3115A, 269 Campus Drive, Stanford, CA 94305, USA; d Department of Medicine Microbiology & Immunology, Division of Gastroenterology and Hepatology, Stanford University School of Medicine, CCSR Building, Rm. 3115A, 269 Campus Drive, Stanford, CA 94305, USA
* Corresponding author.
E-mail address: christopher.koh@nih.gov

virus (HBV) to be a human pathogen.[2] Progression to cirrhosis occurs in 10% to 15% of patients within 2 years and in 70% to 80% within 5 to 10 years.[3,4] Furthermore, HBV-HDV coinfection results in an increased risk of hepatocellular carcinoma[5–11] and mortality[5,7,9,12] compared with HBV monoinfection.

Although HDV infection has historically been thought of as a rare disease, recent estimations have suggested that the global burden of disease may be close to 62 to 72 million.[13] Despite these concerns, HDV does not currently have a US Food and Drug Administration (FDA)-approved therapy. The only treatment that is used outside of clinical trials is pegylated interferon (peginterferon) but this treatment is plagued by significant side effects, such as flu-like symptoms, myalgias, and arthralgias, while having limited efficacy in HDV.[14] Nonetheless, it is currently the only treatment that is endorsed by the major liver societies, such as the American Association for the Study of Liver Diseases[15] and European Association for the Study of the Liver[16] due to its proven effect in reducing fibrosis, decreasing risk of hepatic decompensation, and improving mortality.[17–19] Numerous other treatments, including HBV nucleoside analogues, have been studied in clinical trials over the past several decades with and without interferon therapy without improvements in therapeutic response.[20–26] However, within the past decade, there has been a resurgence of interest in novel therapies in hopes of defeating this rapidly progressive and devastating disease.

This article highlights HDV virology and the viral life cycle, past therapeutic approaches, and current recommended therapies and their associated positive and negative aspects. Investigational therapies, their mechanisms of action, and the current progress and future of HDV therapeutics are discussed.

VIROLOGY AND LIFE CYCLE

The HDV virion is small RNA virus measuring approximately 36 nm in diameter, including an inner nucleocapsid that is made up of a short ($\sim$1.7 kb) single-stranded, circular RNA of negative polarity and approximately 200 molecules of hepatitis D antigen (HDAg).[27–29] This inner nucleocapsid is surrounded by a lipid envelope embedded with all 3 types of hepatitis B surface antigen (HBsAg) proteins obtained from HBV; without HBsAg, HDV is incapable of being a human pathogen.[30] The HDV genome is the smallest among mammalian viruses and shares structural similarity to viroids.[27,28,31] This genome encodes for 1 protein that exists in 2 forms: the small HDAg (S-HDAg) and the large HDAg (L-HDAg).

The HDV viral life cycle begins when the HDV virion binds to the human hepatocyte through interaction between the myristoylated N-terminus of the pre-S1 domain of the large HBsAg and the host receptor (**Fig. 1**), also known as the sodium taurocholate cotransporting polypeptide (NTCP) located on the basolateral membrane of hepatocytes.[32,33] After cell entry and uncoating, the HDV genome is translocated to the nucleus, via HDAg-mediated interactions, where it uses host RNA polymerase II for genome replication. There are no DNA intermediates or archiving events.[34] Instead, HDV replication occurs via a double rolling circle mechanism driven by the catalytic activity of RNA polymerase II with the aid of S-HDAg to create linear multimeric copies of antigenomic RNA from the incoming negative strand circular template genome.[35] These linear multimeric copies then undergo specific cleavage at a unique ribozyme site encoded once in each antigenome. The resulting linear antigenomic monomers are subsequently ligated into antigenomic circles that serve as template for production of linear multimers of opposite polarity genomic RNA. These, in turn, self-process into

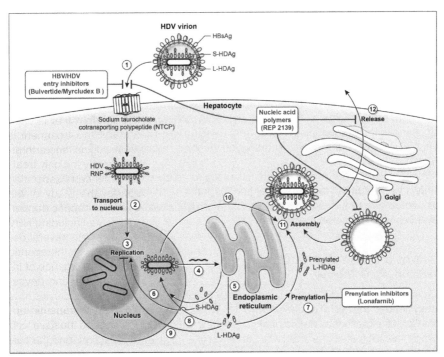

Fig. 1. HDV viral life cycle and sites of investigative drug targets. (1) The HDV virion attaches to the hepatocyte via interaction between HBsAg proteins and the sodium taurocholate co-transporting polypeptide (NTCP). (2) HDV ribonucleoprotein (RNP) is translocated to nucleus mediated by the HDAg. (3) HDV genome replication occurs via a rolling circle mechanism. (4) HDV antigenome is transported out of the nucleus to the endoplasmic reticulum (ER). (5) HDV antigenome is translated in the ER into S-HDAg and L-HDAg. (6) S-HDAg is transported into the nucleus and promotes HDV replication. (7) S-HDAg promotes HDV replication in the nucleus. (7) L-HDAg undergoes prenylation before assembly. (8) New S-HDAg and L-HDAg molecules are transported to the nucleus to prepare for formation of new RNPs. (9) L-HDAg inhibits HDV replication in the nucleus. (10) New HDAg molecules are associated with new transcripts of genomic RNA to form new RNPs that are exported to the cytoplasm. (11) New HDV RNP associates with HBV envelop proteins and assemble into HDV virions. (12) Completed HDV virions are released from the hepatocyte via the trans-Golgi network. Investigative drug and their targets: HBV-HDV inhibitors (bulevirtide/myrcludex B) target the NTCP by competitive binding, nucleic acid polymers (REP 2139-Ca) inhibit HBsAg, subviral assembly and HDV entry, and prenylation inhibitors (lonafarnib) inhibit the process of prenylation of the L-HDAg (the step leading up to assembly).

linear genomic monomers via autocatalytic cleavage at another ribozyme site encoded once in each genomic RNA. The genomic monomers are ligated into circles that can either support additional rounds of replication or be packaged into nascent virions.[36]

A smaller antigenomic sense messenger RNA (mRNA) is also transcribed off of the genomic template. This mRNA codes for the 2 forms of HDAg.[35] The S-HDAg and L-HDAg are identical except that the L-HDAg features an additional 19-amino acid sequence at the C-terminus, resulting from a specific RNA editing event catalyzed by adenosine deaminase acting on RNA 1 (ADAR1) that effects the S-HDAg stop codon.[37,38] This results in translation proceeding to the next downstream stop codon and the addition of the extra 19 amino acids that characterize the L-HDAg. This extra sequence on the L-HDAg contains a CXXX-box motif (C = cysteine, X = 1 of the last 3 amino acids at the carboxyl terminus of the L-HDAg), which then becomes the substrate for host cell farnesyltransferase. The latter covalently attaches a prenyl lipid farnesyl to the cysteine of the CXXX-box. This prenylation event is essential for virion assembly via promoting interaction with HBsAg.[39] In addition, the L-HDAg is a potent transdominant inhibitor of genome replication, whereas the S-HDAg serves to promote genome replication.[40–42] Thus, the RNA editing event catalyzed by ADAR1 that changes the production of HDAg from S-HDAg to L-HDAg serves a key regulatory switch in the virus life cycle, shutting off genome replication and initiating virion assembly.

When the HDV virion is completed, it is ready for release via the trans-Golgi network to infect new hepatocytes. After infection, hepatocyte damage caused by HDV infection can be due to a direct cytopathic effect of HDV or via a still incompletely understood immune-mediated mechanism.[43–45]

HEPATITIS D VIRUS THERAPEUTICS
Interferon-Alpha Therapy

Despite the lack of an FDA-approved therapy for HDV infection, expert guidelines have recommended the use of peginterferon.[16,46] These therapeutic recommendations stem from various experiences dating back to the early 1990s with the first use interferon alfa therapy. Initial experiences evaluated interferon alfa-2a at low doses (3 million IU 3 times a week) compared with high doses (9 million IU 3 times a week) or with no therapy for 1 year.[47] In this study, a complete response, defined as HDV RNA polymerase chain reaction (PCR) negativity with alanine aminotransferase (ALT) normalization, was seen in 21% of those treated with low-dose interferon compared with 50% in those treated with high-dose interferon and 0% in those who did not receive any therapy. However, no subjects demonstrated a sustained virologic response in follow-up up to 48 weeks posttherapy. In this same cohort, a follow-up report of up to 14 years posttherapy with a more sensitive HDV RNA assay revealed that none of the original subjects achieved HDV RNA negativity at the end of the original study. More importantly, long-term outcomes from this study demonstrated improved survival in the high-dose group in those that achieved a greater than or equal to 2 log drop in HDV RNA at the end of treatment (EOT) compared with those in the low-dose group ($P = .019$) and the no treatment group ($P = .003$), both of which were unable to achieve a 2 log drop in HDV RNA at EOT.[18] Interestingly, there was no difference in survival between the low-dose group and controls.

With the efficacy of peginterferon in other viral hepatitis infections, and the initial FDA approval of peginterferon alfa-2b in 2001 for chronic hepatitis C, it was then explored for use in chronic HDV infection. Peginterferon alfa-2b was administered (1.5 µg/kg/wk) for 1 year, which resulted in undetectable HDV RNA in the serum in 8 of 14 (57%) subjects; however after a median posttherapy follow-up of 16 months, the sustained virologic response rate was 43%.[48] Prolonged peginterferon monotherapy has been studied for 72 weeks, which resulted in low-level or undetectable HDV RNA in 34% of subjects at the end of therapy; however, with 24 weeks of posttherapy follow-up, only 21% of subjects had undetectable HDV RNA.[21] Long-term peginterferon alfa-2a with increasing doses up to 360 mcg/wk has been studied for up to 5 years; however, this has not resulted in improved response rates. Only 30% of subjects achieved a complete virologic response, described as HDV RNA negativity and HBsAg seroconversion.[49,50] Thus, in chronic HDV infection, peginterferon seems to be as effective as standard interferon therapy and prolonged therapy does not seem to improve response rates. In fact, HDV RNA levels at 24 weeks of peginterferon therapy may predict response to 1 year of therapy.[51]

Interferon-Alfa Therapy Combinations

Interferon alfa-based therapies have been studied in combination with other medications in chronic HDV infection. Interferon alfa, with and without PEGylation, in combination with ribavirin has been studied in chronic HDV subjects for 1 to 2 years; however, there does not seem be any added value of ribavirin in HDV.[20,21,52] Alternatively, HBV nucleoside analogues have also been evaluated, without much success, in combination with or without interferon alfa, including famicyclovir,[24] lamivudine,[53] adefovir,[26] and tenofovir.[54,55] This is not surprising because such HBV nucleoside analogues can be quite effective at decreasing serum HBV DNA but have no significant effect on HBsAg, which is all that HDV needs to replicate. One of the largest studies of peginterferon in HDV, the Hep-Net/International Delta Hepatitis Intervention Trial (HIDIT-1) study, randomized 90 subjects to adefovir, peginterferon, or the combination. An approximate 2.5 log decline in median HDV RNA was observed at 48 weeks of treatment in both peginterferon arms, with approximately 25% of these subjects achieving HDV RNA negativity at 24 weeks post follow-up. No responses were seen in the adefovir arm.[26] A follow-on study (HIDIT-2), which evaluated switching the nucleoside analogue from adefovir to tenofovir and extending treatment from 48 to 96 weeks, did not show any significant improvement in sustained response rates.[56] In this study, the primary endpoint of undetectable HDV RNA at the end of therapy was not different between the 2 groups (peginterferon plus tenofovir: 28/59 [48%] versus peginterferon plus placebo: 20/61 [33%], $P = .12$). Thus, given these various studies, the combination of nucleoside analogues with interferon does not seem to provide additional benefit in chronic HDV infection.

PAST INVESTIGATIONAL THERAPIES
Thymus-Derived Therapies

Thymosins and their synthetic derivatives are believed to induce T-cell differentiation and maturation, increase T cell function, and restore immune defects. Given the early promising results in chronic HBV monoinfection[57,58] in the early 1990s, it was explored in 2 small pilot studies for HDV.[59,60] However, only 1 of 5 (20%) of subjects became HDV RNA–negative when treated with thymosin-alpha 1900 $\mu g/m^2$ twice weekly for 6 months,[60] and 3 of 11 became HDV RNA–negative when treated with thymic humoral factor-gamma 2 (40 μg) when treated for 24 weeks with 2 of 3 demonstrating a virologic relapse. Since these early studies, further thymosin-focused investigation in HDV has not been described.

CURRENT INVESTIGATIONAL THERAPIES
Peginterferon Lambda-1a

Peginterferon lambda-1a is a type-III interferon that has demonstrated antiviral activity against HBV[61] and HCV.[62] Lambda's antiviral activity was first reported in in vivo models in 2006,[63] and it has been described to use similar interferon-stimulated gene (ISG) induction pathways as interferon alfa, thereby resulting in broad-spectrum antiviral activities and immunomodulatory properties. Lambda binds to type III interferon receptors, which results in dimerization and activation of multiple intracellular signal transduction pathways mediated by the Janus kinase/signal transducer and activator of transcription (JAK/STAT) pathway. Although this is similar to interferon alfa, a type-I interferon, type-III interferon lambda receptors are restricted to cells of epithelial origin, which includes the liver.[64] Thus, initial clinical trials of peginterferon lambda in HBV and HCV demonstrated similar antiviral effects to peginterferon alfa but demonstrated a substantially improved tolerability profile compared with peginterferon alfa.

In HDV, lambda interferon has demonstrated antiviral activity in in vivo human liver chimeric mouse models.[65] In humans, 1 study evaluating peginterferon lambda monotherapy in 33 chronic HDV subjects has recently completed with the end-of-study results presented in the first half of 2019.[66] In this randomized, open-label, multicenter study, peginterferon lambda was administered at doses of 120 or 180 μg weekly for 48 weeks. The end-of-study report has again confirmed that tolerability is improved compared with historical peginterferon alfa data and that both doses of peginterferon lambda have antiviral activity against HDV. Notably, in the high-dose group, 9 out of 14 (64%) subjects achieved either a 2 $\log_{10}$ decline in HDV RNA or had levels below the limit of quantification (BLOQ) at the end of therapy, which was sustained in 7 out of 14 (50%) subjects 24 weeks after therapy. Additionally, 5 out of 14 (36%) subjects demonstrated a durable virologic response after 24 weeks of therapy (ie, HDV RNA–negative at EOT and 24 weeks posttreatment). Given these promising results, peginterferon lambda's improved tolerability may be an attractive option for treating HDV, either as a monotherapy or in combination with other experimental therapies. Currently, an open-label clinical trial exploring lambda interferon in combination with lonafarnib (LNF) (see later discussion) and ritonavir (RTV) for 24 weeks in 26 subjects is being evaluated at the National Institutes of Health Clinical Center (NCT03600714).

Hepatitis B Virus and Hepatitis D Virus Entry Inhibitors

Bulevirtide (myrcludex B), a once daily subcutaneous injection, is a first-in-class HBV and HDV entry inhibitor that targets the human NTCP (hNTCP) transmembrane protein (see **Fig. 1**). The essential factor for receptor binding is the 47 N-terminal amino acids of the pre-S1 domain of the HBsAg envelope protein[67] and competitive binding to hNTCP by bulevirtide, a myristoylated peptide that includes this N-terminal sequence, has demonstrated entry inhibition by HBV and HDV in in vitro and in vivo models.[32,68,69] In an early phase 2, randomized, 3-arm, open-label clinical study, 24 HDV subjects were treated with myrcludex B (2 mg subcutaneous daily) in combination with peginterferon alfa or myrcludex B alone or peginterferon alone for 24 weeks.[70] Although the primary endpoint in this study, change in serum HBsAg levels, was not achieved, subjects who received myrcludex B experienced significant declines in serum HDV RNA and ALT levels. Notably, the combination of myrcludex B and peginterferon group experienced mean HDV RNA declines of 2.6 $\log_{10}$ IU/L, the myrcludex B monotherapy group had a 1.67 $\log_{10}$ IU/L, and the peginterferon group had a 2.2 $\log_{10}$ IU/L decline. HDV RNA became negative in 2 of 8 subjects in both the myrcludex B and peginterferon monotherapy groups and 5 of 7 subjects in the combination therapy group. Myrcludex B was reported to be generally well-tolerated in this study.

Since this study, a multicenter, open-label, randomized, phase 2b clinical trial further exploring the safety and efficacy of myrcludex B has been performed in 120 HDV subjects. Subjects were randomized to subcutaneous daily injectable doses of myrcludex B (2, 5, 10 mg) with oral tenofovir (245 mg/d) for 24 weeks. The primary endpoint of this study was a 2 $\log_{10}$ HDV RNA reduction or negativity in serum. Current end-of-study reports have described median HDV RNA declines in a dose-dependent manner, ranging from 1.6 to 2.7 $\log_{10}$ IU/L, with myrcludex B 10 mg demonstrating the greatest effect.[71] Additionally, ALT normalization was seen in up to 50% of subjects.

HDV RNA relapse occurred in all groups in up to 80% of subjects who responded to myrcludex B therapy by 12 weeks of follow-up.

Additional studies exploring bulevirtide in combination with peginterferon alfa is ongoing in Russia (NCT02888106). This multicenter, randomized, open-label phase 2 study is being performed to further investigate the efficacy and safety of bulevirtide alone and in combination with peginterferon in HDV subjects. In this study, 90 subjects are anticipated to be randomized into 1 of 6 arms: bulevirtide (subcutaneous injection of 5 mg daily or 5 mg twice daily or 10 mg daily) with peginterferon alfa for 48 weeks, or subcutaneous injection of bulevirtide 10 mg with tenofovir for 48 weeks, subcutaneous injection of bulevirtide 2 mg monotherapy for 48 weeks, or peginterferon alfa monotherapy for 48 weeks. The primary endpoint of this study is the achievement of undetectable HDV RNA by PCR 24 weeks after the end of therapy.

In April of 2019, 2 additional clinical trials are expected to begin further exploring bulevirtide. The first is a multicenter, open-label randomized phase 2b clinical trial that will likely enroll 175 subjects from Russia, France, Moldova, and Romania (NCT03852433). Subjects will be randomized to 1 of 4 groups: bulevirtide subcutaneous injection 2 mg/d with peginterferon alfa for 48 weeks followed by bulevirtide 2 mg/d subcutaneous injection monotherapy for an additional 48 weeks, subcutaneous injection of bulevirtide 10 mg/d with peginterferon for 48 weeks followed by subcutaneous injection of bulevirtide 10 mg/d monotherapy for an additional 48 weeks, subcutaneous injection of bulevirtide 10 mg/d monotherapy for 96 weeks, or peginterferon alfa for 48 weeks. All groups will then undergo 48 weeks of posttherapy follow-up. The primary endpoint of this study is undetectable HDV RNA in serum 24 weeks after the EOT.

The second study is a multicenter, open-label, randomized phase 3 clinical trial anticipated to begin assessing the long-term efficacy and safety of bulevirtide in subjects with HDV (NCT03852719). This 3-arm study is estimated to enroll 150 HDV subjects with randomization to observation for 48 weeks followed by therapy with subcutaneous injection of bulevirtide 10 mg/d for 96 weeks, subcutaneous injection of bulevirtide 2 mg/d for 144 weeks, or subcutaneous injection of bulevirtide 10 mg/d for 144 weeks. At the completion of therapy, all groups will undergo 96 weeks of additional follow-up. The primary endpoint of this study is the achievement of undetectable HDV RNA or a greater than or equal to 2 $\log_{10}$ decline from baseline and ALT normalization at 48 weeks of therapy. The rationale for this extended treatment comes from modeling studies that suggest that at least 3 years continuous treatment with bulevirtide might be needed to achieve sustained HDV RNA responses.

Given these early results, bulevirtide has received orphan drug designation for the treatment of HDV infection from the European Medicines Agency (EMA) and from the U.S. FDA. Additionally, the EMA has granted bulevirtide priority medicines (PRIME) scheme eligibility and the FDA has granted it breakthrough therapy designation. Interestingly, the appearance of antibodies to bulevirtide has been demonstrated in some subjects from the phase 2 studies; its significance is unknown and further evaluation is ongoing.[70] A recent study evaluating in vitro and in vivo models of the impact of cell proliferation on HDV persistence demonstrated that even with hNTCP blockage by myrcludex B, clonal cell expansion permitted amplification of HDV infection, which resulted in HDAg- positive hepatocytes to be observed in dividing cells during all study timepoints.[72] Finally, the administration of bulevirtide in healthy volunteers resulted in total plasma bile acids increases by 19.2-fold along with an up to 124-fold increase in taurocholic acid, and an inhibition of uptake transporters OATP1B1 and OATP1B3 cytochrome P450 3A activity.[73,74] However, the clinical importance of these findings has yet to be completely understood.

Hepatitis B Surface Antigen Secretion Inhibitors

Nucleic acid polymers (NAPs) are phosphorothioated oligonucleotides with demonstrated broad-spectrum activities against various infectious agents, including herpes simplex viruses, hepatitis B and C virus, and human immunodeficiency virus.[75–79] NAPs are hypothesized to have antiviral effects through several mechanisms, including blocking viral entry, which depends on NAPs' phosphorothioation or amphipathicity that can interact with hydrophobic surfaces of proteins glycoproteins,[78,80] inhibition of HBsAg release,[79,81] reduction of intracellular HBsAg via inhibition of subviral particle assembly,[82] and (possibly) interactions with the S-HDAg and L-HDAg leading to inhibition of the HDV replication cycle (see **Fig. 1**).[83]

In human clinical studies, REP 2139-Ca is the lead NAP that has been investigated in HDV-infected subjects and is given as a once a week intravenous (IV) infusion. In a phase 2, proof-of-concept study (NCT02233075) treating 12 subjects with REP 2139-Ca monotherapy for 15 weeks weekly IV followed by combination therapy of half dose REP 2139-Ca given weekly IV with peginterferon-alfa for 15 weeks, and then peginterferon-alfa monotherapy for 33 weeks, REP 2139-Ca demonstrated antiviral effects against both HBV and HDV.[84] REP 2139-Ca seems to be the only investigative therapy to reduce HBsAg rapidly, resulting in a 3.5 $\log_{10}$ IU/mL decline in HBsAg from baseline.[84] A similar reduction was also seen in a prior safety and tolerability trial.[85] In subjects who experienced a rapid decline in HBsAg with REP 2139-Ca monotherapy, peginterferon alfa-2a seemed to yield a profound increase in anti-HBsAg concentration. Overall, 6 of the 12 subjects achieved anti-HBsAg titers above 10 mIU/mL by the end of therapy. Moreover, 9 of 12 subjects became HDV RNA–negative in serum by the EOT with a mean HDV RNA decline of 5.34 $\log_{10}$ IU/L. Substantial HDV RNA reduction was present in subjects who had smaller declines in HBsAg, which further suggests that NAPs have more than 1 antiviral mechanism. Moreover, this effect seems persistent because the 5 subjects who achieved functional control of HBV maintained this control through 18 months. In addition, the 7 of the 9 subjects who became HDV RNA–negative maintained their negativity.[86] A follow-up study (NCT02876419) exploring the durability of these responses through 3 years of follow-up is currently ongoing.

REP2139-Ca is generally well-tolerated.[84,85] The most frequently reported side effects with REP 2139-Ca in the initial safety and tolerability study included mild fatigue, dyspepsia, anorexia, dysphagia, dysgeusia, and hair loss. Many of these symptoms were attributed to heavy metal exposure at the trial site and the effect of increased mineral elimination by phosphorothioated oligonucleotides. Similar findings were not described in the more recent trial excluding subjects with heavy metal exposure.[84,87] Commonly seen side effects from REP 2139-Ca in the phase 2 study included pyrexia, chills, thrombocytopenia, and leukopenia.[84] Asymptomatic, self-resolving, substantial aspartate aminotransferase (AST) and ALT flares were commonly seen in HBV monoinfected subjects after reductions of HBsAg raised the possibility of propagating decompensation in patients with advanced liver disease.[85] Smaller flares were also seen in HBV-HDV coinfection.[84] This is concerning because interferon therapy, which is being studied in combination with REP 2139-Ca, can cause similar flares, which prevents its use in decompensated cirrhosis.[85,88–90] One subject in the phase 2 study required discontinuation of the drug due to elevation in ALT and bilirubin after introduction of peginterferon alfa-2a.[84] Thus far, cirrhotic subjects have not been included in studies investigating REP 2139-Ca. However, these flares may potentially be therapeutic because it was described to result in HBV viral load reduction and may be evidence of reactivation of immune response in the liver.[85]

Although promising, the interpretation of the results from these trials are limited by the small size of the trials. Although studies have been done with IV dosing of REP 2139-CA, a subcutaneous formulation, REP2139-Mg, is currently being tested in HBV and a study in HDV is set to begin enrollment in the third quarter of 2019.[91] Good subject tolerability of the subcutaneous formulation will be needed for drug sustainability. Finally, additional evidence of the interplay between interferon therapy and NAPs are needed to determine if there are improved rates of functional control of both HBV and HDV with combination therapy.

Virus Assembly Inhibitors

As previously mentioned in the virology section, prenylation is the process of adding a farnesyl group to the cysteine of the CXXX-box of the L-HDAg and is essential for HDV virion assembly.[39] LNF is an orally available farnesyltransferase inhibitor that has been extensively studied in cancer[92] and progeria,[93] which disrupts the process of prenylation and, in HDV, prevents proper interaction of L-HDAg with HBsAg (see **Fig. 1**).[94] In 2014, a proof-of-concept, randomized, placebo-controlled study demonstrated that oral LNF resulted in a dose-dependent, significant reduction in serum HDV RNA levels compared with placebo.[95] The most common side effects of LNF were noted to be gastrointestinal (GI)-related, including nausea, diarrhea, anorexia, and weight loss, which was also dose-dependent.

This study was followed by the LOnfarnib With and without Ritonavir (LOWR) HDV-1, 2, 3, and 4 studies. RTV, an inhibitor of CYP3A4 that metabolizes LNF, was added to allow for the use of lower doses of LNF compared with the proof-of-concept study, thereby minimizing GI-related side effects in a manner akin to the drug-boosting tactic used with highly active antiretroviral therapy in human immunodeficiency virus.[42] LOWR HDV-1 was a 7-arm, parallel, open-label study of 15 subjects who were treated for up to 12 weeks, which proved that the combination of LNF with RTV improved subject tolerability and achieved higher serum LNF concentrations, and that the addition of peginterferon alfa-2a was possible for future trials.[96]

This was followed by LOWR HDV-2, a dose-optimization, open-label study of various combinations of LNF with RTV with or without peginterferon alfa-2a for 12, 24, or 48 weeks in 55 subjects.[97] At 24 weeks, a dose-dependent response was seen between all oral LNF 25 mg twice daily versus 50 mg twice daily, each with RTV 100 mg twice daily. Addition of peginterferon alfa-2a to either of these regimens demonstrated additive to synergistic effects. The most impressive results thus far with LNF occurred in this study in the low-dose LNF groups (oral 25 or 50 mg twice daily) with low-dose RTV (oral 100 mg twice daily) and peginterferon alfa-2a triple combination therapy. Eight of 9 subjects achieved serum HDV RNA levels BLOQ or a greater than or equal to 2 log_{10} IU/L decline in serum HDV RNA by week 24. Subjects in the 50-mg group experienced an impressive 3.81 log_{10} IU/L decline in HDV RNA at 24 weeks. Finally, LOWR HDV-3 and 4 were 2 additional dose-finding and titration studies that have been recently conducted.[98,99] LOWR HDV-3 demonstrated that once a day LNF of 50 mg with RTV had superior results compared higher doses of LNF (75 mg or 100 mg) with RTV.[98] Meanwhile, LOWR HDV-4 described that dose escalation of up to LNF 100 mg twice daily with RTV was feasible.[99]

It is reassuring that resistance has thus far not been reported with LNF.[95,96] Interestingly, in LOWR-1 and LOWR-2, a subset of subjects who did not achieve HDV RNA negativity on treatment experienced posttreatment, therapeutic, ALT flares with resultant HDV RNA negativity and ALT normalization.[96,97,100] In those subjects who had a liver biopsy before starting treatment, follow-up biopsy performed after LNF-associated flare and ALT normalization revealed regression of fibrosis.[101] Similar to

NAPs, these findings need to be studied further in subjects who are not at risk for decompensation. The main side effects in the LOWR HDV studies with the low doses of LNF (25 mg or 50 mg orally twice daily) to be taken into the phase 3 registration study are mild to moderate GI-related, which can be symptomatically managed with antidiarrheals, proton pump inhibitors, or antiemetics.

Due to these results, LNF has received orphan drug designation for the treatment of HDV infection from the EMA and from the FDA. In addition, LNF in combination with RTV has been granted Breakthrough Therapy designation by the FDA and PRIME designation by the EMA for HDV infection. This has resulted in the first phase 3 study for HDV, which is the randomized, placebo-controlled trial, Delta Liver Improvement and Virologic Response (D-LIVR) (NCT03719313), studying LNF with RTV with or without peginterferon alfa-2a in 400 subjects, which is expected to be fully enrolled by the end of 2019.

Finally, these data have supported the initiation of the first combination study of 2 investigational agents for HDV. As previously mentioned, a smaller phase 2 open-label study evaluating the combination of peginterferon lambda, LNF, and RTV is currently ongoing at the National Institutes of Health Clinical Center (NCT03600714).

SUMMARY

Despite being discovered more than 40 years ago and being known as the most severe form of chronic viral hepatitis, the availability of adequate treatment options continues to an ongoing issue in chronic HDV infection. Although peginterferon alpha can be used with limited efficacy, it is plagued by significant side effects that limits its routine use. Multiple promising investigative therapies are now in clinical trials targeting the ISG-induction pathways (peginterferon lambda), viral entry (bulevirtide, REP2139-Ca), subviral particle assembly or secretion (REP 2139-Ca), and virus assembly (LNF). In the near-term, therapies for patients afflicted with this devastating disease will be through participation in clinical trials and the likely success story will require some form of combination therapy.

REFERENCES

1. Rizzetto M, Canese MG, Arico S, et al. Immunofluorescence detection of new antigen-antibody system (delta/anti-delta) associated to hepatitis B virus in liver and in serum of HBsAg carriers. Gut 1977;18:997–1003.
2. Taylor JM. Structure and replication of hepatitis delta virus RNA. Curr Top Microbiol Immunol 2006;307:1–23.
3. Rizzetto M, Verme G, Recchia S, et al. Chronic hepatitis in carriers of hepatitis B surface antigen, with intrahepatic expression of the delta antigen. An active and progressive disease unresponsive to immunosuppressive treatment. Ann Intern Med 1983;98:437–41.
4. Yurdaydin C, Idilman R, Bozkaya H, et al. Natural history and treatment of chronic delta hepatitis. J Viral Hepat 2010;17:749–56.
5. Kushner T, Serper M, Kaplan DE. Delta hepatitis within the Veterans Affairs medical system in the United States: prevalence, risk factors, and outcomes. J Hepatol 2015;63:586–92.
6. Toukan AU, Abu-el-Rub OA, Abu-Laban SA, et al. The epidemiology and clinical outcome of hepatitis D virus (delta) infection in Jordan. Hepatology 1987;7:1340–5.
7. Romeo R, Del Ninno E, Rumi M, et al. A 28-year study of the course of hepatitis Delta infection: a risk factor for cirrhosis and hepatocellular carcinoma. Gastroenterology 2009;136:1629–38.

8. Tamura I, Kurimura O, Koda T, et al. Risk of liver cirrhosis and hepatocellular carcinoma in subjects with hepatitis B and delta virus infection: a study from Kure, Japan. J Gastroenterol Hepatol 1993;8:433–6.

9. Fattovich G, Giustina G, Christensen E, et al. Influence of hepatitis delta virus infection on morbidity and mortality in compensated cirrhosis type B. The European Concerted Action on Viral Hepatitis (Eurohep). Gut 2000;46:420–6.

10. Ji J, Sundquist K, Sundquist J. A population-based study of hepatitis D virus as potential risk factor for hepatocellular carcinoma. J Natl Cancer Inst 2012;104:790–2.

11. Abbas Z, Abbas M, Abbas S, et al. Hepatitis D and hepatocellular carcinoma. World J Hepatol 2015;7:777–86.

12. Beguelin C, Moradpour D, Sahli R, et al. Hepatitis delta-associated mortality in HIV/HBV-coinfected patients. J Hepatol 2017;66:297–303.

13. Chen HY, Shen DT, Ji DZ, et al. Prevalence and burden of hepatitis D virus infection in the global population: a systematic review and meta-analysis. Gut 2018. https://doi.org/10.1136/gutjnl-2018-316601.

14. Sleijfer S, Bannink M, Van Gool AR, et al. Side effects of interferon-alpha therapy. Pharm World Sci 2005;27:423–31.

15. Terrault NA, Lok ASF, McMahon BJ, et al. Update on prevention, diagnosis, and treatment of chronic hepatitis B: AASLD 2018 hepatitis B guidance. Hepatology 2018;67:1560–99.

16. European Association for the Study of the Liver, European Association for the Study of the Liver. Electronic address: easloffice@easloffice.eu. EASL 2017 clinical practice guidelines on the management of hepatitis B virus infection. J Hepatol 2017;67:370–98.

17. Wranke A, Serrano BC, Heidrich B, et al. Antiviral treatment and liver-related complications in hepatitis delta. Hepatology 2017;65:414–25.

18. Farci P, Roskams T, Chessa L, et al. Long-term benefit of interferon alpha therapy of chronic hepatitis D: regression of advanced hepatic fibrosis. Gastroenterology 2004;126:1740–9.

19. Yurdaydin C, Keskin O, Kalkan C, et al. Interferon treatment duration in patients with chronic delta hepatitis and its effect on the natural course of the disease. J Infect Dis 2018;217:1184–92.

20. Gunsar F, Akarca US, Ersoz G, et al. Two-year interferon therapy with or without ribavirin in chronic delta hepatitis. Antivir Ther 2005;10:721–6.

21. Niro GA, Ciancio A, Gaeta GB, et al. Pegylated interferon alpha-2b as monotherapy or in combination with ribavirin in chronic hepatitis delta. Hepatology 2006;44:713–20.

22. Yurdaydin C, Bozkaya H, Onder FO, et al. Treatment of chronic delta hepatitis with lamivudine vs lamivudine + interferon vs interferon. J Viral Hepat 2008;15:314–21.

23. Lau DT, Doo E, Park Y, et al. Lamivudine for chronic delta hepatitis. Hepatology 1999;30:546–9.

24. Yurdaydin C, Bozkaya H, Gurel S, et al. Famciclovir treatment of chronic delta hepatitis. J Hepatol 2002;37:266–71.

25. Wedemeyer H, Yurdaydin C, Ernst S, et al. Prolonged therapy of hepatitis delta for 96 weeks with pegylated-interferon-2a plus tenofovir or placebo does not prevent HDV RNA relapse after treatment: the HIDIT-2 study. J Hepatol 2014;60:S2–3.

26. Wedemeyer H, Yurdaydin C, Dalekos GN, et al. Peginterferon plus adefovir versus either drug alone for hepatitis delta. N Engl J Med 2011;364:322–31.

27. Sureau C. The role of the HBV envelope proteins in the HDV replication cycle. Curr Top Microbiol Immunol 2006;307:113–31.

28. Bonino F, Heermann KH, Rizzetto M, et al. Hepatitis delta virus: protein composition of delta antigen and its hepatitis B virus-derived envelope. J Virol 1986;58:945–50.

29. Rizzetto M, Canese MG, Gerin JL, et al. Transmission of the hepatitis B virus-associated delta antigen to chimpanzees. J Infect Dis 1980;141:590–602.

30. Polo JM, Jeng KS, Lim B, et al. Transgenic mice support replication of hepatitis delta virus RNA in multiple tissues, particularly in skeletal muscle. J Virol 1995;69:4880–7.

31. Sureau C, Negro F. The hepatitis delta virus: replication and pathogenesis. J Hepatol 2016;64:S102–16.

32. Barrera A, Guerra B, Notvall L, et al. Mapping of the hepatitis B virus pre-S1 domain involved in receptor recognition. J Virol 2005;79:9786–98.

33. Yan H, Zhong G, Xu G, et al. Sodium taurocholate cotransporting polypeptide is a functional receptor for human hepatitis B and D virus. Elife 2012;3:e00049.

34. Hughes SA, Wedemeyer H, Harrison PM. Hepatitis delta virus. Lancet 2011;378:73–85.

35. Chang J, Nie X, Chang HE, et al. Transcription of hepatitis delta virus RNA by RNA polymerase II. J Virol 2008;82:1118–27.

36. Lai MM. The molecular biology of hepatitis delta virus. Annu Rev Biochem 1995;64:259–86.

37. Glenn JS. Prenylation of HDAg and antiviral drug development. Curr Top Microbiol Immunol 2006;307:133–49.

38. Purcell RH, Satterfield WC, Bergmann KF, et al. Experimental hepatitis delta virus infection in the chimpanzee. Prog Clin Biol Res 1987;234:27–36.

39. Guilhot S, Huang SN, Xia YP, et al. Expression of the hepatitis delta virus large and small antigens in transgenic mice. J Virol 1994;68:1052–8.

40. Sato S, Cornillez-Ty C, Lazinski DW. By inhibiting replication, the large hepatitis delta antigen can indirectly regulate amber/W editing and its own expression. J Virol 2004;78:8120–34.

41. Glenn JS, White JM. Trans-dominant inhibition of human hepatitis delta virus genome replication. J Virol 1991;65:2357–61.

42. Chao M, Hsieh SY, Taylor J. Role of two forms of hepatitis delta virus antigen: evidence for a mechanism of self-limiting genome replication. J Virol 1990;64:5066–9.

43. Cole SM, Gowans EJ, Macnaughton TB, et al. Direct evidence for cytotoxicity associated with expression of hepatitis delta virus antigen. Hepatology 1991;13:845–51.

44. Niro GA, Smedile A. Current concept in the pathophysiology of hepatitis delta infection. Curr Infect Dis Rep 2012;14:9–14.

45. Fiedler M, Roggendorf M. Immunology of HDV infection. Curr Top Microbiol Immunol 2006;307:187–209.

46. Terrault NA, Bzowej NH, Chang KM, et al. AASLD guidelines for treatment of chronic hepatitis B. Hepatology 2016;63:261–83.

47. Farci P, Mandas A, Coiana A, et al. Treatment of chronic hepatitis D with interferon alfa-2a. N Engl J Med 1994;330:88–94.

48. Castelnau C, Le Gal F, Ripault MP, et al. Efficacy of peginterferon alpha-2b in chronic hepatitis delta: relevance of quantitative RT-PCR for follow-up. Hepatology 2006;44:728–35.

49. Heller T, Rotman Y, Koh C, et al. Long-term therapy of chronic delta hepatitis with peginterferon alfa. Aliment Pharmacol Ther 2014;40:93–104.
50. Guedj J, Rotman Y, Cotler SJ, et al. Understanding early serum hepatitis D virus and hepatitis B surface antigen kinetics during pegylated interferon-alpha therapy via mathematical modeling. Hepatology 2014;60:1902–10.
51. Keskin O, Wedemeyer H, Tuzun A, et al. Association between level of hepatitis D virus RNA at week 24 of pegylated interferon therapy and outcome. Clin Gastroenterol Hepatol 2015;13:2342–9.e1-2.
52. Kaymakoglu S, Karaca C, Demir K, et al. Alpha interferon and ribavirin combination therapy of chronic hepatitis D. Antimicrob Agents Chemother 2005;49:1135–8.
53. Wolters LM, van Nunen AB, Honkoop P, et al. Lamivudine-high dose interferon combination therapy for chronic hepatitis B patients co-infected with the hepatitis D virus. J Viral Hepat 2000;7:428–34.
54. Wedemeyer H, Yurdaydin C, Ernst S, et al. 96 weeks of pegylated-interferon-alpha-2a plus tenofovir or placebo for the treatment of hepatitis delta: the HIDIT-2 study. Hepatology 2013;58:222A–3A.
55. Wranke A, Heidrich B, Ernst S, et al. Anti-HDV IgM as a marker of disease activity in hepatitis delta. PLoS One 2014;9:e101002.
56. Wedemeyer H, Yurdaydin C, Hardtke S, et al. Peginterferon alfa-2a plus tenofovir disoproxil fumarate for hepatitis D (HIDIT-II): a randomised, placebo controlled, phase 2 trial. Lancet Infect Dis 2019;19:275–86.
57. Mutchnick MG, Appelman HD, Chung HT, et al. Thymosin treatment of chronic hepatitis B: a placebo-controlled pilot trial. Hepatology 1991;14:409–15.
58. Andreone P, Cursaro C, Gramenzi A, et al. A randomized controlled trial of thymosin-alpha1 versus interferon alfa treatment in patients with hepatitis B e antigen antibody–and hepatitis B virus DNA–positive chronic hepatitis B. Hepatology 1996;24:774–7.
59. Rosina F, Conoscitore P, Smedile A, et al. Treatment of chronic hepatitis D with thymus-derived polypeptide thymic humoral factor-gamma 2: a pilot study. Dig Liver Dis 2002;34:285–9.
60. Zavaglia C, Bottelli R, Smedile A, et al. A pilot study of thymosin-alpha 1 therapy for chronic hepatitis D. J Clin Gastroenterol 1996;23:162–3.
61. Chan HLY, Ahn SH, Chang TT, et al. Peginterferon lambda for the treatment of HBeAg-positive chronic hepatitis B: a randomized phase 2b study (LIRA-B). J Hepatol 2016;64:1011–9.
62. Foster GR, Chayama K, Chuang WL, et al. A randomized, controlled study of peginterferon lambda-1a/ribavirin +/- daclatasvir for hepatitis C virus genotype 2 or 3. Springerplus 2016;5:1365.
63. Ank N, West H, Bartholdy C, et al. Lambda interferon (IFN-lambda), a type III IFN, is induced by viruses and IFNs and displays potent antiviral activity against select virus infections in vivo. J Virol 2006;80:4501–9.
64. Lasfar A, Abushahba W, Balan M, et al. Interferon lambda: a new sword in cancer immunotherapy. Clin Dev Immunol 2011;2011:349575.
65. Giersch K, Homs M, Volz T, et al. Both interferon alpha and lambda can reduce all intrahepatic HDV infection markers in HBV/HDV infected humanized mice. Sci Rep 2017;7:3757.
66. Etzion O, Hamid SS, Lurie Y, et al. End of study results from LIMT HDV study: 36% durable virologic response at 24 weeks post-treatment with pegylated interferon lambda monotherapy in patients with chronic hepatitis delta virus infection. J Hepatol 2019;70:e32.

67. Engelke M, Mills K, Seitz S, et al. Characterization of a hepatitis B and hepatitis delta virus receptor binding site. Hepatology 2006;43:750–60.

68. Lutgehetmann M, Mancke LV, Volz T, et al. Humanized chimeric uPA mouse model for the study of hepatitis B and D virus interactions and preclinical drug evaluation. Hepatology 2012;55:685–94.

69. Gripon P, Cannie I, Urban S. Efficient inhibition of hepatitis B virus infection by acylated peptides derived from the large viral surface protein. J Virol 2005;79: 1613–22.

70. Bogomolov P, Alexandrov A, Voronkova N, et al. Treatment of chronic hepatitis D with the entry inhibitor myrcludex B: first results of a phase Ib/IIa study. J Hepatol 2016;65:490–8.

71. Wedemeyer H, Bogomolov P, Blank A, et al. Final results of a multicenter, open-label phase 2b clinical trial to assess safety and efficacy of Myrcludex B in combination with Tenofovir in patients with chronic HBV/HDV co-infection. J Hepatol 2018;68:S3.

72. Giersch K, Bhadra OD, Volz T, et al. Hepatitis delta virus persists during liver regeneration and is amplified through cell division both in vitro and in vivo. Gut 2019;68:150–7.

73. Blank A, Eidam A, Haag M, et al. The NTCP-inhibitor Myrcludex B: effects on bile acid disposition and tenofovir pharmacokinetics. Clin Pharmacol Ther 2018;103:341–8.

74. Blank A, Meier K, Urban S, et al. Drug-drug interaction potential of the HBV and HDV entry inhibitor myrcludex B assessed in vitro. Antivir Ther 2018;23: 267–75.

75. Bernstein DI, Goyette N, Cardin R, et al. Amphipathic DNA polymers exhibit antiherpetic activity in vitro and in vivo. Antimicrob Agents Chemother 2008; 52:2727–33.

76. Guzman EM, Cheshenko N, Shende V, et al. Amphipathic DNA polymers are candidate vaginal microbicides and block herpes simplex virus binding, entry and viral gene expression. Antivir Ther 2007;12:1147–56.

77. Matsumura T, Hu Z, Kato T, et al. Amphipathic DNA polymers inhibit hepatitis C virus infection by blocking viral entry. Gastroenterology 2009;137:673–81.

78. Vaillant A, Juteau JM, Lu H, et al. Phosphorothioate oligonucleotides inhibit human immunodeficiency virus type 1 fusion by blocking gp41 core formation. Antimicrob Agents Chemother 2006;50:1393–401.

79. Noordeen F, Vaillant A, Jilbert AR. Nucleic acid polymers inhibit duck hepatitis B virus infection in vitro. Antimicrob Agents Chemother 2013;57:5291–8.

80. Beilstein F, Blanchet M, Vaillant A, et al. Nucleic acid polymers are active against hepatitis delta virus infection in vitro. J Virol 2018;92 [pii:e01416-17].

81. Noordeen F, Scougall CA, Grosse A, et al. Therapeutic antiviral effect of the nucleic acid polymer REP 2055 against persistent duck hepatitis b virus infection. PLoS One 2015;10:e0140909.

82. Blanchet M, Sinnathamby V, Vaillant A, et al. Inhibition of HBsAg secretion by nucleic acid polymers in HepG2.2.15cells. Antiviral Res 2019;164:97–105.

83. Shamur MP-NR, Mayer R, Vaillant A. Interaction of nucleic acid polymers with the large and small forms of hepatitis delta antigen protein. Hepatology 2017; 66:504A.

84. Bazinet M, Pantea V, Cebotarescu V, et al. Safety and efficacy of REP 2139 and pegylated interferon alfa-2a for treatment-naive patients with chronic hepatitis B virus and hepatitis D virus co-infection (REP 301 and REP 301-LTF): a non-

randomised, open-label, phase 2 trial. Lancet Gastroenterol Hepatol 2017;2: 877–89.

85. Al-Mahtab M, Bazinet M, Vaillant A. Safety and efficacy of nucleic acid polymers in monotherapy and combined with immunotherapy in treatment-naive Bangladeshi patients with HBeAg+ chronic hepatitis B infection. PLoS One 2016;11: e0156667.

86. Bazinet M, Pantea V, Cebotarescu V, et al. Establishment of persistent functional remission of HBV and HDV infection following REP 2139 and pegylated interferon alpha 2a therapy in patients with chronic HBV/HDV co-infection: 18 month follow-up results from the REP 301-LTF study. J Hepatol 2018;68:S509.

87. Mata JE, Bishop MR, Tarantolo SR, et al. Evidence of enhanced iron excretion during systemic phosphorothioate oligodeoxynucleotide treatment. J Toxicol Clin Toxicol 2000;38:383–7.

88. Alfaiate D, Negro F. Nucleic acid polymers: much-needed hope for hepatitis D? Lancet Gastroenterol Hepatol 2017;2:841–2.

89. Janssen HL, Brouwer JT, Nevens F, et al. Fatal hepatic decompensation associated with interferon alfa. European concerted action on viral hepatitis (Eurohep). BMJ 1993;306:107–8.

90. Iacobellis A, Andriulli A. Antiviral therapy in compensated and decompensated cirrhotic patients with chronic HCV infection. Expert Opin Pharmacother 2009; 10:1929–38.

91. Bazinet M PV, Placinta G. Update on safety and efficacy in the REP 401 protocol: REP 2139-Mg or REP 2165-Mg used in combination with tenofovir disoproxil fumarate and pegylated Interferon alpha-2a in treatment naive Caucasian patients with chronic HBeAg negative HBV infection, In International Liver Congress. Amsterdam, Netherlands, April 19–23, 2017.

92. Wong NS, Morse MA. Lonafarnib for cancer and progeria. Expert Opin Investig Drugs 2012;21:1043–55.

93. Gordon LB, Shappell H, Massaro J, et al. Association of lonafarnib treatment vs no treatment with mortality rate in patients with Hutchinson-Gilford progeria syndrome. JAMA 2018;319:1687–95.

94. Bordier BB, Marion PL, Ohashi K, et al. A prenylation inhibitor prevents production of infectious hepatitis delta virus particles. J Virol 2002;76: 10465–72.

95. Koh C, Canini L, Dahari H, et al. Oral prenylation inhibition with lonafarnib in chronic hepatitis D infection: a proof-of-concept randomised, double-blind, placebo-controlled phase 2A trial. Lancet Infect Dis 2015;15:1167–74.

96. Yurdaydin C, Keskin O, Kalkan C, et al. Optimizing lonafarnib treatment for the management of chronic delta hepatitis: the LOWR HDV-1 study. Hepatology 2018;67:1224–36.

97. Yurdaydin C, Idilman R, Keskin O, et al. A phase 2 dose-optimization study of lonafarnib with ritonavir for the treatment of chronic delta hepatitis-end of treatment results from the LOWR HDV-2 study. J Hepatol 2017;66:S33–4.

98. Koh C, Surana P, Han T, et al. A phase 2 study exploring once daily dosing of ritonavir boosted lonafarnib for the treatment of chronic delta hepatitis – end of study results from the LOWR HDV-3 study. J Hepatol 2017;66: S101–2.

99. Wedemeyer H, Port K, Deterding K, et al. A phase 2 study of titrating-dose lonafarnib plus ritonavir in patients with chronic hepatitis D: interim results from the lonafarnib with ritonavir in HDV-4 (LOWR HDV-4) study. Hepatology 2016; 64:121A.

100. Yurdaydin CIR, Kalkan C, Karakya F, et al. The prenylation inhibitor lonafarnib can induce post-treatment Alt flares with viral Cle. Hepatology 2016;64:927A.
101. Yurdaydin C, Idilman R, Kalkan C, et al. The prenylation inhibitor lonafarnib can induce post-treatment viral clearance in patients with chronic delta hepatitis resulting in ALT normalization and regression of fibrosis. J Hepatol 2017;66: S259.

Moving?

Make sure your subscription moves with you!

To notify us of your new address, find your **Clinics Account Number** (located on your mailing label above your name), and contact customer service at:

Email: journalscustomerservice-usa@elsevier.com

800-654-2452 (subscribers in the U.S. & Canada)
314-447-8871 (subscribers outside of the U.S. & Canada)

Fax number: 314-447-8029

Elsevier Health Sciences Division
Subscription Customer Service
3251 Riverport Lane
Maryland Heights, MO 63043

*To ensure uninterrupted delivery of your subscription, please notify us at least 4 weeks in advance of move.

Printed and bound by CPI Group (UK) Ltd, Croydon, CR0 4YY

03/10/2024

01040482-0018